T0093630

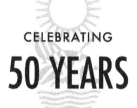

CELEBRATING

50 YEARS

Texas A&M University Press
publishing since 1974

CONSEQUENCES OF COVID-19

CONSEQUENCES OF COVID-19

A One Health Approach to the Responses, Challenges, and Lessons Learned

CHRISTINE CRUDO BLACKBURN
and GERALD W. PARKER

FOREWORD BY PETER HOTEZ

TEXAS A&M UNIVERSITY PRESS | COLLEGE STATION

∞ This paper meets the requirements of ANSI/NISO Z39.48–1993
(Permanence of Paper).
Binding materials have been chosen for durability.
Manufactured in the United States of America.

LIBRARY OF CONGRESS CATALOGING-IN-PUBLICATION DATA

NAMES: Blackburn, Christine Crudo, editor. | Parker, Gerald W., editor. |
   Hotez, Peter J., writer of foreword.

TITLE: Consequences of COVID-19: a One health approach to the responses,
   challenges, and lessons learned / Christine Crudo Blackburn and
   Gerald W. Parker; foreword by Peter Hotez.

DESCRIPTION: First edition. | College Station: Texas A&M University Press, [2024] |
   Includes bibliographical references and index.

IDENTIFIERS: LCCN 2023058468 (print) | LCCN 2023058469 (ebook) |
   ISBN 9781648430305 (hardcover) | ISBN 9781648430312 (ebook)

SUBJECTS: LCSH: COVID-19 Pandemic, 2020– —Social aspects. | COVID-19
   (Disease)—Environmental aspects. | COVID-19 vaccines—Government policy.
   | Pandemics—Prevention. | One health. | BISAC: MEDICAL / Public Health |
   POLITICAL SCIENCE / Public Policy / General

CLASSIFICATION: LCC RA644.C67 C6683 2024 (print) | LCC RA644.C67 (ebook) |
   DDC 362.1962/4144—dc23/eng/20240125

LC record available at https://lccn.loc.gov/2023058468
LC ebook record available at https://lccn.loc.gov/2023058469

Cover design and photo by Noah Van Soest

Contents

Foreword

PETER HOTEZ*

The devastation of the COVID-19 pandemic reminds us of how viruses can convulse our social fabric and destabilize global security. Beyond the specter of six million global COVID-19 deaths and counting, and tens of millions of hospitalizations are the health, economic, and geopolitical effects that will be felt for years or even decades.

There is much to consider both within and outside the health sector. We saw how quickly hospitals and health systems were overwhelmed by COVID-19 surges. Mortality skyrocketed as intensive care units from South Texas to New York City, from London to Madrid, and across India lacked the trained nurses, physicians, and hospital staff to accommodate unprecedented numbers of hypoxic moms, dads, brothers, and sisters. Even once we are past these imminent crises, much more suffering is anticipated downstream. Some estimates indicate that up to 10–30 percent of people infected with SARS-CoV-2 will experience debilitating long-haul COVID-19 symptoms. These include neurological effects, such as brain gray matter degeneration (Douaud et al., 2021). With the delta and omicron variants of the virus, we might expect that tens of millions of people will suffer some form of neurological deterioration in the coming months and years, followed by an uncertain time frame for recovery. Outside of a few dozen well-functioning health systems in North America and Europe, we are at a loss to comprehend how the depleted health systems across the world's

* Hagler Fellow, Hagler Institute for Advanced Study, School of Public Health and College of Medicine, Texas A&M University; Senior Fellow, Scowcroft Institute of International Affairs, Bush School of Government and Public Service, Texas A&M University; National School of Tropical Medicine, Baylor College of Medicine and Texas Children's Hospital

low- and middle-income countries (LMICs) will manage a health crisis of this magnitude. We were all horrified by the potential impact of thousands of neurologically impaired infants born to infected moms in Brazil and elsewhere in the Americas from the 2015–17 Zika virus epidemic. Now, by comparison, the global impact of the Zika virus infection appears almost modest.

The COVID-19 pandemic also exposed fatal flaws in our governance around vaccine production, manufacture, and distribution (Hotez & Narayan, 2021). Up until a few years ago, we felt that we had gotten it right. In 2000, the Gates Foundation together with the major United Nations agencies—including the World Health Organization (WHO), the United Nations Children's Fund (UNICEF), and the World Bank—multinational pharma companies, academic institutions, the Group of Seven (G7), and other national governments came together to create Gavi, the Vaccine Alliance. It was an unqualified success. In the ensuing two decades, deaths from childhood illnesses such as measles, pertussis, tetanus, *Haemophilus influenzae* type b infection, and many others plummeted by more than half, and polio neared elimination. This was a testament to the power of vaccine diplomacy and equity. When COVID-19 emerged from central China at the end of 2019, these organizations, together with a new Coalition for Epidemic Preparedness Innovations (CEPI), felt the vaccine ecosystem had matured sufficiently to establish a COVAX sharing facility for distributing COVID-19 vaccines. But more than a year later, essentially no one on the African continent or those living in most of the world's LMICs have access to high-quality vaccines (Hotez & Narayan, 2021). North America and Europe focused heavily on innovation at the expense of ensuring the availability of low-cost and durable vaccines for global health. This was an epic fail in COVID-19 vaccine diplomacy.

From this experience we are coming to terms with the reality that the world remains unprepared for another pandemic of the magnitude of COVID-19. Beyond the unexpected breakdown in global vaccine governance, there are additional vulnerabilities on multiple fronts.

First, even as COVID-19 vaccines became widely available in the United States, there was no infrastructure in place to counter an aggressive and globalizing antivaccine and antiscience movement (Hotez, 2021a). What began in the new millennium as a response to a retracted scientific paper alleging links between measles vaccinations and autism later grew into a dystopian antiscience disinformation empire. Today, the three major elements of this antiscience empire include well-organized nongovernmental antivax groups learning how to monetize the internet, political action committees (PACs) and parties linked to far-right extremism that adopted antivaccine and antiscience tenets, and even state actors such as the Russian government (Hotez, 2021a). Ultimately, millions died of COVID-19 because of both SARS-CoV-2 and antiscience defiance—defiance against masks, social distancing, and ultimately COVID-19 vaccines. To date, none of the G7 governments or UN agencies have any plans to oppose the antiscience empire and its infodemic. Some of these same antiscience groups further promote conspiracies around the origins of COVID-19, with claims that the virus was manufactured in a laboratory through gain-of-function research. They even allege that the pandemic was the result of the Chinese Communist Party deliberately sending thousands of infected Chinese citizens to enter nations of interest (Hotez, 2021b). In response, the Chinese government has not shown willingness to cooperate with the West.

Yet it is imperative that we fully understand the origins of COVID-19 (Hotez, 2021b). The overwhelming likelihood is that it began in ways that resemble China's earlier SARS epidemic. But elucidating the true origins will require us to apply all our tools in the area of One Health. The field of One Health allows us to integrate bat ecology with secondary animal reservoirs, human contact and spread, climate change, and other factors to fully explain how serious pandemics arise. So far in the twenty-first century, this mix has generated the emergence of SARS in 2002, MERS in 2012, Ebola virus infection in 2014, Nipah virus infection in 2018, and now COVID-19. Unless we identify the social and physical determinants driving these catastrophic zoonoses, we are destined to see future pandemics as dangerous as the current one.

Even before COVID-19 emerged, we started to see aspects of our global health infrastructure unravel or fray from a combination of social determinants, geopolitical factors, and climate change (Hotez, 2021c). For example, civil conflict and other forms of political unrest, urbanization, and climate change brought vaccine-preventable diseases and epidemics of cutaneous leishmaniasis to the Arabian Peninsula, while socioeconomic upheavals together with a prolonged drought brought parasitic and viral infections back to central Latin America, especially in Venezuela and the Honduras–Guatemala–El Salvador triangle.

This current volume brings together experts from across Texas A&M University and other institutions in order to understand how these social and geopolitical forces interact with climate change and other physical factors to promote the emergence of catastrophic infectious diseases. It brings together the multidisciplinary strengths of one of America's largest universities to address disease threats. The timing is important, as the world finally realizes that pandemics represent as great a threat as cyberattacks, nuclear proliferation, or global terrorism. This book launches important discussions on how to begin shaping policies for building an infrastructure to prevent future disease catastrophes.

References

Douaud, G., Lee, S., Alfaro-Almagro, F., Arthofer, C., Wang, C., Lange, F., Andersson, J. L. R., . . . Smith, S. M. (2021). Brain imaging before and after COVID-19 in UK Biobank. *medRxiv*. doi:https://doi.org/10.1101/2021.06.11.21258690

Hotez, P. (2021a). COVID vaccines: Time to confront anti-vax aggression. *Nature*, 592(7856), 661. doi:10.1038/d41586-021-01084-x. PMID: 33907330

Hotez, P. (2021b, June 22). The only way to resolve the Wuhan "lab leak" controversy. *Daily Beast*. https://www.thedailybeast.com/the-only-way-to-resolve-the-wuhan-lab-leak-controversy

Hotez, P. (2021c). *Preventing the next pandemic: Vaccine diplomacy in a time of anti-science*. Baltimore: Johns Hopkins University Press.

Hotez, P. J., & Narayan, K. M. V. (2021). Restoring vaccine diplomacy. *JAMA*, 325(23), 2337–38. doi:10.1001/jama.2021.7439. PMID: 34047758

CONSEQUENCES OF COVID-19

Introduction

ANDREW S. NATSIOS

THIS BOOK ANALYZES THE PUBLIC HEALTH, ECONOMIC, SOCIAL, and developmental consequences of the COVID-19 pandemic so that when a future, possibly more catastrophic pandemic event takes place, we are better prepared. It is important to begin this discussion with a reminder of the major events that occurred over the course of the pandemic. Below is a timeline beginning in January 2020 and running through October 2022 to put into perspective the book's analysis.

> January 9, 2020—The World Health Organization (WHO) announces mysterious coronavirus-related pneumonia in Wuhan, China
>
> January 21, 2020—The Centers for Disease Control and Prevention (CDC) confirms first US coronavirus case in Washington State, and Chinese scientist Zhong Nanshan confirms COVID-19 human transmission
>
> January 23, 2020—Beijing imposes a quarantine on Wuhan
>
> January 31, 2020—WHO issues a global health emergency
>
> February 2, 2020—Global air travel is restricted
>
> February 3, 2020—United States declares a public health emergency
>
> March 11, 2020—WHO declares COVID-19 a pandemic

March 13, 2020—President Trump declares COVID-19 a national emergency, making response funds available, and the United States bans travel of non-US citizens from Europe

March 17, 2020—The Trump administration asks Congress to approve emergency economic stimulus package

March 19, 2020—California becomes the first state to issue a statewide stay-at-home order

March 26, 2020—The US Senate passes the $2 trillion CARES Act to support local governments, nonprofits, and businesses

March 27, 2020—President Trump signs the CARES Act into law

May 1, 2020—Remdesivir receives emergency use authorization (EUA) as a treatment for COVID-19 infection

May 28, 2020—US COVID-19 deaths surpass 100,000

June 10, 2020—US COVID-19 cases reach two million

June 30, 2020—Dr. Anthony Fauci warns new COVID-19 cases could hit 100,000 per day

July 6, 2020—Scientists, citing airborne transmission, ask WHO to revise guidance

July 7, 2020—United States surpasses three million total COVID-19 cases

July 9, 2020—WHO announces COVID-19 can be airborne

July 14, 2020—Early Moderna data suggest vaccine candidate's efficacy

August 12, 2020—Kaiser Permanente announces study finding that severe obesity increases mortality risk from COVID-19

August 17, 2020—COVID-19 becomes the third leading cause of death in the United States

August 28, 2020—First known case of COVID-19 reinfection is reported in the United States

September 16, 2020—Trump administration releases vaccine distribution plan

September 23, 2020—A new, more contagious strain of COVID-19 is discovered

September 28, 2020—Global COVID-19 deaths surpass one million

September 29, 2020—The US Department of Health and Human Services (HHS) distributes 100 million rapid tests to states

October 2, 2020—President Trump and First Lady test positive for COVID-19 and President Trump is hospitalized

October 19, 2020—Global COVID-19 cases top 40 million

October 22, 2020—The Food and Drug Administration (FDA) approves Remdesivir as first COVID-19 drug treatment

November 9, 2020—FDA issues EUA for Eli Lilly's monoclonal antibody treatment

December 11, 2020—FDA issues EUA for the Pfizer-BioNTech COVID-19 vaccine

December 18, 2020—FDA issues EUA for the Moderna COVID-19 vaccine

December 24, 2020—More than one million doses of the of COVID-19 vaccine have been administered in just 10 days

December 29, 2020—The first case of the B.1.1.7/"Alpha" variant (UK variant) is detected in the United States

January 25, 2021—The first case of the P.1/"Gamma" variant (Brazil variant) is detected in the United States

February 21, 2021—US deaths from COVID-19 surpass 500,000

February 27, 2021—FDA issues EUA for the Johnson & Johnson COVID-19 vaccine

April 21, 2021—More than 200 million doses of the COVID-19 vaccine have been administered in the United States

May 10, 2021—FDA expands Pfizer-BioNTech's EUA to include all adolescents aged 12–15 years

June 1, 2021—The B.1.617.2/"Delta" variant is identified and begins the third wave of infections in the United States

October 7, 2021—It is announced that more than 140,000 children have lost their primary or secondary caregiver to the COVID-19 pandemic

December 1, 2021—The first case of the Omicron variant is detected in the United States

April 22, 2022—For the second year in a row, COVID-19 is the third leading cause of death in the United States

May 12, 2022—The number of COVID-19 deaths in the United States reaches one million

June 18, 2022—Pfizer-BioNTech and Moderna receive EUA for their vaccines for children aged six months to five years

October 2022—Worldwide excess deaths likely caused by COVID-19 exceed 22 million

The New Pandemic Challenge

Certainly, one of the most salient and politically explosive issues in observing the consequences of the pandemic is the mortality rates. On September 19, 2021, absolute US deaths from the COVID-19 pandemic reached the same level—675,000 deaths—as the final estimated US mortality in the 1918 Great Influenza (the greatest pandemic of the twentieth century) (Porterfield, 2021). As I write this introduction, deaths in the United States have surpassed one million people. This milestone has led some observers to equate the two pandemics (Sachs, 2021), but such a comparison is inaccurate. While the two crises share some characteristics, comparative mortality is not one of them. The population of the United States in 1918 was 103 million, while today it is over 333 million. Thus, deaths in the United States would have to exceed two million from COVID-19 for a comparable level of devastation between the 1918 influenza pandemic and the COVID-19 pandemic. Known worldwide deaths from COVID-19 exceeded six million as of March 2022 (WHO, 2022), while the upper end of death estimates in 1918 approached 90 million people in absolute numbers, nearly 5 percent of the world's population (CDC, 2019). The six million deaths from COVID-19, however, are somewhat misleading, as many countries do not have sufficient testing capacity. One statistic that may be more useful in measuring the real number of deaths caused by the COVID-19 pandemic is excess mortality. About 22 million more people died worldwide since the pandemic began than had died during a comparable period before the pandemic started (known as excess deaths); this is likely mortality from COVID-19. COVID-19 is certainly one of the worst pandemics since 1918: one million deaths in the United States is a shocking enough level of devastation. This is not to minimize the disastrous consequences of COVID-19, but simply to put it in historical perspective. A future COVID-19 variant could spark mortality on the scale of 1918, but it is also likely that a new unknown disease will appear that will be much worse than the 1918 Great Influenza or COVID-19. It is simply a matter of time before the world faces a new viral crisis.

The Scowcroft Institute of International Affairs at the Bush School of Government and Public Service at Texas A&M University began the Pandemic and Biosecurity Policy Program in 2015 when we held our first Pandemic Policy Summit and issued our first of a series of white papers in 2016. Just as the COVID-19 pandemic was beginning, we published our first book, *Preparing for Pandemics in the Modern World*, edited by Dr. Christine Blackburn. In that book, the authors predicted some of the challenges the world would face from the next pandemic, just as COVID-19 struck (Blackburn, 2020). Many of the observations of that earlier book were prophetic. This second book, the one you are now reading, builds on the first to observe the consequences of the pandemic as it unfolded.

Since it began in 2015, the Scowcroft Institute's Pandemic and Biosecurity Policy Program has brought together scientists from around the world to provide advice on how to prepare for these crises. A challenge from the start of the COVID-19 pandemic response has been the inaccuracy of some experts' analysis of the virus. This was especially true when it first appeared, and knowledge was often portrayed as certain rather than preliminary. These inaccuracies have eroded public trust in science, technology, and public health experts generally, a trend that predated the pandemic and has manifested itself in the antielite and antiexpert rhetoric of ideological extremes of the progressive left and populist right. Full immunization of the world's population may be an unreachable goal because this erosion of trust in science has added fuel to the vaccine hesitancy movement, a subject I will return to later in this introduction. This confusion should lead to reflection and evaluation among the scientific community over what they got wrong, but also what they got right.

To further explain some of the shortcomings of the response within the scientific community, let us examine the following examples: some experts argued early in 2020 that the world would return to the prepandemic state when the circulation of the virus ended (Gallagher, 2020). Scientists underestimated how the availability of so many susceptible hosts would increase mutation emergence (all viruses mutate, but some much more than others); they also did not realize that COVID-19 would behave as did its closest cousin the SARS virus, another coronavirus, which was contained through aggressive public measures within a few months, never to reappear (at least so far) (Achenbach, 2020). COVID-19, however, has a major asymptomatic transmission component that SARS lacked, and many now expect that SARS-CoV-2 will become endemic. Evolutionary pressures are giving rise to new viral variants that have appeared at a troubling rate, and some scientists fear that a future variant could be much worse than what we have experienced thus far. The world may have to learn to coexist with COVID-19 as it has with influenza.

Perhaps the most egregious early scientific error was taken from pandemic models developed at Imperial College London in the United Kingdom, which predicted 500,000 deaths there and 1.2 million deaths in the United States by October 2020 as a result of COVID-19 (Ferguson et al., 2020). As of October 2021, Johns Hopkins University had recorded 139,444 deaths in the United Kingdom and 729,710 deaths in the United States as a result of COVID-19 (Johns Hopkins University, 2021). Harvard epidemiology professor Marc Lipsitch projected in February 2020 that "40–70% of the adult population around the world will be infected" with the COVID-19 virus (Axelrod, 2020). Not until almost two years after this prediction was it believed that more than 40 percent of the world has been infected with COVID-19 (COVID-19 Cumulative Infection Collaborators, 2022). These predictions panicked political leaders across the globe into taking drastic actions to stop the virus by shutting down much of the world's economy and government functions and encouraging people to sequester in their homes. These early models unintentionally exaggerated the expected mortality rates—thank heaven—because they had miscalculated the data, particularly infection and mortality rates, a mistake likely resulting from incomplete data. But massive increases in public debt in many countries, which were needed to fund emergency social safety net measures for the unemployed caused by the economic shutdown, were very real and very damaging to the fiscal health of the countries that enacted them. These massive debt increases and the interest payments needed to fund the debt each year will not disappear even if the pandemic were to end tomorrow.

Additionally, experts predicted that it would take years to develop an effective vaccine for COVID-19, as previous efforts at vaccine development for other diseases had taken an average of more than a decade. In April 2020, the *New York Times* estimated that "our record for developing an entirely new vaccine is at least four years" (Thompson, 2020). Fortunately, the past was not a prologue, at least insofar as vaccine development would go. The first COVID-19 vaccines were developed and tested in less than a year, an extraordinary scientific and technological accomplishment. This book describes Operation Warp Speed (Allison, 2020), the Trump administration's public-private partnership to develop the US vaccines, which turned out to be highly effective. Graham Allison, the former dean of the Kennedy School at Harvard, wrote in the *Wall Street Journal* that this was the Trump administration's one remarkably successful initiative during the pandemic. While the United States was slow in responding to the pandemic in other respects, its efforts in vaccine development were a major success story. But success was also built on a foundation of investments in biodefense, pandemic preparedness, and vaccine platform technologies over the last 20 years. Without evolving policy and operational lessons learned, coupled with past biodefense vaccine technology investments, the accelerated development of COVID-19 vaccines in 11 months would have been impossible.

Many infectious disease experts have argued from the start of the pandemic that herd immunity should be one of the goals in fighting it, a goal that is increasingly elusive (McNeil, 2020). Herd immunity is achieved when the virus, any virus, stops circulating because enough of the population has developed antibody-induced immunity, either from being vaccinated or having had the disease. In the case of COVID-19, people who have been immunized are still getting the disease in milder form but seldom require hospitalization or die from it (Rosenberg et al., 2021). The problem is that the data show that even after getting immunized, one can infect other people, which means vaccination does not offer protection to the unvaccinated, a central component of vaccine-derived herd immunity in the past (CDC,

2021). Even more troubling is that 40–45 percent of the people who are infected have no symptoms (asymptomatic) yet can still infect other people (Oran & Topol, 2020).

Most of these failures took place because scientists attempted, inappropriately, to apply past pandemic history to the COVID-19 virus without knowing what its actual behavior would be based on scientific research. As experiments were completed, scientists appropriately changed their public prognostications based on the results, as any serious expert would do. In fact, one of the most remarkable outcomes of the COVID-19 crisis has been the decentralized worldwide research effort, published in public health and medical journals, by thousands of the world's greatest scientists to inform policymakers and the public about the nature of the virus. No event in modern history has so concentrated the scientific minds of the world on one research undertaking, over such a short period, as the COVID-19 pandemic. Through this research, we knew within months that the elderly, the obese, people with high blood pressure, and those with compromised immune systems were severely at risk. These findings have been validated over and over in subsequent studies. We knew within months that the virus was spread almost entirely through airborne spray or droplets of mucus. We started to learn within months that 27–33 percent of the population would suffer long-term or perhaps even permanent damage to their respiratory, neurological, and circulatory systems, now called "long-haulers" (UC Davis, 2021). We knew within months that a small number of children would suffer from what is called multisystem inflammatory syndrome. We also knew within months that the virus entered the lungs by attaching itself to the ACE2 receptor, and there were many more findings. The free and open publication of these studies for all scientists to review supported the evolution of highly decentralized yet highly effective research coordination that allowed remarkable research progress to be made over a short period. So, while the scientific community made some early mistakes that compromised public trust, when they focused on using scientific research methods to advance our understanding of the virus, they achieved major success. It was when they started speculating without evidence that they got into trouble and damaged their credibility.

Not only has the world community of scientists suffered major set-backs in public trust; so have national governments. The public infighting among US government offices—such as the Centers for Disease Control and Prevention (CDC), the Food and Drug Administration (FDA), the National Institutes of Health (NIH), the Health and Human Services Assistant Secretary for Preparedness and Response (ASPR), and the Biomedical Advanced Research and Development Authority (BARDA)—has now spanned two presidencies. The White House under both Presidents Trump and Biden was unable to effectively coordinate major policy decisions among these competing but subordinate centers of federal executive authority. President Trump openly fought over scientific matters with respected scientists and undermined his own appointees by criticizing them in public. President Biden promised a return to normalcy from the chaotic Trump years, but public disputes among all these competing centers of federal power with the White House have belied these promises of orderly government (*Washington Post*, 2021). While President Biden attempted to take actions that would slow the number of deaths, the spread of the disease, and its mutations, he was unable to make much of a dent in any of these consequences of the pandemic. Disputes over whether to give booster shots, to whom and when, how to make good on repeated US promises to distribute vaccines desperately needed in low-income countries, and the most effective strategy for combating vaccine hesitancy without increasing public resistance, all damaged the Biden administration's credibility, particularly when it appeared to have overruled its own experts, as did President Trump.

It is not only US government institutions that have suffered fallout from the pandemic; international institutions have suffered as well. The institutional weaknesses of the World Health Organization (WHO), which were known to international health professionals, aid officials, and diplomats but not to the public, became apparent in the early weeks, when the director-general, Dr. Tedros Adhanom Ghebreyesus, appeared to be overaccommodating to China, which had refused to cooperate and supply clinical data until it was too late to contain the outbreak. WHO made matters worse by putting people with serious conflicts of interest on a study committee, the IHR Emergency Committee for COVID-19, to determine whether the outbreak in China was a natural occurrence or an accidental release from the BSL-4 or other laboratories in Wuhan (WHO, 2020). The report's findings were widely criticized, even among those who believed the virus was a natural occurrence, because they were based on insufficient access to Chinese data. Even Dr. Tedros questioned the report's conclusions, stating that the committee had made a "premature push" to dismiss other theories (NPR, 2021). The proclamation of findings based on incomplete information further eroded trust in WHO (NPR, 2021).

WHO has structural weaknesses that have little to do with who leads the organization or how they get elected. Little public discussion about these weaknesses has taken place, even though the US government and other donor governments along with senior career WHO leaders have repeatedly attempted unsuccessfully to reform the system over many decades. When WHO was created in 1948 as part of the United Nations, a regional version already existed in the Western Hemisphere, called the Pan American Health Organization (PAHO). It agreed to join the newly created organization only if it could maintain its regional autonomy by reporting to the 30-nation executive council of WHO. The decision was then made to have all the regional offices of WHO report in the same way to the Executive Council—not to the director-general. Thus, the director-general has no direct control over the hiring, firing, or supervising of the field staff of WHO (who are elected by the Executive Council). These regional offices therefore have veto power over any declaration of a pandemic emergency by the director-general in Geneva, Switzerland, and have delayed or stopped declarations in the past, such as the Ebola outbreak declaration in West Africa in 2014. Many countries—both wealthy, advanced, industrial democracies and poor southern countries—do not want a strong director-general, and as a result, the organizational integrity and coherence of WHO has suffered over many years (Liden, 2014).

The Economic Consequences

Next to the human life and health consequences of COVID-19, its economic consequences have been devastating. The economic analysis in this book argues that "falling consumer demand, sharp increase in uncertainty, and disruptions in global supply chains" caused the massive drop in GDP experienced by most economies. While the formal US unemployment rate was 14.6 percent, the real unemployment may have been as high as 26 percent, which would have exceeded the Great Depression peak of 24.75 percent in 1933. Some, though a minority, of scholars and opinion makers have argued that federal and state government policy decisions to shut down large parts of the economy to stop the spread of the virus did economic damage to the livelihoods and family stability of lower-income people that was greater than the public health benefits achieved (Baker, 2020). The evidence in this book suggests it was public fear of the virus, not government actions, that shut down economic activity. This is what happened in 1918, when the federal government was completely missing in action. According to *The Great Influenza* by John Barry, President Woodrow Wilson saw the 1918 influenza pandemic threatening the coherence of the US mobilization for World War I, so he suppressed media coverage of the devastation of the disease. And yet people acted on their own to shut down factories, pull their children from school, and empty the streets. So, the debate over what the government policy should have been in this pandemic may be moot. The question remains as to whether the changes to the economies of the United States and other countries are permanent.

This book describes the single most significant change to the global economy caused by the pandemic, which is the disruption of global supply chains in pharmaceuticals, the world food system, the automotive industry, natural resource extraction, and electronics, among others. As the analysis of this book suggests, multinational corporations are reassessing their supply chain vulnerabilities and are reshoring or nearshoring their industrial processes to reduce risk. Supply chains—focused as they have been almost exclusively on cost reduction and efficiency—remain much more fragile than corporations themselves understood. By October 2021, supply chain disruptions were depressing economic activity and endangering global recovery. An analysis in the *Wall Street Journal* on October 9, 2021, showed that industrialized democracies were recovering faster from the pandemic than low-income countries. These countries, which the world depended on for natural resources and some component parts, were still suffering the ravages of the disease in a severe pandemic time lag (Yap, Boston,

& MacDonald, 2021). COVID-19 has brought all these economic issues into stark relief.

Certainly, Washington policymakers in both parties now understand that pharmaceutical production—just one supply chain—is a national security issue because shortages of lifesaving drugs to treat heart disease, cancer, and diabetes, among other problems, threaten the lives of large swaths of the population. Many Chinese pharmaceutical manufacturing plants, which produce 80 percent of the active pharmaceutical ingredients (APIs) needed by the United States and countries in Europe, are in the greater Wuhan area and were shut down by the Chinese government in the early months of the pandemic to stop the spread of the disease. The US Food and Drug Administration warned of dangerously low supplies of 21 critical drugs by the spring of 2020 (Gibson & Singh, 2021). The availability of these drugs should not be decided by multinational corporations and the marketplace alone, as this is a national security issue much like national defense. We do not know whether these policymakers and the general public are prepared to pay much higher prices for drugs in order to ensure the integrity of supply chains by reestablishing the industry within the United States.

Business supply chains have been profoundly affected by the pandemic, and so have their communications. The massive shift in early 2020 of industrial and office communications from person-to-person interaction to virtual platforms, such as Zoom and Microsoft Teams, has shocked government and business into reconsidering their information systems. Virtual conferences, virtual speeches and lectures, and virtual meetings are here to stay as options for managers and administrators. While they may have existed prior to the pandemic at a modest level, their widespread subsequent use has been a major shift in corporate communications and certainly a positive outcome of COVID-19, as it will increase the efficiency, productivity, and time management of all institutions and organizations. In fact, multinational corporations are now reassessing many of their internal systems to reduce vulnerabilities to pandemics in all areas of activity. We see in this book how one large corporation—ExxonMobil—handled the pandemic and its effects on operations.

Great power rivalry appeared before the pandemic began and has accelerated because of it. China has tried to use its early vaccines as leverage in getting commitments from low-income countries to avoid criticizing China in international bodies for its repression of Tibet, Hong Kong, and the Uighurs, and its threats against Taiwan. The effectiveness of this vaccine diplomacy has diminished, as the efficacy of the Chinese vaccines is now in question (Wee & Meyers, 2021). The aggressive spread of the virus in Russia in late 2021 made its efforts to use the pandemic for strategic purposes a greater failure than Chinese efforts. One study of Russia's attempts to sell its vaccines in Nigeria, the most populous African nation, shows that years of educational exchanges and joint research projects between Nigerian and US scientists, and thousands of Nigerian students getting their doctoral degrees at US universities through USAID scholarships and the State Department Fulbright Program, have made US vaccines the overwhelmingly preferred option in Nigeria. In fact, the Russian antivaccine cyber-warfare campaign over many years, promoting conspiracy theories and disinformation about vaccines, appears to have backfired, as there is more vaccine resistance in Russia than in nearly any other country in the world, according to survey data.

The Impact of Political Systems on Pandemic Response

The Lowy Institute of Australia published a ranking of 116 countries (in January and March 2021) according to how well they managed the pandemic (Lowy Institute, 2021). Autocracies have done no better in their responses than democracies. None of the great powers—the United States, India, Russia, Brazil, France, and the United Kingdom—have done well in the pandemic. China was not ranked at all because it produced insufficient or no data to analyze its response, while the limited data it did provide on absolute deaths and infections were politicized and remarkably unreliable. The Bloomberg news service, using satellite photographs of funeral homes in Wuhan, reported on March 27, 2020, that the images showed a far greater number of burial urns for cremated bodies than deaths reported by the Wuhan health authorities (Bloomberg News, 2020).

Two larger unitary states in Asia did particularly well initially in their responses: Vietnam and Thailand. Countries with federal systems generally ranked more poorly because political authority was decentralized so that subordinate levels of government could legally defy national mandates to manage the pandemic. As federal states, only Australia ranked high, while Canada, Nigeria, Switzerland, and Germany ranked in the middle of the Lowy study. The largest federal states such as the United States, India, Mexico, and Brazil ranked at the very bottom of the 116-country index. Ten small unitary countries that ranked at the top were also island nations: Iceland, Singapore, Cyprus, Malaysia, Sri Lanka, Trinidad and Tobago, Taiwan, Cuba, Malta, and New Zealand. Other smaller unitary countries, such as Bhutan, Israel, and South Korea, also ranked well (at least for the first phase of the pandemic), probably because their borders are oceans or are virtually impermeable, so they benefited from the same geographic isolation as island states. Japan, which is an island country but also a large unitary great power with the world's third largest economy, ranked in the middle of the Lowy study. We may conclude that governance and size both count in pandemic response, but not necessarily in the way in which popular opinion has speculated. Federal democratic states with their systems of checks and balances do not perform well in pandemic response. This is particularly true for large, complex ones. Even if federalism is a superior system in other ways (e.g., promoting diversity of opinion and experimentation, and protecting freedom), it appears to have some drawbacks in public health response. This does not mean that public health response in the United States, or that of other federal systems, should be centralized. In a centralized system, especially in a large, heterogeneous country, one mistaken decision will have cascading impacts across the country.

One explanation for the rapid spread of the disease in the United States, which has not been much studied, is that these high rates may have been a result of the US air transportation system, which is the densest and most integrated of any nation on earth. Over 25 percent of the 144,000 daily flights *in the world* begin in the United States, while it has less than 4 percent of the world's population. Airport terminals are natural accelerators of airborne diseases. Studies have shown the Toronto Pearson International Airport was the means by which the SARS virus outbreak started in Canada, having first departed from China and then traveled to the Mexico City international airport and on to Toronto (*Toronto Star*, 2021). This led to the Canadian government placing travel restrictions for certain destinations for a month (BBC News, 2020).

One simple explanation for the high mortality rates in the United States during the pandemic has little to do with quality of political leadership, equitable access to health care, or the diffuse authority in the federal system. It is the level of obesity in the US population. At 36.47 percent, obesity levels in the United States are the highest in the world (except for 13 very small Pacific island states with populations of under 200,000). According to the CDC, 73 percent of US deaths from COVID-19 were of people who suffered from obesity or were overweight. We have known for years that obesity in the United States is a major health problem, but how to remedy it is another matter entirely and cannot be done in the middle of a pandemic.

Public-Private Partnership between Government and Industry

While much of the US government was engaged in disputes and infighting during the pandemic, one effort, Operation Warp Speed, was remarkably successful, as mentioned previously. This book contains one of the most detailed descriptions in the literature of Operation Warp Speed. The effort worked because it was a public-private partnership that harnessed the best scientific minds, the research and production technology of the US pharmaceutical industry, and the funding and legal authorities of the federal government to provide resources and regulatory support. The United States as a country is comparable to a freight train with 300 cars and four locomotives; it takes a while to accelerate to a high speed, but once it does, it is remarkably powerful.

The speed at which this public-private partnership was organized and became operational provides a case history of what can be done in a crisis. But science, technology, and government leadership (or its failure) are not the whole story regarding containment of COVID-19. The vaccine had to be administered to people at the local level, which involved a highly complex logistical system that was overall successful in getting the vaccines out across the United States in a short time. Senior managers and policymakers, however, had not prepared themselves for the vaccine hesitancy movement. While this movement is not new in history, its worldwide reach, aggressiveness, and entry into US national politics were unusual.

This book also examines the "infodemic": the massive tidal wave of information on the pandemic made possible by the internet and electronic media such as Facebook, Twitter, TikTok, LinkedIn, and others. This term was coined, in the context of SARS, by David Rothkopf of the *Washington Post* in 2003. The infodemic allowed a small number of shadowy cyber operators to manipulate electronic media to spread bizarre conspiracy theories about the disease and vaccines: "they are part of the ancient Illuminati conspiracy," "they are full of mercury to poison the public," "they contain microscopic listening devices to spy on the unknowing public," "the elite is trying to kill off people who they find threatening," or "the infection is spread by the 5G Huawei network," among others. Prior to the pandemic, researchers at George Washington and Johns Hopkins Universities examined the antivaccine messaging sources on Twitter and found that a substantial number were from 10 Russian bots using technology to dramatically expand the number of antivaccine messages. Public health was significantly undermined, especially among the most vulnerable, with around "50% of tweets about vaccination contain[ing] anti-vaccine beliefs" (Broniatowski et al., 2018). Antivaccine messaging from Russian sources accelerated during COVID-19.

The three US epicenters of vaccine hesitancy prior to COVID-19 were Austin, Texas; Detroit, Michigan; and Berkeley, California. The movement was fueled by both left- and right-wing sources and led by Dr. Stephen Wakefield, a disgraced UK doctor; Robert Kennedy Jr., son of the late senator Robert Kennedy; and actor Robert De Niro. They claimed that vaccines caused autism even though no scientific evidence existed to support their theories. Vaccine hesitancy spread among the populist right, promoted by talk show hosts, who peddled conspiracy theory on an epic scale even though it was the Trump administration that had led the development of the vaccines. When Donald Trump spoke at a rally in Alabama in August 2021 and urged everyone to get vaccinated, he was booed by his own supporters and quickly backed down from this message. This incident is astonishing evidence of the depth of paranoia over vaccines among an element of the public (Blake, 2021).

The most dangerous and long-lasting consequence of the COVID-19 pandemic may turn out to be the dramatic expansion of the vaccine hesitancy movement so that the ongoing inoculation of the US population to reach herd immunity for other diseases will become more difficult. A major factor in the rise of US life expectancy in the twentieth century—which rose from about 46 years in 1900 to nearly 80 years in 2019—has been the vaccination of the population against most major diseases (Johnson, 2021). Vaccine hesitancy could undo the progress the United States has made in health and life expectancy, particularly in areas with far-left or far-right ideologies (Higgins, 2021). The same trends are spreading in low-income countries around the world, though they are relatively unstudied at this point.

Unequal availability and distribution of vaccines between wealthy countries and low- and middle-income countries has been legitimately raised as a serious failing in the international system, but what has not risen to the same level of debate is the fact that the vaccine hesitancy movement has affected not only industrialized democracies but also low-income countries. Europe rejected the AstraZeneca vaccine and sent it to Africa, which further inflamed vaccine hesitancy among Africans, who understandably did not want to take a vaccine rejected by Europeans.

The spread of the vaccine hesitancy movement to the poorest and middle-income countries could erase the progress made in the last 50 years in life expectancy and child survival. It would alter demographic patterns, cascading across the world in profound and unpredictable ways over the coming decades. Vaccine hesitancy could accelerate the downward slope of populations caused by declining fertility rates already present before the pandemic in advanced industrial democracies and many middle-income countries.

Wet Markets, Bushmeat, and Zoonotic Diseases

Wealthy countries, focused inwardly during the pandemic, have ignored one of the persistent economic and nutritional challenges in low- and middle-income countries, which has also been the source of many spillover events over the past 40 years: trade in wild animals as a food source.

This book reviews the economics of the bushmeat trade, the disease risks associated with it, and regulatory efforts to contain it. These wet markets are not only difficult to control but are also a critical source of income for poor people and of animal protein in regions of the world with high malnutrition rates. No issue is more important to future risks to both low-income countries and wealthy countries than this bushmeat trade, yet there has been little to no attention given to it except among environmental scientists and development practitioners. Even the United States and other wealthy countries have wet markets where live wild animals are sold for food. In the United States these markets have little regulation and pose a risk. Wealthy country policymakers do not understand the economics or loose regulatory systems that operate in wet markets in their own countries, let alone in low- and middle-income countries. Many of these wet markets are in densely populated urban areas, which makes disease crossover from animals to people even more dangerous.

The pandemic has affected different demographic groups at highly variable rates, but none as severely as undocumented migrants moving northward from countries in the Southern Hemisphere. This book documents these effects. The pandemic has also affected education, schools, and children in unanticipated ways that have implications for the mental health of children and have led to conflicts among teachers, unions, school administrators, and parents. This book describes the effects of the pandemic in grades K–12 and in colleges and universities.

Investigating the Origin of COVID-19

Perhaps no pandemic issue has elicited more emotion and debate than the investigation into the origin of SARS-CoV-2. Determining the origin of the virus is not just an academic question; it will affect efforts to prepare for the next pandemic. In 2021, a 34-member UN team of international scientists was sent to China to investigate the origin of the virus but concluded, without sufficient evidence to support any side of the debate, that the pandemic resulted from natural spillover (UN News, 2021). Commentators discussing the origin of the virus have reported two source theories—a natural occurrence, and an accidental Wuhan lab–associated release—while in fact there are four theories (Folmer et al., 2021).

The first was suggested by the *Epoch Times*, a newspaper published by the Buddhist Falun Gong movement, proposing that this was a deliberate release of a biological weapon (Fang, 2021). Falun Gong has a conflict of interest in that its members have been brutally persecuted, tortured, and executed by the Chinese government. They have produced a documentary presenting evidence for their theory, which is ultimately unconvincing.

The second hypothesis is that the Wuhan Institute of Virology—which has a BSL-4 lab (the most secure category of virology laboratories for the study of the most dangerous pathogens) and is part of the Chinese Academy of Sciences and the Chinese Center for Disease Control and Prevention Laboratory in Wuhan—collected samples of SARS-CoV-2 from bats in caves 900 miles south of Wuhan and were performing gain-of-function experiments. (An example of gain-of-function research is a study in which scientists alter the RNA of a virus to make it more virulent in order to understand what makes it so dangerous and then create vaccines or treatments to treat the illness [*Wall Street Journal*, 2021]). Then a laboratory accident caused the release of the modified virus (Page, McKay, & Hinshaw, 2021). The Obama administration had suspended NIH grant-making for gain-of-function research in October 2014 while it investigated complaints from scientists about the dangers of this kind of research, but in December 2017 the suspension was lifted and the funding streams were opened again (NIH, 2017). Critics of the lab-release theory have confused the debate by focusing only on the BSL-4 lab in Wuhan, where there is also a BSL-2 lab at which bat virus research was also being conducted. The leak may well have taken place at this lab, not the BSL-4 lab (Qin & Buckley, 2021).

The investigative news service Results released 900 pages of documents (which it received from a Freedom of Information appeal) from the National Institutes of Health. Some of these documents were proposals submitted for funding by the EcoHealth Alliance to the Defense Advanced Research Projects Agency (DARPA), the famous Defense Department research center that funded the creation of, among other things, the internet. DARPA denied the proposal, but we have no way to know whether the work was done anyway; the EcoHealth Alliance receives US funding from several federal funding agencies, and the Wuhan Institute of Virology likewise receives funding from the Chinese government, and all included the creation of potentially dangerous chimerical viruses not seen in nature. Dr. Peter Daszak, the president of the EcoHealth Alliance, had previously denied that anyone was involved in gain-of-function research at the BSL-2 and BSL-4 labs in Wuhan, where his NGO was working with Chinese virologists collecting virus samples. However, his organization had submitted proposals to fund gain-of-function research (Natsios, 2020), showing the NGO's intent to perform such studies.

A February 2020 article from the *South China Morning Post*, the oldest and largest English-speaking paper in Hong Kong (owned by Chinese billionaire and former CEO of Alibaba, Jack Ma Yun), stated that Chinese scientists Botao Xiao and Lei Xiao wrote a blog arguing that the virus was accidentally released from the Wuhan lab, which was posted to the website of their university, the South China University of Technology. Thus, it was Chinese scientists, not US political figures or US journalists, who first described the source of the virus as an accidental release. The Chinese scientists' blog was taken down almost immediately, and their names were removed from the university website.

Yanzhong Huang, senior fellow for global health at the Council on Foreign Relations, writing in *Foreign Affairs* on March 5, 2020, reported in detail on the trial of a famous Chinese scientist, Li Ning, who was convicted of selling wild animals, which had been used in viral experiments, at wet markets for food. He made $1.46 million on these illegal sales. While there is no evidence that any of these animals were being used specifically for COVID-19 virus research, the fact that a prominent scientist would put the Chinese public at risk by selling lab animals for human consumption was shocking enough to get him sentenced to 12 years in prison (Huang, 2020). While not definitive proof, the previous grant submissions by EcoHealth Alliance, the blog posted by Chinese scientists, and the history of illegal lab animal management certainly make it possible that the virus could have originated in the Wuhan lab.

The third hypothesis is that the scientists who were searching for bat virus specimens in caves were infected by the virus and carried

it back to Wuhan, or they became infected in labs before any experiments on the virus had begun. We have reports that the bats had bitten
scientists collecting them for research. In this source hypothesis, the
virus had not yet been altered in gain-of-function research and thus
was a wild virus, which through natural mutation became efficient at
infecting people.

Relevant to both the second and third hypotheses, it is known
that the US Embassy in Beijing sent US scientists to the Wuhan lab
on an assessment mission in late 2017 and early 2018 because the
US government had been providing technical support to the labs as
part of NIH grants to EcoHealth Alliance. The cable they sent back
to Washington on March 27, 2018, was alarming because it "warned
about safety and management weaknesses" at the lab, and there was
a risk of accidental release. The *Washington Post* published a story on
April 14, 2020, on the cable after the State Department leaked it on
June 10, 2020 (Rogin, 2020).

The fourth official explanation for the source of the virus is natural
spillover, which was the explanation given by the Chinese government
at the beginning of the pandemic (Novel Coronavirus Pneumonia
Emergency Response Epidemiology Team, 2020). Beijing announced
that the virus was naturally occurring, having been spread from a
wet animal market (the Huanan market) 8.5 miles from the Wuhan
lab (Woodward, 2020). The Wuhan wet market as the original spillover point, however, was fatally undermined by Chinese scientists (it
would appear deliberately) when they published a report in *Lancet* on
January 24, 2020, showing that 13 of the 41 earliest infections were of
people who had no connection to the wet market. This article demonstrated that the Chinese government was not being truthful about the
origins and raised questions about where the original spillover event
could have occurred, if not in the wet market. In October 2021 an article in *Nature* reported the discovery of a highly similar coronavirus in
bat caves in Laos (Mallapaty, 2021). The virus taken from the caves in
Laos was more similar to SARS-CoV-2 than the virus taken from the
caves in China. While this report has been used to support the natural-
release theory, it does not provide enough evidence to prove that the
COVID-19 pandemic began with a natural spillover event. Questions
have been raised about how the virus got from Laos to Wuhan without

infecting anyone in between, an argument raised by Nicholson Baker in his *New York Magazine* article (described below).

In November 2021, one news service released emails from the National Institutes of Health that had been made public through a Freedom of Information request, which showed that bat virus samples with RNA highly similar to that of SARS-CoV-2 had been collected in Laos and sent to Wuhan for analysis. Such a finding again raises alarm about a possible lab accident as the origin.

Some scientists who are critical of the second and third hypotheses appear to want to avoid open criticism of the Chinese government, perhaps believing that these attacks would damage the government's credibility, or else feeling concerned that determination of a lab accident origin could suppress important life science research. While the evidence for both a lab accident and a natural spillover is not definitive, circumstantial evidence uncovered during the debate into the origins of the virus offers significant support for the third hypothesis of an accidental release of an unaltered naturally occurring virus. Nicholson Baker, a respected science writer from the *New York Times*, published an article in the *New York Magazine* on January 4, 2021, which broke the mainstream media wall on the Wuhan lab-leak hypothesis (Baker, 2021). He argued that the accidental lab release was the most plausible explanation for the origin, though for all four theories there remains only circumstantial evidence. As Baker argued in his thorough examination of the source of the virus, the lack of evidence of any human infections between the bat caves, where the closest relatives of the virus appear to have originated, and central Wuhan—a 900-mile journey— is difficult to reconcile. Why were no other infections detected between the two critical points separated by 900 miles?

The lab-leak hypothesis was politicized by the Trump administration when it attacked the Chinese government starting in April 2020 for allowing the release of the virus through shoddy safety protocol enforcement (Miller, 2020). The Trump administration's support for the lab-release theory meant that no self-respecting liberal mainstream media outlet could take the theory seriously until several left-leaning journals investigated the matter and wrote detailed analyses supporting the lab-release argument. This was followed by articles in *Newsweek*, the *Wall Street Journal*, and the *Washington Post* all arguing for the accidental-release theory. An *Intercept* investigation of the DARPA grant proposal was published on September 6, 2021 (Lerner & Hvistendahl, 2021). *Science* magazine sponsored a face-to-face debate, published on September 30, 2021, among scientists from different sides of the issue (Enserink, 2021).

Additionally, the previously mentioned NIH email release raised several important questions about the work being conducted in the Wuhan lab. Perhaps the most damaging of the released NIH emails from early 2020 were those indicating that Dr. Anthony Fauci and Dr. Francis Collins thought that the so-called "furin cleavage site," which appeared on the initial version of the SARS-CoV-2 virus, was unlikely to have occurred in nature and was very likely to have been created in a lab. Though they changed their position later, it demonstrated a concern that the virus might not be the result of natural spillover.

The *South China Morning Post* reported on February 17, 2020, several weeks after the outbreak, that President Xi Jinping had announced to a closed meeting with top leaders of the Chinese Communist Party a proposed new law based on the US public health system to increase the accountability of their research, safety measures, and data reporting systems (Cai & Pinghui, 2020). He could have done this for one of two reasons: (1) the senior leadership in Beijing knew that an accidental lab release had taken place and wanted to reduce the chance of reprisal, or (2) they realized their system was inadequate for pandemics in general. In September 2021, Xi gave a public speech warning Chinese scientists that regular inspections would be made to ensure that adequate lab safety measures in virology labs were being followed in order to avoid accidents in the future (Baptista, 2021). This serves as further circumstantial evidence regarding the origins of the SARS-CoV-2 virus.

Risky Research

This raises one final issue in this introduction, one that must soon be addressed by policymakers worldwide, before another viral disaster takes place. Since the COVID-19 pandemic struck, governments around the world have been funding the construction of BSL-4 labs so that their national scientists can do research on dangerous pathogens, presumably to protect their own people from worse disease outbreaks in the future. In theory, this appears to be a prudent policy. In practice, it may be the exact opposite, as these labs may increase the likelihood of a new pandemic should an accident take place, irrespective of what policymakers believe the origin of COVID-19 to be, particularly if samples of animal viruses are collected to do gain-of-function research. The United States probably has the most highly developed system of accountability in all spheres of endeavor of any nation in history, so much so that it has become an impediment in many disciplines (Natsios, 2010). And yet, US institutions themselves have had some breaches of biosafety protocols (GAO, 2016). If the United States has had breaches despite its strong institutions, its highly developed legal system to prosecute offenders, and its extraordinary levels of accountability, the risks for countries without any of these institutions if they build BSL-4 labs and conduct gain-of-function research on dangerous new pathogens almost ensure that we will face another lab leak. The proliferation of these BSL-4 labs and gain-of-function research may be more dangerous than nuclear proliferation: they represent a viral time bomb waiting to explode across the entire globe. Policymakers must ask this question before it is too late: Does "risky research" (which my colleague Dr. Gerry Parker coined) on extremely dangerous pathogens provide scientific benefits that exceed the extraordinary potential cost?

References

Achenbach, J. (2020, March 24). Coronavirus isn't mutating quickly, suggesting a vaccine would offer lasting protection. *Washington Post*. https://www.washingtonpost.com/health/the-coronavirus-isnt-mutating-quickly-suggesting-a-vaccine-would-offer-lasting-protection/2020/03/24/406522d6-6dfd-11ea-b148-e4ce3fbd85b5_story.html

Allison, G. T. (2020, December 23). Who made the vaccine possible? Not WHO. *Wall Street Journal*. https://www.wsj.com/articles/who-made-the-vaccine-possible-not-who-11608744603?page=1

Axelrod, J. (2020, March 2). Coronavirus may infect up to 70% of the world's population. *CBS News*. https://www.cbsnews.com/news/coronavirus-infection-outbreak-worldwide-virus-expert-warning-today-2020-03-02/

Baker, G. (2020, April 3). We only ever fight threats when they're upon us. *Wall Street Journal*. https://www.wsj.com/articles/we-only-ever-fight-threats-when-theyre-upon-us-11585932107

Baker, N. (2021, January 4). The lab-leak hypothesis. *New York Magazine*. https://nymag.com/intelligencer/article/coronavirus-lab-escape-theory.html

Baptista, E. (2021, September 30). Xi Jinping warns that Chinese laboratories handling deadly pathogens will face closer scrutiny. *South China Morning Post*. https://www.scmp.com/news/china/science/article/3150777/xi-jinping -warns-chinese-laboratories-handling-deadly-pathogens

BBC News. (2020, January 29). Covid travel restrictions: Canada suspends flights to Caribbean and Mexico. https://www.bbc.com/news/world-us-canada-55863882

Blackburn, C. C. (Ed.). (2020). *Preparing for pandemics in the modern world*. College Station: Texas A&M University Press.

Blake, A. (2021, August 23). Trump and top ally get booed by the monster Trump's GOP created. *Washington Post*. https://www.washingtonpost.com/politics/2021/ 08/23/trump-booed-gop-vaccines/

Bloomberg News. (2020, March 27). Urns in Wuhan prompt new questions of virus's toll. https://www.bloomberg.com/news/articles/2020-03-27/stacks-of-urns-in -wuhan-prompt-new-questions-of-virus-s-toll

Broniatowski, D. A., Jamison, A. M., Qi, S., Al Kulaib, L., Chen, T., Benton, A., Quinn, S. C., & Dredze, M. (2018). Weaponized health communication: Twitter bots and Russian trolls amplify the vaccine debate. *American Journal of Public Health*, *108*(10), 1378–84.

Cai, J., & Pinghui, Z. (2020, February 17). China to fast-track biosecurity law in corona-virus aftermath. *South China Morning Post*. https://www.scmp.com/news/china/ politics/article/3051045/china-fast-track-biosecurity-law-coronavirus-aftermath

CDC (Centers for Disease Control and Prevention). (2019, March 20). 1918 pandemic (H1N1 virus). https://www.cdc.gov/flu/pandemic-resources/1918-pandemic -h1n1.html

CDC (Centers for Disease Control and Prevention). (2021, September 7). Possibilities of COVID-19 illness after vaccination. https://www.cdc.gov/coronavirus/ 2019-ncov/vaccines/effectiveness/why-measure-effectiveness/breakthrough -cases.html

COVID-19 Cumulative Infection Collaborators. (2022, June 25). Estimating global, regional, and national daily and cumulative infections with SARS-CoV-2 through Nov 14, 2021: A statistical analysis. *Lancet*, *399*(10344): 2351–80.

Enserink, M. (2021, September 30). "Lab-leak" and natural origin proponents face off—civilly—in forum on pandemic. *Science*. https://www.science.org/content/ article/lab-leak-and-natural-origin-proponents-face-civilly-forum-pandemic -origins

Fang, F. (2021, March 15). Pandemic may have been caused by bioweapon research accident in China: Former State Department investigator. *Epoch Times*. https:// www.theepochtimes.com/pandemic-may-have-been-caused-by-bioweapon -research-accident-in-china-former-state-department-investigator_3733595 .html

Ferguson, N., Laydon, D., Nedjati Gilani, G., Imai, N., Ainslie, K., Baguelin, M., . . . Ghani, A. (2020). *Report 9: Impact of non-pharmaceutical interventions (NPIs) to reduce COVID19 mortality and healthcare demand*. Imperial College London. doi:10.25561/77482.

Folmer, K., Salzman, S., Pezenik, S., Abdelmalek, M., & Bruggeman, L. (2021, June 14). Natural-based or lab leak? Unraveling the debate over the origins of COVID-19. *ABC News.* https://abcnews.go.com/US/nature-based-man-made-unraveling-debate-origins-covid/story?id=78268577

Gallagher, J. (2020, November 9). Covid vaccine: First "milestone" vaccine offers 90% protection. BBC News. https://www.bbc.com/news/health-54873105

GAO (Government Accountability Office). (2016, August 30). High-containment laboratories: Improved oversight of dangerous pathogens needed to mitigate risk. https://www.gao.gov/assets/gao-16-642.pdf

Gibson, R., & Singh, J. P. (2021). *China Rx: Exposing the risks of America's dependence on China for medicine.* New York: Prometheus Books.

Higgins, Eoin. (2021, September 23). Opinion: Notable and quotable: Antivaxx. *Wall Street Journal.* https://www.wsj.com/articles/antivaxxer-liberals-conservatives-upstate-new-york-covid-19-11632426624

Huang, C., Wang, Y., Li, X., Ren, L., & Zhao, J. (2020). Clinical features of patients infected with 2019 novel coronavirus in Wuhan, China. *Lancet.* https://doi.org/10.1016/S0140-6736(20)30183-5

Huang, Y. (2020, March 5). U.S.–Chinese distrust is inviting dangerous coronavirus conspiracy theories. *Foreign Affairs.* https://www.foreignaffairs.com/articles/united-states/2020-03-05/us-chinese-distrust-inviting-dangerous-coronavirus-conspiracy

Johns Hopkins University. (2021, October 20). Coronavirus Resource Center. https://coronavirus.jhu.edu/map.html

Johnson, S. (2021, July 21). How humanity gave itself an extra life. *New York Times.* https://www.nytimes.com/2021/04/27/magazine/global-life-span.html

Learner, S., & Hvistendahl, M. (2021, September 6). New details emerge about coronavirus research at Chinese lab. *Intercept.* https://theintercept.com/2021/09/06/new-details-emerge-about-coronavirus-research-at-chinese-lab/

Liden, J. (2014). The World Health Organization and global health governance: Post-1990. *Public Health,* 128(2), 141–47.

Lowy Institute. (2021, March 13). Covid Performance Index. https://interactives.lowyinstitute.org/features/covid-performance/

Mallapaty, S. (2021, September 24). Closest known relatives of virus behind COVID-19 found in Laos. *Nature.* https://www.nature.com/articles/d41586-021-02596-2

McNeil, D. G. (2020, December 24). How much herd immunity is enough? *New York Times.* https://www.nytimes.com/2020/12/24/health/herd-immunity-covid-coronavirus.html

Miller, Z. (2020). Trump speculates that China released virus in lab "mistake." AP News. https://apnews.com/article/understanding-the-outbreak-intelligence-agencies-asia-pacific-technology-wuhan-c9499f7b8ab2ae7097c8588f1ccdddea

Natsios, A. S. (2010). The clash of the counter-bureaucracy and development. Center for Global Development. http://www.cgdev.org/content/publications/detail/1424271

Natsios, A. S. (2020, July 14). Predicting the next pandemic—the United States needs an early warning system for infectious disease. *Foreign Affairs.* https://www.foreignaffairs.com/articles/united-states/2020-07-14/predicting-next-pandemic

NIH (National Institutes of Health). (2017, December 19). NIH lifts funding pause on gain-of-function research. https://www.nih.gov/about-nih/who-we-are/nih -director/statements/nih-lifts-funding-pause-gain-function-research

Novel Coronavirus Pneumonia Emergency Response Epidemiology Team. (2020). The epidemiological characteristics of an outbreak of 2019 novel coronavirus diseases (COVID-19)—China, 2020. *China CDC Weekly*, 2(8), 113–22.

NPR (National Public Radio). (2021, July 15). WHO's chief says it was premature to rule out a lab leak as the pandemic's origin. https://www.npr.org/2021/07/15/ 1016436749/who-chief-wuhan-lab-covid-19-origin-premature-tedros

Oran, D. P., & Topol, E. J. (2020). Prevalence of asymptomatic SARS-CoV-2 infection. *Annals of Internal Medicine*. https://doi.org/10.7326/M20-3012

Page, J., McKay, B., & Hinshaw, D. (2021, May 25). The Wuhan lab leak debate: Disused mine at center stage—not predominant hypothesis, yet scientists call for deeper probe. *Wall Street Journal*. https://www.wsj.com/articles/ wuhan-lab-leak-question-chinese-mine-covid-pandemic-11621871125

Porterfield, C. (2021, September 20). 675,000 American deaths: Coronavirus now deadlier than the Spanish Flu. *Forbes*. https://www.forbes.com/sites/ carlieporterfield/2021/09/20/675000-american-deaths-coronavirus-now -deadlier-than-the-spanish-flu/?sh=d2c7510720a1

Qin, A., & Buckley, C. (2021, June 14). A top virologist in China, at center of a pandemic storm, speaks out. *New York Times*. https://www.nytimes.com/2021/06 /14/world/asia/china-covid-wuhan-lab-leak.html.

Rindsberg, A. (2021, November 15). The lab leak fiasco. *Tablet*. https://www.tabletmag .com/sections/news/articles/lab-leak-fiasco

Rogin, J. (2020, April 14). State Department cables warned of safety issues at Wuhan lab studying bat coronaviruses. *Washington Post*. https://scholar.harvard.edu/ files/kleelerner/files/20200414_wapo_-_state_department_cables_warned_of_ safety_issues_at_wuhan_lab_studying_bat_coronaviruses_-_the_washington_ post.pdf

Rosenberg, E. S., Holtgrave, D. R., Dorabawila, V., Conroy, M., Greene, D., Lutterloh, E., . . . Zucker, H. A. (2021). New COVID-19 cases and hospitalizations among adults, by vaccination status—New York, May 3–July 25, 2021. *Morbidity and Mortality Weekly Report*, *70*, 1306–11. doi:http://dx.doi.org/ 10.15585/mmwr.mm7037a7

Rothkopf, D. J. (2003, May 11). When the buzz bites back. *Washington Post*. https:// www.washingtonpost.com/archive/opinions/2003/05/11/when-the-buzz -bites-back/bc8cd84f-cab6-4648-bf58-0277261af6cd/

Sachs, J. (2021, September 22). The real reason this pandemic is the deadliest to ever hit the US. CNN. https://www.cnn.com/2021/09/22/opinions/staggering -selfishness-pandemic-surpasses-deaths-1918-sachs/index.html

Soy, A. (2020, October 8). Coronavirus in Africa: Five reasons why Covid-19 has been less deadly than elsewhere. BBC News. https://www.bbc.com/news/ world-africa-54418613

Thompson, S. A. (2020, April 30). How long will a vaccine really take? *New York Times*. https://www.nytimes.com/interactive/2020/04/30/opinion/coronavirus -covid-vaccine.html

Toronto Star. (2021, March 24). Toronto airport loses $383 million in 2020 as passenger numbers plunge due to COVID. https://www.thestar.com/business/2021/03/24/toronto-airport-loses-383-million-in-2020-as-passenger-numbers-plunge-due-to-covid.html

UC Davis. (2021, March 30). Studies show long-haul COVID-19 afflicts 1 in 4 COVID-19 patients, regardless of severity. UC Davis Health. https://health.ucdavis.edu/health-news/newsroom/studies-show-long-haul-covid-19-afflicts-1-in-4-covid-19-patients-regardless-of-severity/2021/03

UN News. (2021, March 30). COVID-19 origins report inconclusive: We must "leave no stone unturned"—WHO chief. https://news.un.org/en/story/2021/03/1088702

Wall Street Journal. (2021, September 13). Where the Covid origin inquiry goes now; Congress can focus on U.S. funding for gain-of-function research. https://www.wsj.com/articles/where-the-covid-origin-inquiry-goes-now-china-wuhan-institute-of-virology-lab-leak-theory-11631223271

Washington Post. (2021, September 13). Opinion: The Biden administration must clear up the confusion over booster shots. https://www.washingtonpost.com/opinions/2021/09/13/biden-administration-must-clear-up-confusion-over-booster-shots/

Wee, S. L., & Meyers, S. L. (2021, August 20). As Chinese vaccines stumble, U.S. finds new opening in Asia. *New York Times.* https://www.nytimes.com/2021/08/20/business/economy/china-vaccine-us-covid-diplomacy.html

WHO (World Health Organization). (2020, July 31). WHO-convened global study of the origins of SARS-CoV-2. https://www.who.int/publications/m/item/who-convened-global-study-of-the-origins-of-sars-cov-2

WHO (World Health Organization). (2022, April 4). WHO Coronavirus (COVID-19) Dashboard. https://covid19.who.int/

Woodward, A. (2020, April 15). An unsubstantiated theory suggests the coronavirus accidentally leaked from a Chinese lab—here are the facts. *Business Insider.* https://www.businessinsider.com/theory-coronavirus-accidentally-leaked-chinese-lab-2020-4

Yap, C. W., Boston, W., & MacDonald, A. (2021, October 8). Global supply-chain problems escalate, threatening economic recovery. *Wall Street Journal.* https://www.wsj.com/articles/supply-chain-issues-car-chip-shortage-covid-manufacturing-global-economy-11633713877

PART 1

DISEASE EMERGENCE AND SPILLOVER

CHAPTER 1

The Human-Wildlife Nexus

COVID-19 and Preventing the Next Pandemic

LILIANA K. WOLF AND LESLIE E. RUYLE

Introduction

A PANDEMIC RESULTING IN THE DEATHS OF MILLIONS OF PEOPLE and crushing economic hardship can begin with just a single event. Roughly 61 percent of human pathogens and 75 percent of novel disease outbreaks are zoonotic in origin (Taylor, Latham, & Woolhouse, 2001). It takes only one instance of human contact with wildlife for a pathogen to jump into the human sphere and set off a chain of events leading to a pandemic, and yet many people around the world rely on wildlife and wildlife products for food and medicine. Generations of hunters have brought their kills home to feed their families or sell to others in markets around the world. One day in the fall or winter of 2019, we can imagine that there was a hunter, transporter, market worker, or consumer who came into contact with an animal that carried a virus with zoonotic potential. This person likely would not have noticed symptoms until a week later when a nagging cough and/ or a fever developed. This person probably continued about his or her business, seeing customers and visiting family. We do not know whether patient zero survived this infection, but we know that hundreds of thousands of others around the world did not.

Zoonotic spillover is a term that describes the method by which an infectious agent from an animal population—or zoonosis—makes the jump to infecting humans. The likelihood of a spillover event leading to a pandemic may be enhanced by risky human activity, but a spillover incident needs to happen just once to initiate a catastrophic outbreak. This singular event is unpredictable and indistinguishable from identical actions that could just as easily have ended in a case of zoonotic spillover—but did not. Because so many potential instances of spillover end without incident, it may seem that this one time a virus did infect the human population was a matter of bad luck. But in fact, when we consider the increasing rate at which humans are destabilizing wild ecosystems and coming into contact with wildlife, it is apparent that this outcome was inevitable. With an understanding of the increasing potential for spillover, the fact that previous events ended without consequence should be considered only a matter of good luck.

One such example happened in the late twentieth century, when Malaysia experienced a period of rapid economic growth and a subsequent boom in population. As the country developed, farming practices shifted away from traditional family enterprises in favor of large-scale commercial farms. In order to meet the demand of the country's increasing appetite for meat, natural rain forest was cleared away to create space for pig farms and other agricultural land use. Pigs on these farms lived in edge habitat—the areas of agricultural human-dominated landscape and forest still frequented by wildlife. In these areas, pigs came into contact with wild fruit bats. Bats would fly overhead, sometimes dropping bits of half-eaten fruit into the pig enclosures, which the pigs would happily gobble up. Humans would then slaughter and eat the pigs. In 1998 an outbreak of a mysterious illness was documented in areas around these pig farms. Patients suffered from encephalitis, vomiting, dizziness, and coma. Subsequent outbreaks had an average mortality rate of a staggering 75 percent. Nipah virus, as the pathogen went on to be named, was listed by the World Health Organization (WHO) as one of the top 10 most important diseases to monitor and prepare countermeasures for in order to prevent a pandemic, and it served as the inspiration for the 2011 film *Contagion*.

Instances of zoonotic spillover have been increasing in number and severity since the latter half of the twentieth century (Cunningham, Daszak, & Wood, 2017; Daszak, Cunningham, & Hyatt, 2001). Drivers of this increase include (1) expanding land-use change, (2) range shifts of pathogens and hosts because of a changing climate, and (3) increasing movement of goods, humans, and livestock that creates conduits for pathogens and hosts to travel across previous geographic and spatial barriers (Cunningham, Daszak, & Wood, 2017; Karesh & Noble, 2009; Wolfe et al., 2005; Ostfeld & Keesing, 2000). In the case of Nipah virus, wild land was increasingly converted into agricultural fields, causing humans and livestock to come into contact with wild animals. This increased contact between wildlife, domestic animals, and humans allowed the Nipah virus to infect hosts (domestic pigs, and later humans) that it had rarely encountered previously. Other examples of such transmission include the Ebola virus in sub-Saharan Africa, which made the jump from bats to humans in multiple isolated events as humans became increasingly present in wild forest areas (Baize et al., 2014; Olival & Hayman, 2014; Olson et al., 2012; Leroy, Gonzalez, & Pourrut, 2007) The SARS virus, which is thought to have originated in colonies of horseshoe bats in eastern Asia (Wang et al., 2006; Li et al., 2005); HIV, which is believed to have first been transmitted to humans from chimpanzees in forested regions of south-central Africa (Heeney, Dalgleish, & Weiss, 2006; Sharp and Hahn, 2011); and Marburg virus, which is asymptomatically present in African fruit bats but causes high mortality rates in infected human and nonhuman primates (Bente et al., 2009; Swanepoel et al., 2007), are all examples of deadly spillover events.

When these infectious diseases spill from wild animal populations to humans, the host human immune system has no experience with the pathogen, and the potential for a severe reaction and illness is high. Therefore, it is paramount to limit the potential for spillover events as part of a pandemic preparedness plan.

One facet of the modern world that incorporates the multiple aforementioned risks of zoonotic spillover is the wildlife trade. The wildlife trade is a global, often illicit market for wild plants and animals. Created by a demand for wildlife products, this market encourages suppliers to have increased contact with wild animals, and the intercontinental shipment routes of live animals and animal parts create new conduits for zoonoses to travel. When they are trafficked and brought to market, species that do not commonly interact are stored in close containers in unsanitary conditions. Additionally, stress is a known trigger for weakening immune systems and causing viral shedding. All these factors combined can create a perfect natural laboratory for diseases to mutate and jump between species.

Why Do Wildlife Markets Exist?

Wildlife is traded for many purposes, and markets cater to a variety of customers. In some rural communities, wildlife, in this instance known as bushmeat, offers a valuable source of protein. This is especially true in regions where endemic infectious cattle disease and harsh terrain make domestic animal farming and cattle ranching difficult. However, the greatest environmental disruption and threat to biodiversity is caused by the demand for wildlife products as luxury items and traditional medicine.

Traditional Chinese medicine (TCM) is a practice of Eastern medicine based on a third-century BCE written account, the *Huangdi neijing*, although records of TCM practices exist from as early as 2,000 years BCE (Kong, 2010). TCM is still widely used in modern times and has been expanding in popularity as a consequence of growing global Chinese influence. Adherents of TCM use healing exercises such as tai chi and acupuncture, as well as traditional herbal mixtures and holistic curative compounds containing plants and animal parts (Kong, 2010; Tang, Liu, & Ma, 2008). While there is some scientific evidence to suggest that TCM practices such as acupuncture and tai chi are useful in relieving stress and pain, evidence supporting the usefulness of herbs, plants, and animal products is lacking, and many of the ailments people seek to treat with these cures are more efficiently treated with modern medicine. Nonetheless, strict adherents of TCM are socially and culturally inclined to continue their use of TCM products, and they often supplement or replace expensive or regionally unavailable modern medicine with TCM practices and products. On the other hand, wealthier adherents of these practices view the more-difficult-to-obtain "cures" as status symbols and a way to flaunt wealth. As the income of the average Chinese citizen has increased, so has the conspicuous consumption of expensive exotic animal parts. Famous examples include soup made from the fetus of a pangolin in order to aid fertility (Yue, 2009; Sutter, 2015), and powdered rhino horn promoted as a treatment for ailments ranging from cancer to impotence, as well as a powerful status symbol (Dang Vu & Nielsen, 2018; Truong, Dang Vu, & Hall, 2016).

As global Chinese diasporas expand, so do the influence of Chinese culture and the demand for TCM products. In this way, modern TCM practices are variable and change frequently with demand (Brown, 2017). The concept of *ye wei*, or "wild taste," refers to the desire to consume wild species, and it drives demand for the expansion of this market (Brown, 2017). Species that are charismatic or well marketed as being charismatic are particularly desirable for conspicuous consumption as well as for the pet trade. The Chinese Belt and Road Initiative creates easier avenues for the trade of difficult-to-obtain species while also providing more entry points to make wildlife hunting more accessible (Bush, Baker, & Macdonald, 2014; Espinosa, Branch, & Cueva, 2014; Farhadinia et al., 2019). Roads built in previously wild areas allow access for human hunting activities (Espinosa, Branch, & Cueva, 2014). Further, the expansion of Chinese culture in these areas creates a TCM demand for new species. A prime example of the dangers of demand expansion is the story involving the vaquita porpoise (*Phocoena sinus*) and the totoaba fish (*Totoaba macdonaldi*) in the Gulf of California.

Totoaba have no history in TCM, but early Chinese immigrants in the region recognized the similarities between these large, ancient-looking fish and the giant yellow croaker (*Bahaba taipingensis*), a common staple in TCM that is found off the southern coast of China (Joyce, 2016). The swim bladder from such large fish is prized in TCM as a medicinal ingredient thought to alleviate symptoms of arthritis and pregnancy complications (Martínez & Martínez, 2018). By 2011, a totoaba swim bladder could cost as much as $130,000 on the Hong Kong market, and a fisherman supplier could net nearly $3,000 to $4,000 for a single bladder. As demand for this ingredient exploded in China, so did the draw for fishermen in the Gulf of California to catch as many fish as possible using gill nets, thereby making their fortunes (Navarro, 2018). Gill nets are indiscriminate killers—they infamously catch and strangle unintended large animals such as sea turtles, dolphins, and sharks. The deployment of such fishing tools in the Gulf of California has led to the near extinction of the vaquita, which is the smallest porpoise in the world, measuring just four to five feet in length as an adult (Navarro, 2018). Despite the adoption of a gill net ban in 2015, the vaquita has continued to experience a precipitous decline in population size. Studies of acoustic activity suggest a 34 percent decline per year between 2011 and 2015 (Jaramillo-Legorreta et al., 2017). An approximate halving of the wild population each following year has left an estimated population of between just 6 and 22 vaquita in the wild. The decrease in the prevalence of totoaba has only increased the demand and price for the product, making any chance of vaquita population recovery seem slim, at best.

In the realm of environmental conservation, TCM practices offer a substantial obstacle to progress. The use of wild animals in TCM creates markets in poor communities, and suppliers are often presented with a means of economic mobility that is impossible to refuse. A recent story in the *New York Times* told of Mr. Mao, a bamboo rat farmer who used the demand for bamboo rats to lift himself and his family out of poverty (Myers, 2020). Over two decades, he expanded his business to acquire multiple bamboo rat farms. However, in the wake of the COVID-19 pandemic, his and other wildlife farms are being shuttered, and he stands on the edge of financial ruin. It is important to remember the lives of all people involved in the wildlife trade when offering up solutions to decrease demand. Some players are unfairly enriching themselves at the expense of ecological, environmental, and public health, but many are desperate and in fragile economic conditions. These people make difficult decisions to sustain their lives and the lives of their families. With this in mind, no progressive plan against the wildlife trade is complete without robust economic stabilization efforts for suppliers in order to reduce both supply and demand for wildlife products.

Wildlife Trafficking—the Perils of Oversight

The issues of wildlife markets and trafficking are often compounded by the dangers posed by the organized crime groups that oversee international trade in these illicit wildlife products. For all the known public health hazards posed to humans by wild animals, it seems sensible that governments should go to great lengths to limit contact between their citizens and wildlife. However, as we will discuss, decreasing the supply of and demand for wildlife products and enforcing bans on sales of these products is a complex, multifaceted issue and can often produce counterproductive results. Further, policing trade often does not address the issues of systemic poverty and corruption, which make wildlife trade appealing to participants at the base of the supply chain. Furthermore, in order to address this illicit global trade network, one must first acknowledge how a long history of imperial colonialism has shaped attitudes toward wildlife use and management in tropical countries. To be effective, actions to stymie the trade of wildlife must address the basic needs of people who live alongside the natural resources that feed this market.

Combating wildlife trade is a critical component of pandemic preparedness (Dobson et al., 2020; Smith et al., 2009). The global illicit market for wildlife products is vast, and it is complicated by the diversity of regions and players that contribute to it. To combat wildlife trade, these complexities must be acknowledged so that effective and intuitive policies can be developed.

When we consider issues of wildlife markets and international wildlife trade, it is important to understand that not all wildlife trade is illegal. The authority on the legality of international trade in wild animal and plant resources is the Convention on International Trade in Endangered Species of Wild Fauna and Flora (CITES). Under this 1974 international convention, only trade that does not threaten the survival of a species in the wild is permitted. As of this writing, CITES is made up of a total of 183 signatory countries and grants protections of varying levels to over 35,000 species of wild plants and animals. The levels of protection granted under CITES are indicated by the appendix level accorded to a species. For example, Appendix I species, such as orangutans (*Pongo pygmaeus*) and Bengal tigers (*Panthera tigris tigris*), are highly endangered and threatened with extinction in the wild without immediate intervention. All trade of these species is completely illegal for commercial purposes (although exemptions can be made for purposes of scientific research). Appendix II species may not necessarily be threatened with extinction, but trade must be controlled to avoid utilization incompatible with their survival. Examples of such species include American black bears (*Ursus americanus*) and zebras (*Equus quagga*). Products from these species may be traded with the proper trade permits. These permits are highly controlled and are issued only when granting authorities are confident that the trade in the species will not be detrimental to its survival in the wild. Appendix III species are protected by national legislation in at least one country that has requested assistance in controlling its international trade.

The absence of a CITES appendix listing for a species does not imply that the species is sustainably harvested and traded. In fact, a species is often added to the CITES list after many years of overexploitation have threatened its survival in the wild. Still, species of all appendix levels are often trafficked to fill demand in illicit markets around the world. Further, demand for products from each trade is driven by different consumer desires. Buyers of internationally traded wildlife products do not consume wildlife as a necessity but rather see the products as a status symbol. This offers more flexibility for intervention, and some successful campaigns against the consumption of wildlife have been launched with the intent of changing public perception of wildlife consumption. Examples include public service announcements featuring Chinese celebrities such as Yao Ming, Michelle Yeoh, and Jackie Chan denouncing the consumption of dishes made from shark fins, Chinese tigers, and pangolins. Yao Ming's public campaign against shark fin soup was particularly successful, bringing the consumption of sharks in China down by an estimated 80 percent.

When considering intervention strategies, we must also recognize the different drivers within the market for wildlife consumption. There are two distinct groups: (1) those who consume wildlife for subsistence, and (2) those who conspicuously consume wildlife to display prestige. Those who consume wildlife for subsistence are often poor, live in rural areas, and rely on local bushmeat markets for necessary protein. Suppressing these markets pushes demand underground without lessening it, as people need the product for survival. By contrast, the market for wildlife as a luxury product is driven by wealthy consumers and is often supplied by international trade (as exotic procurements are more highly sought after). In this market, species rarity increases demand, causing species from unsustainable populations and fragmented land to be more intensely hunted. Species in this category are more likely to be unhealthy and harbor disease, thereby increasing the chances of zoonotic spillover.

While subsistence markets for wildlife protein also create the potential for zoonotic spillover, these markets are typically more localized. They rely on community demand for protein that can be satiated by sustainable hunting practices. By contrast, international luxury markets demand "interesting" foods and do not rely on the continued integrity of the ecosystems from which they are sourced. Further, international laws that regulate hunting at the supplier level are often reminiscent of former colonial laws that restricted land use by native peoples. In this respect, these laws can be perceived by the community as illegitimate, making them difficult to enforce, at best. Certainly, preventing poor, marginalized communities from utilizing natural resources for subsistence and marginal profit is ethically problematic, and potentially politically unsustainable. A more effective means to combat poaching at the supplier level is through community-based natural resource management. This style of conservation prioritizes the rights and needs of local communities in areas of conservation concern by allowing individual communities to govern their own natural resources. However, natural resource policy is a complex intertwining of the fields of ecology, market economy, and local and state government, and the effectiveness of conservation methods is often hotly debated.

A Note on Culling

While decreasing the contact humans have with wildlife is necessary to lessen the risk of zoonotic spillover, efforts to cull wildlife populations to control disease are not recommended. Wildlife culls conducted to control the spread of disease have proven mostly ineffectual; they often increase infection rates in humans, threaten biodiversity, and disrupt ecosystems and ecosystem services (Florens & Baider, 2019; Olival, 2016). While it seems intuitive that decreasing the number and density of potential hosts and/or vectors should decrease transmission, increased human-animal interaction during the process of culling often amplifies exposure between infected organisms and susceptible humans and can therefore be counterproductive. Further, data on cost-benefit analyses of culling as a management practice are often lacking, or they show that the cost of the cull exceeds the revenue from reduced disease prevalence (Miguel et al., 2020; Florens & Baider, 2019; Olival, 2016; Harrison et al., 2010).

Politics, rather than science, can direct the call for wildlife culls. For example, Mauritius is the only remaining Mascarene Island that is home to an intact population of bats known as flying foxes (*Pteropus niger*). In what conservationists believed to be an effort to shore up popular political support, the Mauritius parliament disregarded scientific evidence and instituted a culling campaign against thousands of flying foxes. The plan was presented to the public as a means to increase yields from lychee and mango farms where the bats are perceived as pests. The actual damage that bats cause to crops in the island nation is highly contested, and the lack of robust studies on the subject hampers mitigation efforts (Tollington et al., 2019). Most crop damage can likely be attributed to invasive species such as rats and parakeets, while nets have been shown to be effective against crop damage by fruit bats (Tollington et al., 2019; Florens & Vincenot, 2018; Oleksy, 2015). The proposed cull sought a 20 percent reduction of the island population, but inflated estimates of the baseline population of this endangered species likely resulted in a 40 percent cull. Contrary to the claims made by the Mauritius parliament when the policy was proposed, the bat cull had little to no effect on damage to mango and lychee crops. In fact, according to the Mauritius Food and Agricultural Research and Extension Institute, there has been an estimated *decrease* in fruit crop yield since the cull began. Flying foxes are responsible for dispersing an estimated 53 percent of seeds for forest trees in Mauritius—this is the most significant contribution of a single bat species to a forest ecosystem that is scientifically known (Florens et al., 2017). It will be years before the full impact this cull has had on the forests of Mauritius will be evident.

Culling has been used to control both domestic and wildlife populations to stem the spread of disease. A sad example of such a domestic cull during the COVID-19 pandemic involves mink farms in the Netherlands. The first cases of mink coronavirus infection became apparent in April 2020 (Enserink & Kupferschmidt, 2020). Mink at two farms in the Netherlands began to show symptoms of nasal discharge and difficulty breathing—more of them also began to die than usual. In November 2020, Denmark found over 200 mink farms to be infected with SARS-CoV-2 and decided to cull over 17 million mink (Kesslen,

2021). Mink are closely related to ferrets, which can contract human influenza viruses and are often used as a model in laboratory studies on influenza epidemiology. While mortality rates at the two infected farms in the Netherlands were low (from a negligible amount at one farm to 10 percent at the other), two cases of human infection were traced back to the farms (Enserink, 2020). The alarmed government then called for a cull of millions of farmed mink since host reservoirs are known to be able to amplify virulence of zoonoses. Indeed, one of the facets that makes bird influenza so dangerous is its ability to be amplified among new hosts—especially poultry. Although SARS-CoV-2 did undergo noticeable mutations as it spread through Dutch mink populations, its virulence showed no signs of increasing (Enserink & Kupferschmidt, 2020; Oreshkova et al., 2020). These mink farms were destined to be phased out in 2024 for ethical reasons. Farmers may choose to reopen if they can prove their mink are uninfected, but for three years of profit in an uncertain market, it may seem hardly worth the effort, and many mink farmers have been left devastated.

Suggestions for the Future

Changes meant to mitigate the instances of zoonotic spillover should focus on combating the trade of wild species, preserving natural areas, and addressing social and economic disparities that allow risky activities to persist. Regulations should restrict the trade of all wildlife but specifically prevent the capture, movement, and trade of species of zoonotic interest (specifically primates, bats, pangolins, civets, and rodents) (Dobson et al., 2020).

Zoonotic spillover can occur at any point in the wildlife supply chain, but international markets garner more of our attention; the demand for wildlife as an exotic experience is entirely superfluous and offers no benefit to consumers. This is in opposition to local wildlife markets in poor rural communities, where bushmeat makes up the majority of protein available (Fa, Currie, & Meeuwig, 2003; Fa, van Vliet, & Nasi, 2016; Friant et al., 2020), and barriers to domestic meat raising make alternative protein sources difficult to establish (Tongue & Ngapagna, 2019). The majority of wildlife traded to international markets finds its destination in the United States, China, and other East Asian countries, where it is consumed both as a status symbol and as an ingredient in traditional medicinal practices. In an early effort to control the spread of diseases such as COVID-19, China officially banned the buying, selling, and transportation of wild animals in markets, restaurants, and online marketplaces throughout the country in February 2020 (Mallapaty, 2020). This ban extended to farms that bred and transported nondomestic animals in captivity, and while the ban was originally announced to last until the end of the COVID-19 pandemic, it is now permanent.

Although this ban has been widely hailed as a win for conservationists and epidemiologists who believe decreased contact with wild animals promotes better public health, others have been quick to voice their concerns about its efficacy and legitimacy. Those who are opposed point out that much of China's wildlife trade was already illegal, but a corrupt system and pervasive loopholes within the wording of the law allowed vast inconsistencies in enforcement. Furthermore, the ban penalizes previously legal producers for continuing their business and creates the choice of complying with the new law and returning to a life of poverty, or driving their business underground where they will no longer feel compelled to comply with regulations (Mallapaty, 2020). Certainly, many wildlife farmers must view this new law as illegitimate.

To understand the scale of the effect this ban could have on suppliers, note that the wild-meat industry in China is valued at $7.1 billion and employs approximately one million people. A comprehensive study conducted by the Chinese Academy of Engineering in 2017 suggests that the wild fur and meat industry in China could be valued at as much as $74 billion and employ 14 million workers (Chinese Academy of Engineering, 2017). Finally, this is not the first time a ban has been implemented on the wildlife trade in China as an attempt to stem the spread of zoonoses. After the outbreak of SARS-CoV-1 in 2003, China banned the trade of 54 species of animals believed to be potential reservoirs for the virus. However, after WHO announced that the virus had been cleared from the human population worldwide, the ban was reversed. Reversing this ban so soon seems to show a lack of foresight and understanding of zoonotic spillover—perhaps if the ban had remained in place, readers of this book would have spent the last several years attending parties and working in cafés, and at least six million more people would still be alive.

Seemingly the most effective way to control the amount of contact humans have with zoonoses should involve changes in policy to control wildlife trade along with enforcement strategies to carry them out. However, each commonly proposed policy has pitfalls that must be considered. Not all wildlife trade is illegal, and historically, some legal markets have been crucial in facilitating poaching and illegal movement of banned and protected species (Brown, 2017). One interesting example of this phenomenon involves a 2019 joint proposal from Israel and Kenya to include woolly mammoths (*Mammuthus primigenius*) as a CITES Appendix II species (Bending, 2019). Woolly mammoths are, of course, extinct and have been for thousands of years. However, there was concern that elephant ivory could be laundered as mammoth ivory as a way to circumvent trade restrictions. The proposal was ultimately withdrawn, but delegates agreed to revisit it in three years, after a study had been completed on the effect of mammoth ivory on the global elephant ivory market.

Policy changes rely on effective implementation and enforcement, which are particularly difficult in corrupt systems and where policies are deemed illegitimate by the resident population. This is especially true when enforcement units are underfunded, which they often are. Interdiction is the measurement most often cited as an example of law enforcement effectiveness in illicit trade. Seizures of illegal wildlife shipments including pangolin scales, ivory, or live animals such as baby sea turtles are examples of success. However, there are problems with using interdiction as the baseline indicator of enforcement success. Interdiction is meant to reduce supply and discourage demand. It essentially imposes a "tax" on smugglers—forcing them to lose profit and product as a consequence of conducting illicit trade. It also increases cost to the consumer, which has variable effects depending on the product. Interdiction is extremely difficult to implement effectively, however, and even when carried out appropriately, it can have counterproductive effects.

Research into drug trafficking is well resourced and can provide us with a benchmark from which to assess the effectiveness of wildlife trafficking enforcement policies (Brown, 2017). This research suggests that interdiction in illicit commodities often fails to curtail supplies and instead demands an increase in production from the supplier. In the world of drugs, an increase in commodity supply is troubling, but not completely counterproductive to the mission of enforcement. Drugs are not inherently rare or valuable—their worth is derived from their illegality. Production of drug products can be increased at the source to meet demand, and losses from interdiction can be sustained.

Conversely, wildlife is a depletable resource, and increasing the poaching and trafficking of wild animals to offset losses from interdiction creates the undesirable effect of increased defaunation while heightening the level of contact between humans and zoonoses. Further, research on the various effects of drug policies shows that prohibition can have complex effects on prices and demand. Parrot smugglers in Indonesia expect to lose over 90 percent of their product to law enforcement during shipment, so they instead put the parrots in plastic tubes and drop them into the ocean to be collected ashore. Recovery and survival of live parrots is only about 10 percent—comparable to what it would be through other means of transportation—but with a lesser risk of legal trouble. This cruel practice depletes the parrot population and allows smugglers to increase the cost of their product to offset the costs of their operation. Further, classifying a species as endangered or implementing a trade ban could actually have the counterproductive effect of increasing the desirability of that species (Rivalan et al., 2007). Overall, the effects of wildlife bans on conservation have been variable and complex. For effective policy implementation, high levels of communication and cooperation are necessary between scientists, policymakers, and law enforcement to ensure there is no or minimal lapse in implementation from the time a policy is announced to the time it is enforced.

While issues of enforcement must be considered and mitigated, interdiction and law enforcement are also important weapons against wildlife trafficking when used correctly. In addition to raising prices for products, interdiction and law enforcement efforts also create barriers for suppliers who do not have the will to attempt trade when stakes are higher. Similarly, when a product is illegal, the flow of the product is more constrained. This limits consumer uptake and potential market innovation. This holds true for illicit wildlife markets. Driving the market for wildlife products underground puts barriers between consumer and product, which ultimately decreases demand. This is especially true in the case of conspicuous consumption of wildlife as a status symbol. When luxury products cannot be consumed in the open, the desire for those products lessens substantially.

Finally, although law enforcement is at times at odds with values held by a community, the steady presence of enforcement can change cultural norms and motivate compliance. For law enforcement to become socially legitimized, it must be designed to collaborate with the community it polices and minimize deleterious social and environmental effects. Interdiction, bans, and law enforcement are designed to constrict supply, but ultimately the greatest value they bring to the table is the change in normative rules they establish in a population.

References

Ahn, M., Anderson, D. E., Zhang, Q., Tan, C. W., Lim, B. L., Luko, K., . . . Ng, J. H. J. (2019). Dampened NLRP3-mediated inflammation in bats and implications for a special viral reservoir host. *Nature Microbiology, 4*(5), 789–99.

Altizer, S., Bartel, R., & Han, B. A. (2011). Animal migration and infectious disease risk. *Science, 331*(6015), 296–302.

Baize, S., Pannetier, D., Oestereich, L., Rieger, T., Koivogui, L., Magassouba, N. F., . . . Tiffany, A. (2014). Emergence of Zaire Ebola virus disease in Guinea. *New England Journal of Medicine, 371*(15), 1418–25.

Banerjee, A., Rapin, N., Bollinger, T., & Misra, V. (2017). Lack of inflammatory gene expression in bats: A unique role for a transcription repressor. *Scientific Reports, 7*(1), 1–15.

Bending, Z. (2019, August 28). Why we need to protect the extinct woolly mammoth. *The Conversation.* https://theconversation.com/why-we-need-to-protect-the -extinct-woolly-mammoth-122256

Bente, D., Gren, J., Strong, J. E., & Feldmann, H. (2009). Disease modeling for Ebola and Marburg viruses. *Disease Models & Mechanisms, 2*(1–2), 12–17.

Brown, V. F. (2017). *The extinction market: Wildlife trafficking and how to counter it.* Oxford: Oxford University Press.

Burdette, D. L., Monroe, K. M., Sotelo-Troha, K., Iwig, J. S., Eckert, B., Hyodo, M., . . . Vance, R. E. (2011). STING is a direct innate immune sensor of cyclic di-GMP. *Nature, 478*(7370), 515–18.

Bush, E. R., Baker, S. E., & Macdonald, D. W. (2014). Global trade in exotic pets 2006–2012. *Conservation Biology, 283*, 663–76.

Calisher, C. H., Childs, J. E., Field, H. E., Holmes, K. V., & Schountz, T. (2006). Bats: Important reservoir hosts of emerging viruses. *Clinical Microbiology Reviews, 19*(3), 531–45.

Castañeda-Álvarez, N. P., Khoury, C. K., Achicanoy, H. A., Bernau, V., Dempewolf, H., Eastwood, R. J., . . . Müller, J. V. (2016). Global conservation priorities for crop wild relatives. *Nature Plants, 2*(4), 1–6.

CDC (Centers for Disease Control and Prevention). (2019, October 15). History of Ebola disease outbreaks. https://www.cdc.gov/vhf/ebola/history/chronology.html

Chinese Academy of Engineering. (2017). *Report on sustainable development strategy of China's wildlife farming industry.* Consulting Research Project of the Chinese Academy of Engineering [in Chinese].

Cunningham, A. A., Daszak, P., & Wood, J. L. (2017). One Health, emerging infectious diseases and wildlife: Two decades of progress? *Philosophical Transactions of the Royal Society B: Biological Sciences, 372*(1725), 20160167.

Dang Vu, H. N., & Nielsen, M. R. (2018). Understanding utilitarian and hedonic values determining the demand for rhino horn in Vietnam. *Human Dimensions of Wildlife, 23*(5), 417–32.

Daszak, P., Cunningham, A. A., & Hyatt, A. D. (2001). Anthropogenic environmental change and the emergence of infectious diseases in wildlife. *Acta Tropica, 78*(2), 103–16. https://doi.org/10.1016/s0001-706x(00)00179-0

Dobson, A. P., Pimm, S. L., Hannah, L., Kaufman, L., Ahumada, J. A., Ando, A. W., . . . Kinnaird, M. F. (2020). Ecology and economics for pandemic prevention. *Science, 369*(6502), 379–81.

Drexler, J. F., Corman, V. M., Müller, M. A., Maganga, G. D., Vallo, P., Binger, T., . . . Seebens, A. (2012). Bats host major mammalian paramyxoviruses. *Nature Communications, 3*(1), 1–13.

DutchNews. (2020, August 17). Coronavirus found on more mink farms, pressure mounts on minister to close them all. Accessed August 18, 2020. https://www.dutchnews.nl/news/2020/08/coroanvirus-found-on-more-mink-farms-pressure-mounts-on-minister-to-close-them-all/

Enserink, M., & Kupferschmidt, K. (2020). With COVID-19, modeling takes on life and death importance. *Science, 367*(6485), 1414–15. https://doi.org/10.1126/science.367.6485.1414-b

Erisman, J. W., van Eekeren, N., de Wit, J., Koopmans, C., Cuijpers, W., Oerlemans, N., & Koks, B. J. (2016). Agriculture and biodiversity: A better balance benefits both. *AIMS Agriculture and Food, 1*(2), 157–74.

Espinosa, S., Branch, L. C., & Cueva, R. (2014). Road development and the geography of hunting by an Amazonian indigenous group: Consequences for wildlife conservation. *PLoS ONE, 9*, e114916.

Fa, J. E., Currie, D., & Meeuwig, J. (2003). Bushmeat and food security in the Congo Basin: Linkages between wildlife and people's future. *Environmental Conservation, 30*(1), 71–78.

Fa, J. E., van Vliet, N., & Nasi, R. (2016). Bushmeat, food security, and conservation in African rainforests. In A. A. Aguirre & R. Sukumar (Eds.), *Tropical conservation: Perspectives on local and global priorities* (pp. 331–44). Oxford: Oxford University Press.

Farhadinia, M. S., Maheshwari, A., Nawaz, M. A., Ambarli, H., Gritsina, M. A., Koshkin, M. A., . . . Macdonald, D. W. (2019). Belt and Road Initiative may create new supplies for illegal wildlife trade in large carnivores. *Nature Ecology & Evolution, 3*(9), 1267–68.

Florens, F. B. V., & Baider, C. (2019). Mass-culling of a threatened island flying fox species failed to increase fruit growers' profits and revealed gaps to be addressed for effective conservation. *Journal for Nature Conservation, 47*, 58–64.

Florens, F. B. V., Baider, C., Marday, V., Martin, G. M. N., Zmanay, Z., Oleksy, R., ... Kingston, T. (2017). Disproportionately large ecological role of a recently mass-culled flying fox in native forests of an oceanic island. *Journal for Nature Conservation, 40*, 85–93.

Florens, F. B. V., & Vincenot, C. E. (2018). Broader conservation strategies needed. *Science, 362*(6413), 409.

Food and Agriculture Organization. 2012. *H5N1 HPAI global overview, January–March 2012*. http://www.fao.org/docrep/015/an388e/an388e.pdf

Friant, S., Ayambem, W. A., Alobi, A. O., Ifebueme, N. M., Otukpa, O. M., Ogar, D. A., ... Rothman, J. M. (2020). Eating bushmeat improves food security in a biodiversity and infectious disease "hotspot." *Ecohealth, 17*(4), 1–14.

Gaff, H., Burgess, C., Jackson, J., Niu, T., Papelis, Y., & Hartley, D. (2011). Mathematical model to assess the relative effectiveness of Rift Valley fever countermeasures. *International Journal of Artificial Life Research (IJALR), 2*(2), 1–18.

Gulbudak, H., & Martcheva, M. (2013). Forward hysteresis and backward bifurcation caused by culling in an avian influenza model. *Mathematical Biosciences, 246*(1), 202–12.

Harrison, A., Newey, S., Gilbert, L., Haydon, D. T., & Thirgood, S. (2010). Culling wildlife hosts to control disease: Mountain hares, red grouse and louping ill virus. *Journal of Applied Ecology, 47*(4), 926–30.

Heeney, J. L., Dalgleish, A. G., & Weiss, R. A. (2006). Origins of HIV and the evolution of resistance to AIDS. *Science, 313*(5786), 462–66.

Hensley, L. E., Alves, D. A., Geisbert, J. B., Fritz, E. A., Reed, C., Larsen, T., & Geisbert, T. W. (2011). Pathogenesis of Marburg hemorrhagic fever in cynomolgus macaques. *Journal of Infectious Diseases, 204*(suppl. 3), S1021–31.

Hing, S., Narayan, E. J., Thompson, R. A., & Godfrey, S. S. (2016). The relationship between physiological stress and wildlife disease: Consequences for health and conservation. *Wildlife Research, 43*(1), 51–60.

Jaramillo-Legorreta, A., Cardenas-Hinojosa, G., Nieto-Garcia, E., Rojas-Bracho, L., Ver Hoef, J., Moore, J., ... Taylor, B. (2017). Passive acoustic monitoring of the decline of Mexico's critically endangered vaquita. *Conservation Biology, 31*(1), 183–91.

Joyce, C. (Host). (2016, February 9). Chinese taste for fish bladder threatens rare porpoise in Mexico. NPR. https://www.npr.org/sections/goatsandsoda/2016/02/09/466185043/chinese-taste-for-fish-bladder-threatens-tiny-porpoise-in-mexico

Karesh, W. B., & Noble, E. (2009). The bushmeat trade: Increased opportunities for transmission of zoonotic disease. *Mount Sinai Journal of Medicine: A Journal of Translational and Personalized Medicine, 76*(5), 429–34.

Kesslen, B. (2020, December 1). Here's why Denmark culled 17 million minks and now plans to dig up their buried bodies. The Covid mink crisis, explained. NBC News. https://www.nbcnews.com/news/animal-news/here-s-why-denmark-culled-17-million-minks-now-plans-n1249610

Kilpatrick, A. M., Salkeld, D. J., Titcomb, G., & Hahn, M. B. (2017). Conservation of biodiversity as a strategy for improving human health and well-being. *Philosophical Transactions of the Royal Society B: Biological Sciences, 372*(1722), 20160131.

Kong, Y. C. (2010). *Huangdi neijing: A synopsis with commentaries.* Hong Kong: Chinese University of Hong Kong Press.

Lambert, A. J., & Brand, M. D. (2009). Reactive oxygen species production by mitochondria. In J. A. Stuart (Ed.), *Mitochondrial DNA: Methods in Molecular Biology,* vol. 554. Totowa, NJ: Humana Press.

Leroy, E., Gonzalez, J. P., & Pourrut, X. (2007). Ebolavirus and other filoviruses. In J. E. Childs, J. S. Mackenzie, & J. A. Richt (Eds.), *Wildlife and emerging zoonotic diseases: The biology, circumstances and consequences of cross-species transmission* (pp. 363–87). Berlin: Springer.

Li, W., Shi, Z., Yu, M., Ren, W., Smith, C., Epstein, J. H., . . . Zhang, J. (2005). Bats are natural reservoirs of SARS-like coronaviruses. *Science, 310*(5748), 676–79.

Luis, A. D., Hayman, D. T., O'Shea, T. J., Cryan, P. M., Gilbert, A. T., Pulliam, J. R., . . . Fooks, A. R. (2013). A comparison of bats and rodents as reservoirs of zoonotic viruses: Are bats special? *Proceedings of the Royal Society B: Biological Sciences, 280*(1756), 20122753.

Luis, A. D., O'Shea, T. J., Hayman, D. T., Wood, J. L., Cunningham, A. A., Gilbert, A. T., . . . Webb, C. T. (2015). Network analysis of host–virus communities in bats and rodents reveals determinants of cross-species transmission. *Ecology Letters, 18*(11), 1153–62.

Mallapaty, S. (2020, February 21). China set to clamp down permanently on wildlife trade in wake of coronavirus. *Nature.* https://doi.org/10.1038/d41586-020-00499-2

Martínez, I. A., & Martínez, E. R. (2018). Trafficking of totoaba maw. In I. Arroyo-Quiroz & T. Wyatt (Eds.), *Green crime in Mexico: A collection of case studies* (pp. 149–70). Cham, Switzerland: Palgrave Macmillan.

McLeod, A. (2010). Economics of avian influenza management and control in a world with competing agendas. *Avian Diseases, 54*(suppl. 1), 374–79.

Miguel, E., Grosbois, V., Caron, A., Pople, D., Roche, B., & Donnelly, C. A. (2020). A systemic approach to assess the potential and risks of wildlife culling for infectious disease control. *Communications Biology, 3*(1), 1–14.

Myers, S. L. (2020, June 7). China vowed to keep wildlife off the menu, a tough promise to keep. *New York Times.*

Navarro, C. (2018). Environmentalists warn about further drop in numbers of endangered porpoises in Mexico. SourceMex. https://digitalrepository.unm.edu/sourcemex/6424

Oleksy, R. (2015). *The impact of the Mauritius fruit bat* (Pteropus niger*) on commercial fruit farms and possible mitigation measures.* Report to the Rufford Foundation. https://www.rufford.org/projects/dr-ryszard-oleksy/the-impact-of-the-mauritius-fruit-bat-pteropus-niger-on-commercial-fruit-farms-and-possible-mitigation-methods/

Olival, K. J. (2016). To cull, or not to cull, bat is the question. *Ecohealth, 13*(1), 6–8.

Olival, K. J., & Hayman, D. T. (2014). Filoviruses in bats: Current knowledge and future directions. *Viruses, 6*(4), 1759–88.

Olson, S. H., Reed, P., Cameron, K. N., Ssebide, B. J., Johnson, C. K., Morse, S. S., . . . Joly, D. O. (2012). Dead or alive: Animal sampling during Ebola hemorrhagic fever outbreaks in humans. *Emerging Health Threats Journal*, *5*(1), 9134.

Omrani, A. S., Al-Tawfiq, J. A., & Memish, Z. A. (2015). Middle East respiratory syndrome coronavirus (MERS-CoV): Animal to human interaction. *Pathogens and Global Health*, *109*(8), 354–62.

Oreshkova, N., Molenaar, R. J., Vreman, S., Harders, F., Munnink, B. B. O., Honing, R. W. H. V., . . . Tacken, M. (2020, April). SARS-CoV2 infection in farmed mink, Netherlands. *bioRxiv*.

O'Shea, T. J., Cryan, P. M., Cunningham, A. A., Fooks, A. R., Hayman, D. T., Luis, A. D., . . . Wood, J. L. (2014). Bat flight and zoonotic viruses. *Emerging Infectious Diseases*, *20*(5), 741.

Ostfeld, R. S., & Keesing, F. (2000). Biodiversity series: The function of biodiversity in the ecology of vector-borne zoonotic diseases. *Canadian Journal of Zoology*, *78*(12), 2061–78.

Pamela, C., Kanchwala, M., Liang, H., Kumar, A., Wang, L. F., Xing, C., & Schoggins, J. W. (2018). The IFN response in bats displays distinctive IFN-stimulated gene expression kinetics with atypical RNASEL induction. *Journal of Immunology*, *200*(1), 209–17.

Patil, R. R., Kumar, C. S., & Bagvandas, M. (2017). Biodiversity loss: Public health risk of disease spread and epidemics. *Annals of Tropical Medicine and Public Health*, *10*(6), 1432.

Pushpangadan, P., George, V., Ijinu, T. P., & Chithra, M. A. (2018). Biodiversity, bioprospecting, traditional knowledge, sustainable development and value added products: A review. *Journal of Traditional Medicine & Clinical Naturopathy*, *7*(1), 1–7.

Rivalan, P., Delmas, V., Angulo, E., Bull, L. S., Hall, R. J., Courchamp, F., . . . Leader-Williams, N. (2007). Can bans stimulate wildlife trade? *Nature*, *447*(7144), 529–30.

Sharp, P. M., & Hahn, B. H. (2011). Origins of HIV and the AIDS pandemic. *Cold Spring Harbor Perspectives in Medicine*, *1*(1), a006841.

Smith, G. C., & Cheeseman, C. L. (2002). A mathematical model for the control of diseases in wildlife populations: Culling, vaccination and fertility control. *Ecological Modelling*, *150*(1–2), 45–53.

Smith, K. F., Behrens, M., Schloegel, L. M., Marano, N., Burgiel, S., & Daszak, P. (2009). Reducing the risks of the wildlife trade. *Science*, *324*(5927), 594–95.

Subudhi, S., Rapin, N., & Misra, V. (2019). Immune system modulation and viral persistence in bats: Understanding viral spillover. *Viruses*, *11*(2), 192.

Sutter, J. D. 2015. The most trafficked mammal you've never heard of. CNN: Change the List. Accessed September 1, 2016. http://edition.cnn.com/interactive/2014/04/opinion/sutter-change-the-list-pangolin-trafficking/

Swanepoel, R., Smit, S. B., Rollin, P. E., Formenty, P., Leman, P. A., Kemp, A., . . . Zeller, H. (2007). Studies of reservoir hosts for Marburg virus. *Emerging Infectious Diseases*, *13*(12), 1847.

Tang, J. L., Liu, B. Y., & Ma, K. W. (2008). Traditional Chinese medicine. *Lancet*, *372*(9654), 1938–40.

Taylor, L. H., Latham, S. M., & Woolhouse, M. E. (2001). Risk factors for human disease emergence. *Philosophical Transactions of the Royal Society B: Biological Sciences*, *356*(1411), 983–89.

te Beest, D. E., Hagenaars, T. J., Stegeman, J. A., Koopmans, M. P., & van Boven, M. (2011). Risk based culling for highly infectious diseases of livestock. *Veterinary Research*, *42*(1), 81.

Tollington, S., Kareemun, Z., Augustin, A., Lallchand, K., Tatayah, V., & Zimmermann, A. (2019). Quantifying the damage caused by fruit bats to backyard lychee trees in Mauritius and evaluating the benefits of protective netting. *PloS ONE*, *14*(8), e0220955.

Tongue, L. K., & Ngapagna, A. N. (2019). Emerging vector-borne diseases in central Africa: A threat to animal production and human health. In D. Claborn, S. Battacharya, & S. Roy (Eds.), *Current topics in the epidemiology of vector-borne diseases*. IntechOpen.

Towner, J. S., Pourrut, X., Albariño, C. G., Nkogue, C. N., Bird, B. H., Grard, G., . . . Leroy, E. M. (2007). Marburg virus infection detected in a common African bat. *PloS ONE*, *2*(8), e764.

Truong, V. D., Dang Vu, H. N., & Hall, C. M. (2016). The marketplace management of illegal elixirs: Illicit consumption of rhino horn. *Consumption Markets & Culture*, *19*(4), 353–69.

Wang, L. F., Shi, Z., Zhang, S., Field, H., Daszak, P., & Eaton, B. T. (2006). Review of bats and SARS. *Emerging Infectious Diseases*, *12*(12), 1834.

Wolfe, N. D., Daszak, P., Kilpatrick, A. M., & Burke, D. S. (2005). Bushmeat hunting, deforestation, and prediction of zoonotic disease. *Emerging Infectious Diseases*, *11*(12), 1822.

Xie, J., Li, Y., Shen, X., Goh, G., Zhu, Y., Cui, J., . . . Zhou, P. (2018). Dampened STING-dependent interferon activation in bats. *Cell Host & Microbe*, *23*(3), 297–301.

Xu, Y. (2006). DNA damage: A trigger of innate immunity but a requirement for adaptive immune homeostasis. *Nature Reviews Immunology*, *6*(4), 261–70.

Yue, Z. 2009. Conservation and trade control of pangolins in China. In S. Pantel & S. Y. Chin (Eds.), *Proceedings of the workshop on trade and conservation of pangolins native to South and Southeast Asia* (pp. 66–74). Singapore: TRAFFIC.

CHAPTER 2

The Anatomy of a Wildlife
Infectious Disease Spillover

MIKE CRANFIELD

Introduction

THE PHENOMENON OF A DISEASE "SPILLOVER" OR "EVOLUTIONARY jump" refers to the transmission of a pathogen from a natural (reservoir) animal host to a novel host(s), leading to infection in the new host(s). This can occur in a number of ways, including by chance, novel exposure, repeated exposure, or a genomic change enabling the pathogen to infect the new host (Plowright et al., 2017). Zoonotic disease emergence from animals to humans is a complex process usually involving a series of external drivers that allow some pathogens to expand and adapt to a new niche. The drivers are mostly ecological, but political, economic, and social forces operating at local, national, regional, and global levels may also play a role (National Research Council [US] Committee on Achieving Sustainable Global Capacity for Surveillance and Response to Emerging Diseases of Zoonotic Origin et al., 2009). Recent recognition that most emerging infectious disease events have wildlife origins highlights the need for a deep understanding of the type of contact between wild animals and people that enables disease transmission (Kreuder Johnson et al., 2015). This chapter will focus on viruses that spill over from wildlife to humans but can involve humans and animals simultaneously, as with Ebola virus, which spilled over from an animal reservoir (bats) to both great apes and humans. This spillover caused an epidemic with devastating losses to populations of chimpanzees and gorillas in West Africa (Reed et al., 2014), in addition to the human toll.

Human exposure to novel viruses is common and results in two scenarios. The first scenario is dead-end exposure and/or spillover that causes no human-to-human viral transmission (Wolfe et al., 2005). These events can result in elimination of the pathogen (e.g., simian foamy viruses known to infect bushmeat hunters), or health issues including death in the human host (e.g., rabies). The second scenario is that the spillover organism can initiate human-to-human transmission, with varying health effects on the new host and host community.

The emergence of a disease originating from wildlife often involves interactions among populations of wildlife, livestock, and people within a rapidly changing environment. Emerging diseases are distinguished from established infectious diseases, which have been endemic long enough to establish predictable levels of illness and death. Reemerging diseases are established diseases with new features, such as the ability to survive in a new geographic region, or another factor favoring their relationship with humans. Diseases do not always stay in one category. In time, a zoonotic emerging disease can become an established disease and possibly evolve into a reemerging disease (e.g., West Nile virus). Spillover transmission occurs when an animal pathogen successfully infects a human. The probability of zoonotic spillover is determined by interactions among several factors, including the dynamics of the disease within the animal, the way the human is exposed to the pathogen, and the factors that affect an individual human's susceptibility to infections. These factors describe all major routes of transmission. Emerging infectious diseases (EIDs) such as COVID-19 have proven to be a significant and growing threat to global health, economies, and security. Our awareness and knowledge of EIDs and their causes are growing, and it appears that their emergence is on the increase.

Although many of the individual determinants of spillover are subjects of intensive study, each is often addressed in isolation in a specialized discipline. For example, reservoir hosts (animals) or vectors (organisms that carry diseases between organisms, such as mosquitoes) are often targeted for control before the cause of the spillover is understood. This can sometimes lead to inefficient or even counter-productive interventions. In other cases, factors are lumped together, which makes it difficult to determine which factor or factors are truly driving the spillover risk (Plowright et al., 2017).

The nature of spillover events reveals a true need for a multidisciplinary approach to disease detection and prevention. It also necessitates cooperation through practical applications of One Health, which recognizes the importance of the interconnection between people, animals, and their shared environment in maintaining global health. One Health is theoretically well accepted, but there are few robust examples of the concept in action.

This chapter describes the various factors that make disease spillover between wildlife and human populations more likely. These factors include, but are not limited to, land conversion, climate change, bushmeat consumption, and viral dynamics. It also discusses previous disease detection and prevention programs, before suggesting strategies for strengthening spillover prevention. Such strategies, if implemented, could minimize the chance of the next pandemic.

Wildlife Health and Environmental Factors

When natural ecosystems like forests remain intact, interactions between major human population groups, their livestock, and wildlife are limited. With rapid human expansion along with the agricultural activities needed to support that growth, however, there has been a rapid increase in land conversion and use. This has done several things. It has decreased the size of habitats directly, modified and fragmented habitats, and increased the areas in which humans and wildlife interact (Pfeifer et al., 2017). Such interactions increase the risk of spillover.

The risk of a spillover event is neither geographically nor socially equal. The highest risk is usually near the equator in biodiversity hot spots with dense human and/or domestic animal populations, often in resource-poor countries. Land conversion and disturbance for agriculture has been driven mainly by three commodities: beef, soy, and palm oil. Land conversion via deforestation occurs at a rate of about 2–3 percent of global forests per year. Some species may take advantage of human activities and cohabitate with humans or their livestock. Species that cannot will be forced to compete for ever-decreasing resources, which often results in loss of biodiversity. As a result of extensive land conversion, about 70 percent of forests globally are now within one kilometer of a forest edge (Pfeifer et al., 2017), meaning that the animals have greater likelihood of interaction with humans. Land conversion with irrigation can provide increased suitable habitat for disease vectors such as mosquitoes. Large-scale environmental changes can alter migration patterns, feeding behavior, and the dynamics of viral transmission to promote the emergence of pathogens. For example, fruiting trees planted next to hog containment facilities in Malaysia provide feeding and roosting sites for fruit bats harboring Nipah virus, which can infect pigs and humans (Epstein et al., 2020). These actions led to the first human exposures to Nipah virus.

Human-Wildlife Interface

The boundary between human-altered and natural habitats is often called an edge or the human-wildlife interface. Habitat fragmentation increases the amount of edge, which then also increases interactions between wildlife and humans. This interaction poses a serious threat to wildlife conservation and the health of humans and wildlife. Several studies have found that humans living near a forest edge harbored more pathogens similar to those in local primates than humans farther from the edge (Rwego et al., 2008). There is strong evidence of other microbes flowing between wildlife and humans at the forest edge (Nizeyi, Cranfield, & Graczyk, 2002; Graczyk et al., 2002).

With few exceptions, such as migratory birds, the human-wildlife interface is where EID spillovers occur. The intensity of the potential spillover is increased with higher human and domestic animal densities as well as the density and species of wildlife at or near the interface. Environmental conditions near boundaries usually vary more strongly than conditions in the ecosystem interior, and this can have important consequences for both host and pathogen species. For example, relative humidity and ultraviolet exposure are important determinants of the survival of many pathogens and can vary dramatically at ecosystem boundaries (Gortazar et al., 2014). Permeability, or the frequency and distance of movement across the human-wildlife interface, also affects the likelihood of spillover. Generally, the more porous or permeable the interface, the more interactions occur between wildlife and humans. Humans may enter the natural habitat for resources such as food, water, and fuel, or recreational activities such as global ecotourism. Wildlife such as bats, rodents, and birds may enter the human-modified habitat for food or even permanent shelter as they become peridomestic.

There are several mechanisms by which pathogen transmission may occur. Direct or close contact with wildlife can result in the exposure of humans to bodily fluids of wildlife through bites, scratches, butchering, or poorly cooked food. The second mode of transmission is through a vector such as mosquitoes, ticks, or an intermediate domestic animal host. The third is contact with environmental fecal or water contamination. The rate of spillover across ecosystem boundaries depends on the likelihood that source and recipient hosts, as well as the pathogen, are present in or near a boundary region at the same time. It can also depend on factors such as seasonal rainfall and temperatures as well as breeding seasons and associated stress in reservoir species. Bats in Python Cave in Uganda show a twice-yearly spike in their shedding of Marburg virus during birthing seasons, which has resulted in the disease spilling over to humans (Amman et al., 2012).

The size and shape of an ecosystem and its boundaries also have an impact on the density of wildlife populations and the prevalence of diseases that can spill over into the human population. Overall, species richness tends to be higher along ecosystem boundaries than in the interior (Plowright et al., 2017). The presence of pathogens along boundaries varies because of a number of factors, such as climate factors that impact the survival of the pathogen (Plowright et al., 2017). Primates have been extensively studied in land conversion sites and compared with the same species in undisturbed areas. Researchers found increased parasitism in primates in disturbed habitats, and this increased parasitism is the result of increased disease susceptibility because of low food availability, which causes the primates to be nutritionally stressed and immunocompromised (Chapman et al., 2015). These factors increase the risk of transmission of infectious diseases since the immunocompromised animal sheds significantly higher amounts of disease-causing agents into the environment.

Human Activities and Cultural Occurrences

The rise in the human population and consumerism has now placed the planet in an ecological predicament of unsustainable patterns of production and consumption. These patterns escalate human activities in previously undisturbed habitats. Examples of human activities that affect wildlife-human interactions are bushmeat hunting, wet markets, and the trade of wildlife and wildlife products.

Bushmeat is the product of hunting or trapping wildlife for butchering, or selling wildlife for personal use or commercial gain. It is often consumed as an inexpensive source of protein or as a sought-after delicacy (Wolfe et al., 2005). Bushmeat hunting occurs in most countries but is riskier in areas that have high biodiversity but low biosecurity measures. Bushmeat consumption, specifically, has been linked to zoonotic diseases such as HIV and Ebola (Wolfe et al., 2005). The demand for bushmeat is driven by cultural factors as well as wild game availability, poverty, food insecurity, and increased demand for protein. Active bushmeat hunters and butchers are at the greatest risk for contracting zoonotic diseases, and as food insecurity increases, the bushmeat market becomes more essential and more lucrative, creating more opportunities for the transmission of pathogens to humans (Wolfe et al., 2005).

If distances from the point of killing or trapping wildlife to the bushmeat market are short, the products are often sold freshly killed or alive at a wet market. A wet market, or traditional market, sells fresh meat, fish, produce, and other perishable goods. There is a mixing of wildlife and domestic products, often in extremely crowded conditions, which enhances contamination by pathogens and the likelihood of possible spillovers. Wet markets often have low biosecurity, resulting in food contamination because of a lack of handwashing and cleaning of tables, and generally poor market cleanliness (Morales, 2009). These trends have major implications for the emergence of zoonotic diseases. Wet markets are a major route for bushmeat to get to intermediate-sized communities and sometimes attract tourists, which sets up a potential for an international event.

Another important factor is the global wildlife trade. This is hard to quantify, but its value is estimated in the billions of dollars annually. Some analysts identify the United States, the People's Republic of China, and the European Union as the areas with the greatest demand,

driven by the need for zootherapeutics, human consumption, symbols of wealth (e.g., hunting trophies), and exotic pets. The United
States purchases nearly 20 percent of all legal wildlife products on the
global market (Institute of Medicine and National Research Council,
2009). Source countries of both legal and illegal exports tend to
include low-income countries with rich biological diversity (Institute
of Medicine and National Research Council, 2009). A recent study by
the Consortium for Conservation Medicine showed that more than
half a million shipments containing more than one billion live animals
were imported into the United States between 2000 and 2006 (Smith
et al., 2008). In countries across income levels, the legislative authority
and responsibility for the impacts of the wildlife trade on human and
ecosystem health are unclear and/or poorly coordinated. Additionally,
wildlife reservoirs of zoonotic pathogens often show no clinical signs
of disease, so they are likely to be missed by US Fish and Wildlife
Service (USFWS) screenings of shipments. Furthermore, the focus of
the agency is conservation, not disease prevention and detection. The
USFWS physically inspects an average of only 25 percent of all wildlife
shipments (Smith et al., 2008).

Taken together, bushmeat hunting and consumption, along with
the global wildlife trade, further elevate the risk of disease spillover
between animals and humans and increase the likelihood of a pandemic event.

Biodiversity

Biodiversity is the number of different species of plants, animals, and
microorganisms in a specified environment. Biodiversity enables habitats to withstand and mitigate ecological threats. One of the simple
analogies to biodiversity is known as the portfolio effect, which compares biodiversity to stock holdings. With the portfolio effect, diver-
sification minimizes the volatility of the investment, or in this case,
the risk of instability of ecosystem services. This is related to the idea
of response diversity, where a suite of species will exhibit differential
responses to a given environmental perturbation. When considered
together, they create a stabilizing function that preserves the integrity
of a service (Tilman, Lehman, & Bristow, 1998).

With a loss of biodiversity comes a decrease in the health of an ecosystem. The resulting less-resilient ecosystem loses its ability to respond to ever-increasing threats from human activity and protect the health of the environment and living organisms within its boundaries. As described earlier, biodiversity loss and its contributing factors are actively driven by human activities that change ecosystems. Certain areas in the world with high biodiversity (biodiversity hot spots) are often also hot spots for spillover events. These hot spots are usually near the equator and are frequently in low- and middle-income countries. As humans encroach on these areas, there is a higher probability of encountering a unique animal species carrying novel bacteria and viruses, increasing the chance of spillover.

Massive changes in land use for agriculture and increased fossil fuel use for human activities have transformed large ecosystems and biodiverse areas into what are essentially monocultures. Combined, these factors are drivers of climate change. The main and most universal of these changes is increased warming, which in turn has changed weather patterns. The direct influence of this temperature change has changed the distribution of disease vectors such as mosquitoes and ticks. These changes can impact transmission dynamics and increase the likelihood of disease outbreaks.

Reservoir Host Characteristics

The reservoir for EIDs is generally wildlife and can be defined as a species that is usually (although not necessarily) the primary carrier of a pathogen and that may transmit the infection to another species. Knowing the ecology of reservoir species and the main route of interspecies transmission is central to any preventive program.

Characteristics of the reservoir host that have been found to enhance spillover are its geographic location in a biodiverse hot spot, its abundance within that location, the viral load and diversity of pathogens it is carrying, and its relatedness to the new host. Stress, poor nutrition, and the presence of concurrent disease or pathogen infestation are common problems that increase the risk of transmission of infectious disease and the likelihood that infected animals will shed significant amounts of disease-causing agents into the environment.

Large and dense reservoir populations may be predictive of a large pathogen load and virulence. Because of this, certain species of bats and birds are being increasingly recognized as major reservoirs for several viruses. Remarkably, it has been reported that bats can serve as reservoir hosts of greater viral diversity than other host species, for example rodents. Reservoir capabilities of bats may arise, first, because of their roosting behavior in large and dense congregations that greatly promote transmission within the population; second, because of their unique physiology resulting from the evolution of flying capabilities; and third, because of ample home ranges that may allow them to move viruses across large geographic regions (Carrasco-Hernandez et al., 2017).

Host traits that increase the probability of occupying or crossing ecosystem boundaries may lead to such species functioning as *bridge hosts*. Bridge host traits can include being a generalist consumer, having high tolerance of different habitats, or being an edge-habitat specialist. The presence of bridge hosts can be particularly important for spillover between two other host species for which the boundary has low permeability (Borremans et al., 2019).

Hosts with broad environmental tolerance and generalist resource use are more likely to be able to cross ecosystem boundaries than specialists. Ecosystem boundary areas may therefore support a larger proportion of generalist species than ecosystem interiors. Additionally, as generalists tend to move through a more diverse range of ecosystems than specialists, they may be more likely to encounter, and become infected with, a wider range of pathogens, elevating both spillover diversity and spillover rate near boundaries. Alternatively, some host species specialize in edge habitat, and such edge-specific hosts might be disproportionately more likely to be involved in spillover near ecosystem boundaries (Borremans et al., 2019).

Recipient Host Characteristics That Enhance Spillover from Wildlife to Humans

For viruses, host phylogenetic distance (genetic relatedness) is less important than geography in explaining pathogen flow. After cross-species exposure of a recipient host, the within-host barriers and their interactions with the strain of pathogen will determine the functional relationship between the pathogen dose and the likelihood that an infection will establish. Within-host barriers to infection vary widely and depend on the specific combination of pathogen, host species, and individual receptivity (Plowright et al., 2017). Researchers found that bats in Uganda and Rwanda shed coronaviruses that were phylogenetically more closely related to SARS coronavirus 1 than to SARS coronavirus 2 (COVID-19), but the viruses were not able to use human ACE2 receptor sites and therefore were not able to infect humans (Wells et al., 2021). Interferon-induced and other innate immune responses may be triggered after the initial infection of a cell, resulting in protection. The genetic, immunological, and physiological state of the host can also modulate the dose-response relationship. Pathogen dose can play an important role in overpowering the new host immune system (Plowright et al., 2017).

Viral Characteristics That Enhance Spillover from Wildlife to Humans

The proportion of zoonotic viruses is higher for RNA viruses (159 of 382, 41.6 percent) than DNA viruses (29 of 205, 14.1 percent). RNA viruses show remarkable capabilities to adapt to new environments and confront the different selective pressures they encounter. Selective pressures on viruses include not only their host's immune system and defense mechanisms but also the current artificial challenges devised by the biomedical community (i.e., antiretroviral drugs or vaccines) (Carrasco-Hernandez et al., 2017). Thus, from an evolutionary perspective, it appears that RNA viruses benefit from random mutations.

Additionally, spillover of pathogens that have short environmental survival times (for example, influenza A virus when transmitted through the respiratory route) may require close interactions between reservoir and recipient hosts. By contrast, if pathogens survive for sufficient periods outside their reservoir host, they may be dispersed beyond the home range of the host. In this case, the release of a pathogen from its reservoir host and human exposure to the pathogen may become disconnected in space and time (Plowright et al, 2015).

Globalization and Containment

Globalization increases movement and exchange of people, goods, services, capital, technologies, and cultural practices over the planet. One effect of globalization is that it promotes and increases interactions between different regions and populations around the globe. The current era of globalization is intensifying trends that have occurred throughout history. Never before have pathogens had such ample opportunity to spread via airplanes, people, and products. No geographic or political location is immune to the growing global threat that can be posed by an isolated outbreak of infectious disease, even in a remote area. On the positive side, this intensification of connectedness also comes with more sharing of information and health initiatives. A growing network of such efforts, combined with the global proliferation of technology and information, continues to strengthen the global public health capacity to prevent and control the spread of emerging and reemerging pathogens (Institute of Medicine [US] Forum on Microbial Threats et al., 2006).

Disease Detection and Prevention

Disease and pathogen discovery was thought to be the route to the prediction and prevention of EIDs. One early attempt at this approach was the Emerging Pandemic Threats (EPT) program of USAID. It was well thought out and involved 20 countries that had a history of spillovers or conditions conducive to such an event. It was a multipronged approach that surveyed for viruses in bats, rodents, and primates known to be involved in many of the previous spillovers at the human-wildlife interface. It was felt that knowing which viruses were present would help predict pathways of a spillover and possibly prevent it.

Another part of the program aimed to boost the capacity of animal and human laboratories in both physical infrastructure and human training. That way, early detection could be achieved in the country with the spillover, which would allow a faster response and flatten the curve. The program also taught the One Health concept and held many multidisciplinary workshops to promote collaboration in identifying and responding to an issue.

Finally, it helped support response efforts when a suspected emerging threat was identified. During the 10 years of the program, it trained 6,800 people in the One Health workforce. It optimized 60 laboratories so they could perform PCR tests on human, domestic animal, and wildlife samples, and it increased biosecurity. Wildlife and human surveillance teams sampled 164,000 animals and people at the human-wildlife interface in dwellings, markets, trade value chains, bushmeat events, and in situations where conservation efforts were focused on animals in areas of land conversion or with a history of close contact with people. Humans with fevers of unknown origin coming from these same environments were also tested for viruses. Each animal was sampled for multiple body fluids, which were chosen as appropriate for the species and were most likely to be involved in a transmission event. From these samples, 217 viruses expected to be present in the sampled species were detected, and 949 novel viruses were detected. This doubled the number of known mammalian viruses in the world in a short period. The program proved that there were a lot more viruses in wildlife than previously thought and showed that with the multitude of viruses present, we need to delineate which are important as potential human pathogens and which are just circulating in a reservoir host (Kelly, 2020).

The Way Forward

The COVID-19 pandemic and outbreaks of other novel and deadly viruses underscore the world's vulnerability to emerging diseases, many of which have massive health and economic impacts.

Humans will need to make large-scale social changes in economics, population growth, and lifestyle that reduce resource use, produce less waste, and stop the increase of land-use modification. This will reduce the loss of biodiversity and maintain the remaining healthy ecosystems to provide the services necessary to sustainably support the total diversity of the planet. These changes will be slow, and other, more immediate and focused mitigations should also be sought.

Surveillance, technological development, and capacity building should be prioritized for RNA viruses, but not to the exclusion of DNA viruses and other pathogens. Additionally, the continuous monitoring of viral genetics and phenotypes in wildlife reservoirs and in people with fevers of unknown origin is also crucial in identifying pathogens early to flatten the epidemic curve and not overwhelm health care systems in the face of an outbreak.

The Global Virome Project (Morse et al., 2012) has been proposed to look at the viral density and richness in wildlife on a massive scale to identify the bulk of this viral threat and provide timely data for public health interventions against future pandemics. This would be a Herculean-scale undertaking since sampling wildlife is not easy or efficient, and it is costly. It could even be counterproductive to conservation efforts for some species.

Efforts in wildlife surveillance must be tempered with knowledge from the EPT work that (1) RNA viruses are present in larger numbers than previously thought, and (2) there will be further spillovers regardless of the extent of the data on viruses that presently exist. RNA virus biological diversity and rapid adaptive rates necessitate continuous development of pharmaceutical and medical technology. Perhaps the best strategy against RNA viral diseases is to design preventive survey programs that evaluate the most vulnerable sectors, their high-risk behaviors, and their geographic regions. Where needs are identified, high-capacity laboratories as well as human capacity should be built in these areas to identify pathogens early in a zoonotic outbreak. More research needs to be done on the ecology of interfaces and the human behaviors that enhance the ability of pathogens to spill over. Results from these studies should be used to make risky interfaces less permeable via changes in the biosecurity of domestic animals and, where possible, the use of effective physical barriers to wildlife such as buffer zones. Efforts should be made to educate people living on and using interfaces so that appropriate social and individual behavioral changes will take place. Computer applications can help estimate the threat of a virus spillover event if certain data points are known. One such application is called SpillOver (Grange et al., 2021).

Public health needs to place additional focus on the health care needs of mobile populations. Unless the capacity to monitor mobile populations is strengthened, we will see foreign pathogens continuing to enter new geographic locations. Enhanced global public health forces will enhance the capacity for proper contact tracing and containment before a disease reaches urban populations and overwhelms local and international health care systems.

Better diagnostics and treatments should be developed and general vaccine technology improved to quickly develop responses when a pathogen is identified. Conservation policies that control the disturbance of natural ecosystems are also essential.

The One Health approach needs to move from a conceptual idea to regular on-the-ground activity. Because wildlife is an essential component in the epidemiology of many zoonoses, wildlife should be prioritized in any risk analysis. Training and education are prerequisites to enable the personnel involved at the various stages, from field to laboratory, to be trained to detect zoonoses.

Easier permitting and better biosecurity for transport of wildlife samples are needed so that when a source country lacks infrastructure, samples can be quickly transported to appropriate labs elsewhere. Information and communication are key components in any prevention and control strategy. Restrictions on anthropogenic animal movement is another important preventive measure. For vector-borne zoonoses, vector control should be an integral part of any intervention strategy.

There is a need for global resource mapping so financial aid can be sent to priority areas and places where there are extreme gaps in the ability to fight emerging pandemic threats. Without such a global approach in this era of globalization on an ecologically stressed planet, all countries will be at risk of huge financial and human loss from the next pandemic.

Acknowledgments

The author would like to thank Dr. Leslie Ruyle for constructive editing and suggestions for this chapter.

References

American Veterinary Medical Association, & Mahr, R. (2008, July). *One Health: A new professional imperative*. American Veterinary Medical Association. https://www.avma.org/sites/default/files/resources/onehealth_final.pdf

Amman, B. R., Carroll, S. A., Reed, Z. D., Sealy, T. K., Balinandi, S., Swanepoel, R., . . . Towner, J. S. (2012). Seasonal pulses of Marburg virus circulation in juvenile

Rousettus aegyptiacus bats coincide with periods of increased risk of human infection. *PLoS Pathogens, 8*(10), e1002877. https://doi.org/10.1371/journal .ppat.1002877

Borremans, B., Faust, C., Manlove, K. R., Sokolow, S. H., & Lloyd-Smith, J. O. (2019). Cross-species pathogen spillover across ecosystem boundaries: Mechanisms and theory. *Philosophical Transactions of the Royal Society B: Biological Sciences, 374*(1782), 20180344. https://doi.org/10.1098/rstb.2018.0344

Carrasco-Hernandez, R., Jácome, R., López Vidal, Y., & Ponce De León, S. (2017). Are RNA viruses candidate agents for the next global pandemic? A review. *ILAR Journal, 58*(3), 343–58. https://doi.org/10.1093/ilar/ilx026

CDC (Centers for Disease Control and Prevention). (2002). Identifying reservoirs of infection: A conceptual and practical challenge. *Emerging Infectious Diseases, 8*(12), 1468–73. https://doi.org/10.3201/eid0812.010317

Chapman, C. A., Schoof, V. A. M., Bonnell, T. R., Gogarten, J. F., & Calmé, S. (2015). Competing pressures on populations: Long-term dynamics of food availability, food quality, disease, stress and animal abundance. *Philosophical Transactions of the Royal Society B: Biological Sciences, 370*(1669), 20140112. https://doi.org/ 10.1098/rstb.2014.0112

COVID-19 Cumulative Infection Collaborators. (2022). Estimating global, regional, and national daily and cumulative infections with SARS-CoV-2 through Nov 14, 2021: A statistical analysis. *Lancet, 399*(10344): P2351–80. doi:https://doi.org/ 10.1016/S0140-6736(22)00484-6

de Merode, E., & Cowlishaw, G. (2006). Species protection, the changing informal economy, and the politics of access to the bushmeat trade in the Democratic Republic of Congo. *Conservation Biology, 20*(4), 1261–71. https://doi.org/10.1111/ j.1523-1739.2006.00425.x

Duffy, S., Shackelton, L. A., & Holmes, E. C. (2008). Rates of evolutionary change in viruses: Patterns and determinants. *Nature Reviews Genetics, 9*(4), 267–76. https://doi.org/10.1038/nrg2323

Epstein, J. H., Anthony, S. J., Islam, A., Kilpatrick, A. M., Ali Khan, S., Balkey, M. D., . . . Daszak, P. (2020). Nipah virus dynamics in bats and implications for spill-over to humans. *Proceedings of the National Academy of Sciences, 117*(46), 29190–201. https://doi.org/10.1073/pnas.2000429117

Gortazar, C., Reperant, L. A., Kuiken, T., de la Fuente, J., Boadella, M., Martínez-Lopez, B., . . . Mysterud, A. (2014). Crossing the interspecies barrier: Opening the door to zoonotic pathogens. *PLoS Pathogens, 10*(6), e1004129. https://doi .org/10.1371/journal.ppat.1004129

Graczyk, T. K., Nizeyi, J. B., da Silva, A. J., Moura, N. S., Pieniazek, N. J., Cranfield, M. R., & Linquist, H. D. (2002). A single genotype of *Encephalitozoon intestinalis* infects free-ranging gorillas and people sharing their habitats in Uganda. *Parasitology Research, 88*(10), 926–31. https://doi.org/10.1007/ s00436-002-0693-5

Grange, Z. L., Goldstein, T., Johnson, C. K., Anthony, S., Gilardi, K., Daszak, P., . . . Mazet, J. A. K. (2021). Ranking the risk of animal-to-human spillover for newly discovered viruses. *Proceedings of the National Academy of Sciences, 118*(15), e2002324118. https://doi.org/10.1073/pnas.2002324118

Institute of Medicine and National Research Council. (2009, September 22). *Sustaining global surveillance and response to emerging zoonotic diseases.* Washington, DC: National Academies Press. http://www.nap.edu/catalog/12625/ sustaining-global-surveillance-and-response-to-emerging-zoonotic-diseases

Institute of Medicine (US) Forum on Microbial Threats, Knobler, S., Mahmoud, A., Lemon, S., & Pray, L. (Eds.). (2006). *The impact of globalization on infectious disease emergence and control: Exploring the consequences and opportunities* (Bookshelf ID: NBK56589). Washington, DC: National Academies Press. https://doi.org/10.17226/11588

Kelly, T. R. (2020, January 10). Implementing One Health approaches to confront emerging and re-emerging zoonotic disease threats: Lessons from PREDICT. *One Health Outlook.* https://onehealthoutlook.biomedcentral.com/articles/ 10.1186/s42522-019-0007-9

Kreuder Johnson, C., Hitchens, P. L., Smiley Evans, T., Goldstein, T., Thomas, K., Clements, A., . . . Mazet, J. K. (2015). Spillover and pandemic properties of zoonotic viruses with high host plasticity. *Scientific Reports, 5*(1). https://doi.org/ 10.1038/srep14830

Millennium Ecosystem Assessment. (2005). *Ecosystems and human well-being: Synthesis.* 1st ed. Millennium Ecosystem Assessment Series. Washington, DC: Island Press.

Morales, A. (2009). Public markets as community development tools. *Journal of Planning Education and Research, 28*(4), 426–40. https://doi.org/10.1177/ 0739456X08329471

Morse, S. S., Mazet, J. A., Woolhouse, M., Parrish, C. R., Carroll, D., Karesh, W. B., Zambrana-Torrelio, C., Lipkin, W. I., & Daszak, P. (2012). Prediction and prevention of the next pandemic zoonosis. *Lancet, 380*(9857), 1956–65. https://doi .org/10.1016/s0140-6736(12)61684-5

National Research Council (US) Committee on Achieving Sustainable Global Capacity for Surveillance and Response to Emerging Diseases of Zoonotic Origin, Keusch, G. T., Pappaioanou, M., Gonzalez, M. C., Scott, K. A., & Tsai, P. (Eds.). (2009). *Sustaining global surveillance and response to emerging zoonotic diseases.* Washington, DC: National Academies Press.

Nizeyi, J. B., Cranfield, M. R., & Graczyk, T. K. (2002). Cattle near the Bwindi Impenetrable National Park, Uganda, as a reservoir of *Cryptosporidium parvum* and *Giardia duodenalis* for local community and free-ranging gorillas. *Parasitology Research, 88*(4), 380–85. https://doi.org/10.1007/s00436-001-0543-x

Olival, K. J., Hosseini, P. R., Zambrana-Torrelio, C., Ross, N., Bogich, T. L., & Daszak, P. (2017). Host and viral traits predict zoonotic spillover from mammals. *Nature, 546*(7660), 646–50. https://doi.org/10.1038/nature22975

Pfeifer, M., Lefebvre, V., Peres, C. A., Banks-Leite, C., Wearn, O. R., Marsh, C. J., . . . Ewers, R. M. (2017). Creation of forest edges has a global impact on forest vertebrates. *Nature, 551*(7679), 187–91. https://doi.org/10.1038/nature24457

Plowright, R. K., Eby, P., Hudson, P. J., Smith, I. L., Westcott, D., Bryden, W. L., . . . McCallum, H. (2015). Ecological dynamics of emerging bat virus spillover. *Proceedings of the Royal Society B: Biological Sciences, 282*(1798), 20142124. https://doi.org/10.1098/rspb.2014.2124

Plowright, R. K., Parrish, C. R., McCallum, H., Hudson, P. J., Ko, A. I., Graham, A. T., & Lloyd-Smith, J. O. (2017). Pathways to zoonotic spillover. *Nature Reviews Microbiology, 15*(8), 502–10. https://doi.org/10.1038/nrmicro.2017.45

Reed, P. E., Mulangu, S., Cameron, K. N., Ondzie, A. U., Joly, D., Bermejo, M., . . . Sullivan, N. J. (2014). A new approach for monitoring Ebolavirus in wild great apes. *PLoS Neglected Tropical Diseases, 8*(9), e3143. https://doi.org/10.1371/journal.pntd.0003143

Rwego, I. B., Isabirye-Basuta, G., Gillespie, T. R., & Goldberg, T. L. (2008). Gastro-intestinal bacterial transmission among humans, mountain gorillas, and live-stock in Bwindi Impenetrable National Park, Uganda. *Conservation Biology, 22*(6), 1600–1607. https://doi.org/10.1111/j.1523-1739.2008.01018.x

Smith, K. F., Behrens, M. D., Max, L. M., & Daszak, P. (2008). U.S. drowning in unidentified fishes: Scope, implications, and regulation of live fish import. *Conservation Letters, 1*(2), 103–9. https://doi.org/10.1111/j.1755-263x.2008.00014.x

Suter, W., Bollmann, K., & Holderegger, R. (2007a). Landscape permeability: From individual dispersal to population persistence. In F. Kienast, O. Wildi, & S. Ghosh (Eds.), *A changing world* (Landscape Series vol. 8, pp. 157–74). https://doi.org/10.1007/978-1-4020-4436-6_11

Tilman, D., Lehman, C., & Bristow, C. (1998). Diversity-stability relationships: Statistical inevitability or ecological consequence? *American Naturalist, 151*(3), 277–82. https://doi.org/10.1086/286118

Wells, H. L., Letko, M., Lasso, G., Ssebide, B., Nziza, J., Byarugaba, D. K., . . . Anthony, S. J. (2021). The evolutionary history of ACE2 usage within the coronavirus sub-genus *Sarbecovirus*. *Virus Evolution, 7*(1). https://doi.org/10.1093/ve/veab007

Wolfe, N. D., Daszak, P., Kilpatrick, A. M., & Burke, D. S. (2005). Bushmeat hunting, deforestation, and prediction of zoonotic disease. *Emerging Infectious Diseases, 11*(12), 1822–27. https://doi.org/10.3201/eid1112.040789

World Health Organization, & Rozenbaum, M. (2020). The increase in zoonotic diseases: The WHO, the why and the when? https://www.understanding animalresearch.org.uk/news/research-medical-benefits/the-increase-in -zoonotic-diseases-the-who-the-why-and-the-when/

PART 2

COVID-19 RESPONSE

CHAPTER 3

Prison Break

How Applying the Prisoner's Dilemma to COVID-19 Mitigation May Predict Climate Change Response

ERIN NGUYEN AND LESLIE E. RUYLE

What Do Climate Change, COVID-19, and the Prisoner's Dilemma Have in Common?

WE LIVE IN AN ERA OF UNPRECEDENTED GLOBAL CHANGE (WEST, 2017). Advances in technology, connectivity, and medicine have increased the quality of people's lives; however, we have also altered the composition of our atmosphere, fractured our landscapes, and polluted our lands. These changes can, in some ways, exacerbate the conditions that allow pandemics to occur. The infection of millions by the COVID-19 pandemic can be linked to these changes, and the potential for future pandemics is unlikely to decrease as our ecosystems are impacted by climate change and our world becomes even more connected. These challenges to twenty-first-century humanity have had devastating effects and promise more harm unless we learn from our past mistakes. The problems posed by a pandemic and those resulting from ecological destruction are deeply intertwined and will require consensus solutions.

First, both challenges have global implications—every person and every nation, without exception, is affected by both problems as well as the response (or lack thereof) of other actors to these problems. Second, both problems will require immense amounts of resources, capital, research, and human effort to overcome—far beyond the capacity of any one country, institution, or entity. Third, though the effects of both problems are felt by all, neither the causes nor the effects are proportionately distributed (Levy and Patz, 2015). Fourth, the costs and benefits associated with each problem operate on different timescales. In both cases, a future payoff requires high up-front costs in the present. This time lag may account for why a rational actor may choose to discount the future good in favor of a present material benefit. The four parallels between actions on climate change and future pandemics suggest that the successful eradication of either problem will require swift global cooperation—but why is this so difficult to achieve?

We propose that some clues may lie in the paradigm of the Prisoner's Dilemma (Pittel and Rübbelke, 2010; DeCanio and Fremstad, 2013). The Prisoner's Dilemma is a thought experiment derived from game theory wherein two rational actors must make a decision to cooperate or not cooperate with each other, all while possessing incomplete knowledge of how the other actor will respond. The catch of the problem is this—each actor's choice impacts the final payoff of both parties. In a simplified model, there are three potential scenarios with the following potential payoffs: if both parties cooperate, the payoff is medium and equal (each partner gains x benefits); if both parties abstain and choose not to cooperate, the payoff is low but equal (each partner loses x benefits); however, should one party cooperate while the other does not, then the payoff results in an uneven distribution such that the cooperator bears the brunt of the cost but the uncooperative partner receives the highest payoff (cooperator loses x benefits, defector gains x benefits). With these three possible outcomes of fully cooperative, fully uncooperative, or a mixed response, the Prisoner's Dilemma offers useful and intuitive categories capable of characterizing the broad and diverse policies (or lack thereof) of different actors regarding global threats.

If we assume humans to be rational actors such that both individuals and aggregates of individuals in a society should each seek to advance self-interest, the logical choice is the one that yields the highest gain while minimizing personal cost. Applying the Prisoner's Dilemma paradigm to both climate change and pandemics may allow a better understanding of the Other Actor and why each may act with a rational, albeit conflicting strategy. Given the parallels between the two challenges, we hypothesize that the decision-making of rational actors (whether individuals or nations) in response to a short-term cooperative challenge like the COVID-19 pandemic may be indicative of how the same actor will respond to a long-term cooperative challenge like climate change. Only in being able to describe complex human responses to COVID-19 or climate change can we hope to foster cooperation and overcome such challenges. Only in understanding the crux of human behavior and motivation through the Prisoner's Dilemma can we attempt a prison break. We recognize that measuring the cause and effect of these ideas is difficult, but we believe there is value in putting these wicked problems into a framework to help us better understand behavior and possibly identify interesting solutions.

COVID-19 and the Prisoner's Dilemma

In late 2019, a novel coronavirus similar in structure to severe acute respiratory syndrome (SARS) was identified as SARS-CoV-2 (Fauci, Lane, & Redfield, 2020). The virus causes the disease named COVID-19 and is believed to be the result of zoonotic spillover, likely originating in a bat species before eventually making the leap to humans and other species such as mink and cats (Contini et al., 2020; Reynolds, 2020). The first major outbreak of the disease is widely considered to have been at a wet market in Wuhan, China, in December 2019, with some limited evidence suggesting there may have been isolated cases elsewhere (Li et al., 2020). COVID-19 then spread rapidly, appearing in Thailand, the United States, Italy, France, Germany, Japan, Vietnam, Algeria, and Egypt. The World Health Organization (WHO) launched a pandemic response to contain the disease. Because COVID-19 is spread predominantly via respiratory droplets from human-to-human contact, much research has since confirmed that a combination of quarantining, social distancing, and wearing face coverings is the most effective measure to reduce exposure and prevent spread (Manikandan, 2020).

As of August 2020, COVID-19 had infected approximately 21 million and killed over 750,000—but the distribution of these deaths was not proportionately distributed across all nations of the world (Manikandan, 2020). To understand why some individuals cooperatively combated the pandemic while others did not, we apply the question of COVID-19 to the Prisoner's Dilemma paradigm, which predicts three potential outcomes (Kaushik, 2020; Mulaney, 2020). In the first possible scenario, if all individuals cooperate to eliminate COVID-19, the payout to each individual is high and equal. Although there are up-front costs to this scenario (actions like social distancing, quarantining when infected, wearing face coverings, etc.), these costs will result in a future, but greater, benefit—the reduction of COVID-19 cases. In the second possible scenario, if no individuals cooperate to reduce COVID-19 infections, then personal freedoms such as unrestricted travel, commerce, and trade are enjoyed by all but with the long-term payout of higher rates of infection and death, such that cases would overwhelm health care infrastructure and result in more preventable losses of life—there are no winners here. In the third possible scenario, if some individuals cooperate but others do not, we can expect mixed outcomes that are disproportionately distributed such that cooperators are worse off but noncooperators enjoy a greater benefit than they might otherwise if all other actors chose to not cooperate. An example of this is individuals in susceptible categories exhibiting greater caution and self-restricting activities, but individuals whose perceived risk is lower not doing so. Because the cooperators who engage in COVID-19 containment measures reduce overall rates of community spread, those who do not cooperate will actually receive two benefits: first, not restricting personal freedom; and second, still benefiting from reduced spread. Such a scenario may generate lingering levels of COVID-19 because of the incomplete cooperation of individuals in a society.

From a collective standpoint, there are also three potential Prisoner's Dilemma scenarios for COVID-19 (Kaushik, 2020; Mulaney, 2020). In the first potential scenario, if every nation cooperates to contain the pandemic, the up-front costs are high, but the payouts are justifiably greater and universal. Costs like initial investments in health and protective gear, financial losses incurred from enforced closures of nonessential businesses or reduced hours, and losses of personal freedom, comfort, and travel are meant to be secondary to the eventual benefit of a return to normalcy. The second potential scenario suggests that if no countries cooperate to contain COVID-19 and continue travel and trade per usual, the losses will be equal but universal.

If all nations continue to engage in global commerce, profits may not be impacted, but once community spread overwhelms all, the threats to human health and life will overwhelm all nations such that financial losses will be incurred and will likely impact the entire global economy for longer than the COVID-19 pandemic may last. Finally, the third potential scenario suggests that some countries may implement steps to contain COVID-19 at higher costs to their own economies than those of nations that do not. An example of this can be seen in how countries like New Zealand that have greatly reduced COVID-19 deaths have had novel cases reintroduced by travelers from other nations where COVID-19 is still prevalent. This suggests that such cooperative countries positively contributed to the reduced risk enjoyed by uncooperative countries but incurred losses in their own economy, trade, and travel that were not experienced by those same, uncooperative countries. Similar to the outcomes observed at the individual scale, the anticipated outcome of this scenario is that COVID-19 will continue to spread and infect, albeit at varying rates, across the entire globe.

Climate Change and the Prisoner's Dilemma

Climate change refers to long-term changes to the earth's natural climate patterns and processes as a result of anthropogenic release of large volumes of greenhouse gases into the atmosphere (IPCC, 2014). Although the earth's climate has historically varied over geological time, with documented periods of global warming and cooling, the current rapid rate of warming is unprecedented. Since the mid-twentieth century, industrial revolutions across the world have led to the large-scale production and emission of carbon dioxide and other pollutants. The concurrence of these events—industrialization and global warming—demonstrates that climate change is the result of anthropogenic activity on the planet (IPCC, 2014).

Beyond the general increase in global temperatures, a swath of other changes indicate the extent to which humans have disrupted natural climate processes. In recent decades, the frequency, duration, and magnitude of extreme weather phenomena have all increased. Events in recent collective memory such as the wildfires of Australia and Brazil, Hurricanes Maria and Katrina, Typhoon Lekima, and Tropical

Cyclone Idai are all reminders of the devastation of life and property possible from even a handful of such tragedies. The annual cost of mitigating climate and weather disasters like these may be upward of several billion US dollars, depending on the nation and its existing infrastructure and vulnerability to extreme climate change events (Regan, 2016). Left unchecked, climate change is predicted to cost the world a hefty price tag of US$1.9 trillion by 2100—and many scientists fear this number to be an underestimate (Ackerman & Stanton, 2008). Beyond the financial costs, however, are the very real costs to human life and health. In the aforementioned events alone, over 6,000 individuals died, nearly 1.5 million were displaced, and over 20 million were impacted (EM-DAT, 2020). Climate change also exacerbates other human-induced landscape alterations like water use (Mehran et al., 2017), forest clearing (DeFries et al., 2010), and strip mining (Odell, Bebbington, & Frey, 2018), such that extracting natural resources will require increasing amounts of input and effort for rapidly diminishing returns (West, 2017). Climate change–induced decreases in resource availability, particularly fresh water, are linked to increased migration, which in turn leads to conflict, overcrowding, and resource shortages that weaken or directly kill vulnerable populations (Klare, 2019).

Climate change also has less direct but still insidious effects on human and wildlife health. Warmer temperatures lead to range expansions as organisms migrate to cooler climates to compensate for rising temperatures (Goudarzi, 2020). This disruption in physical habitat ranges as well as migration routes and times may increase opportunities for non-coevolved organisms to encounter each other's pathogens and enhance the likelihood of zoonotic spillover (Goudarzi, 2020), and thus another pandemic. Additionally, as climate change reduces and fragments existing wildlife habitat, more and more organisms are forced into human areas of occupation, furthering the likelihood that a novel infectious disease may infect a human host or a species of livestock critical to our food supply.

Despite the real danger posed by climate change, the variable behaviors exhibited by both individuals and their collective societies suggest that human responses to the threat of climate change are still poorly understood. To answer the question of why some individuals cooperate to mitigate climate change but others do not, we first consider the three outcomes of the Prisoner's Dilemma at the level of the individual consumer (Kaushik, 2020). In the first possible scenario, if all individuals within a society cooperate to reduce emissions, the highest payoff is attained, wherein consumers reduce personal emissions but also have adequate critical mass to demand climate change mitigation from their lawmakers. This scenario will yield the highest return in the long run through preservation of natural resources, protection of global and individual health, development of new technology and jobs, and prevention of natural disasters, among other benefits. However, this scenario also requires the highest up-front cost by demanding that consumers undergo radical lifestyle changes and incur losses of personal freedom, convenience, and finances through choices like taking public transport, eliminating single-use products, and purchasing locally grown foods for higher prices. In the second possible scenario, no individuals in a society cooperate to reduce emissions and each seeks to maximize his or her own comfort, convenience, and capital, often at the expense of increased carbon emissions. For a short time, some individuals may enjoy greater degrees of freedom or financial return until all nonrenewable resources are permanently depleted. The third possible scenario is the one currently seen, wherein some individuals will work to reduce climate change but others will not. Those who cooperate will incur the brunt of the up-front costs, while those who do not cooperate will continue to benefit from the status quo. An example of this can be seen in the current market prices for food items that are imported versus locally grown or in the price differential between red meat versus meat-substitute products; the former products have worse implications for climate change, and they are cheaper and therefore preferred by most consumers, who value primarily present financial savings over future abstract goods like ecological restoration or natural resource conservation. This perpetuates an endless cycle wherein demand for a less ecologically friendly product is high because it is cheaper, which encourages production of the same product, which drives and maintains low prices that continue to draw consumers.

The Prisoner's Dilemma may also explain the actions taken by a collective. We next consider the three potential outcomes of the Prisoner's Dilemma at the level of national governance. In the first possible scenario, if all countries cooperate to reduce emissions, the highest payoff is attained such that the threat of climate change is mitigated, if not entirely eliminated. Although this scenario generates the highest overall payout in terms of economics, human health, and quality of life, it also requires the highest up-front cost because swift legislation and enforcement as well as capital and research are needed to combat climate change on a relevant and effective timescale. In the second possible scenario, if all countries choose to prioritize their own payoff, typically in the form of short-term economic gains, then the end result is that climate change is exacerbated such that all nations receive the worst payout from economic, human health, and quality-of-life standpoints in the long term. In the third possible scenario, if there is a mixed response by the actors, then the distribution of risks and responsibilities is likewise disparate. For example, in the climate change scenario, nations like Germany and Sweden are leading the world in carbon emission reductions, whereas nations like the United States and India have done very little in the way of formal legislation to limit such emissions (Keating 2017; Beck 2011). The payoff, however, is substantially different between the former and the latter sets of countries—while the United States and India continue to financially benefit from continued industrialization, Germany and Sweden are financially burdened with the cost of climate alleviation and incur economic losses during the period of transition to clean energy sectors and green industries. Furthermore, because of factors like geographic location and infrastructure strength, some industrialized nations are so buffered from the effects of climate change that their citizens may even reject claims of the crisis (Fischer, 2019). Instead, observable effects of climate change in the form of more frequent and more ferocious natural disasters like tropical storms, hurricanes, and heat waves are most keenly experienced by small island nations that collectively average less than 2 percent of all greenhouse gas emissions.

Comparing Responses: Does COVID-19 Response Predict Climate Change Mitigation Success?

Whether the problem to be resolved is climate change, COVID-19, or some other difficulty, in our increasingly globalized world, cooperative action should be not just lauded but required, because the choices of one individual and the policies (or lack thereof) of one nation can have a cascading impact that is globally felt. With the advent of satellites, the internet, commercial airlines, and more, no one country can reasonably expect to exist wholly isolated from other sovereign nations and their decisions. Isolationism is ineffective toward eradicating COVID-19 because the imposition of a national total lockdown would result in economic ruin. Isolationism is also wholly ineffective toward resolution of climate change because of the nonexcludable nature of most natural resources (Ostrom, 1990; Ostrom et al., 1999). Goods like air, rainwater, and the ozone layer are nonexcludable; therefore, problems like air pollution, water scarcity, and carbon emissions must be borne equally as well. Cooperation is needed to overcome problems of such global scale, and we anticipate that the crucible of the COVID-19 pandemic will demonstrate which nations are most adept at cooperation for a relatively short-term challenge; conversely, COVID-19 responses will also predict which nations will be most successful at cooperating in the long-term experiment of combating climate change.

We compared responses to both COVID-19 and climate change for seven countries to assess which of the three possible Prisoner's Dilemma outcomes a particular nation has chosen and what factors in the nation may have influenced this choice. We expect that countries with a successful response to COVID-19 will have the most progressive policies toward combating climate change; we also expect its correlate to hold true, that countries with a poor response to COVID-19 will have the least progressive policies toward climate change mitigation. Our case study examines the individual responses to COVID-19 and climate change by seven nations: New Zealand, Germany, Taiwan, China, Brazil, Italy, and the United States. To assess the effectiveness of each nation's COVID-19 response, we relied on WHO daily reports for records of confirmed cases as well as the number of deaths related to COVID-19, alongside a growing body of literature and news reports on each nation's policy actions. To assess the effectiveness of these same seven nations' climate change mitigation, we relied predominantly on the 2018 rankings generated by the Notre Dame Global Adaptation Initiative (ND-GAIN), which assesses 181 sovereign nations against 36 metrics of climate vulnerability and 9 metrics of climate adaptability/ readiness, in addition to climate change reports detailing existing climate-related policies per country (Chen et al., 2015). By considering each country's choices and policies passed in light of the Prisoner's Dilemma paradigm, we hope to understand what factors are imperative for successfully taking cooperative actions, and whether there is any relationship between the ability to respond to a short-term cooperative challenge like COVID-19 and the ability to respond to a long-term cooperative challenge like climate change mitigation.

New Zealand

Two months before its first confirmed COVID-19 case, New Zealand established a National Health Coordination Centre (NHCC) and implemented travel bans from nations designated to be high-risk areas for the novel coronavirus. Within two weeks of COVID-19 being confirmed in the island nation, New Zealand imposed a complete lockdown, implemented aggressive contact tracing, invested heavily in distance learning, and provided support packages to New Zealanders during lockdown. In June 2020, the nation had lifted all quarantine restrictions and reported no new cases, save a few from travelers to the country. Although concerns remain about how New Zealand's tourism-heavy economy will recover from the quarantine measures, Prime Minister Ardern's approval ratings have skyrocketed in the wake of her handling of the COVID-19 pandemic (Menon, 2020). Likewise, New Zealand's response to climate change is almost unrivaled in its success: ND-GAIN (2018) ranks New Zealand as second out of 181 nations in terms of climate readiness, and the best-prepared nation of the seven compared here. Existing measures to reduce carbon emissions include the establishment of an independent Climate Change Commission to oversee the country's progress toward a zero-carbon emission plan, which saw support from both liberal and conservative parties in the New Zealand Parliament. This commission's self-professed mission is to "deliver independent, evidence-based advice," suggesting that New Zealand's climate change policies rely heavily on the interdisciplinary cooperation of both environmental science and policy (CCC, 2020). Thus, New Zealand as a nation tends toward the Prisoner's Dilemma outcome that proactively seeks cooperation in pursuit of a long-term, highest good. On a more individual level, about a third of the people of New Zealand currently consider climate change to be a problem, and nearly two-thirds support more ambitious emissions targets but show limited willingness to implement lifestyle changes, suggesting that the populace may exhibit a mixed cooperative-uncooperative Prisoner's Dilemma strategy. As demonstrated by the relative return to normalcy enjoyed by New Zealand in the wake of COVID-19, as well as the large strides made by the country toward mitigating climate change, it appears as though decisive but empathetic leadership rooted in scientific evidence ensures a greater degree of policy success (Beaubien, 2020). In the words of Prime Minister Ardern, New Zealand is characterized by "going hard and going early" to combat COVID-19, but the same sentiment holds true for climate change mitigation as well (Masola, 2020). Such a cooperative position is most beneficial to the nation in the long term if other nations follow suit to mitigate either challenge, but it also recognizes that the country faces financial costs now as well as potential opportunity costs in the near future because of the relatively short timescales that political leaders facing reelection prospects typically consider.

Germany

Much like New Zealand's success story, much of Germany's handling of COVID-19 was characterized by decisive and immediate government action. Although the nation could not adequately prevent the outbreak, once confirmed, Germany proceeded to develop one of the first diagnostic tests for COVID-19 and implement a strict regime of testing and contact tracing at no cost to its citizens, coupled with a "no-contact" ban that forbade public gatherings beyond two people with social distancing (Tabari et al., 2020). Although not as stringent as a full lockdown, the measures nonetheless proved effective, reducing the number of cases from a peak count of over 6,000 to about 600 in a given day, as of July 2020 (Manikandan, 2020). The decrease in cases was praised by most but garnered some limited criticism by those who believe the measures to have been overstringent given that COVID-19 was not severe in the nation (Muno, 2020). Such responses suggest that at the individual level, there may be a mixed response wherein most individuals are cooperative and a minority are (vocally) uncooperative yet have still managed to benefit from Germany's reduced infection rates. Chancellor Merkel's training as a scientist was credited as part of her strong and successful response to containing the pandemic in Germany (Beaubien, 2020). This same emphasis on scientifically informed policy may also be a common linkage behind Germany's high ranking of 10th out of 181 nations, the second highest ND-GAIN (2018) ranking of the seven nations assessed here. Germany has consistently polled as one of the most concerned regarding issues of climate change, a value reflected in the nation's ambitious plans to reduce its carbon emissions by 55 percent in the next 10 years, suggesting that at both the individual and collective levels, Germany has adopted a cooperative strategy in mitigating climate change. Germany has invested a staggering US$60 billion in a carbon emission pricing system, suggesting that in pursuit of the eradication of climate change and its effects, the nation is assuming a leadership role to bear some of the up-front costs that may be a key component of other nations' unwillingness to cooperate (Thompson, 2019). The challenges of both COVID-19 and climate change suggest that Germany is well poised as a world leader on matters requiring global cooperative strategies, which we anticipate will occur with increasing frequency.

Taiwan

Despite being about 160 kilometers away from the outbreak center of COVID-19 and having nearly 5 percent of its workforce commuting to China frequently, Taiwan was remarkably successful in containing COVID-19, tallying a total of 480 cases between when the disease was first detected in January 2020 and August 2020. The nation's success may be partly a result of its past experience with the 2003 SARS epidemic and the 2009 H1N1 flu (Chen, 2020), which enabled it to leverage its unique real-time electronic health database in contact tracing (Emanuel, Zhang, & Glickman, 2020). By utilizing data science in powerful ways to complement established pandemic protocols, Taiwan learned from its past failures and acted quickly to negate the risk posed by COVID-19. These immediate actions included aggressive testing, enforced quarantine for travelers, and transparency in government operations, as well as a societal willingness to use face masks to reduce spread, suggesting an individual-level commitment to cooperation. President Ing-wen's success in containing the outbreak has been attributed to her centralized government, use of data science, and knowledge base developed from past epidemics (Beaubien, 2020). That same ingenuity and rapid deployment of strategies proven to be effective are not limited to Taiwan's handling of COVID-19 but have also emerged under the threat of climate change. Although not ranked by ND-GAIN, in the past 10 years, Taiwan has increased its climate change legislation, passing a number of plans and acts that target reducing emissions in energy production, manufacturing, transportation, construction, and agriculture. At present, the country is working toward cutting half of all national carbon emissions by 2050 through a mixed methodology involving a carbon tax on fossil fuels as well as increased development of sustainable energy sources. On the global stage, Taiwan seeks to participate in international climate mitigation agreements but has often been excluded because of questions of the nation's independence from mainland China. These responses suggest that where possible, Taiwan prioritizes preemptive, cooperative actions to combat both the COVID-19 pandemic and the impending threat of climate change.

Italy

As the European epicenter of COVID-19, Italy had confirmed cases by the end of January 2020 but responded predominantly through localized action as opposed to a coordinated, nationwide effort, in part because of some initial skepticism by both politicians and the populace regarding the severity of the impending pandemic. Within two months, however, it was apparent that COVID-19 was far more contagious than anticipated, and the country's health centers were rapidly inundated as both infections and death tolls rose. Italy then began to implement increasingly aggressive containment measures including travel bans, more testing, and a gradual to complete lockdown of the nation (Tabari et al., 2020). Italy's tepid response was in part the result of a lack of appropriate health care infrastructure amid warring political parties that promoted further distrust by the public. Prime Minister Conte began implementing extensive lockdown protocols, with resulting decreases in the number of daily cases reported in Italy, suggesting that the nation reversed course from an uncooperative or mixed-cooperation Prisoner's Dilemma model to one of cooperation with international efforts to stymie COVID-19. This same hesitation to act, followed by a rapid attempt to reverse course once death tolls increased, may potentially characterize the climate change responses of Italy and other nations with a mixed-cooperation strategy. Italy was ranked 32nd out of 181 nations by ND-GAIN (2018) in terms of climate change readiness and mitigation policy, in part because the assessment noted two weaknesses in Italy's existing structure. The first item of concern was that the nation relied heavily on imported energy sources, and the second was that Italy had been experiencing a decline in medical staff—a trend noted two years before that would severely impact the nation's COVID-19 response in 2020. While the nation has established a climate change plan and implemented an informal carbon tax based on usage, critics have suggested that the tax is not sufficiently high to substantially reduce carbon emissions, despite about a 20-year trend indicating that Italy's carbon emissions are generally falling (Mongelli, Tassielli, & Notarnicola, 2009).

Brazil

In August 2020, Brazil had just over three million confirmed cases of COVID-19, with over 100,000 dead (Andreoni, 2020). Despite past success in mitigating AIDS and Zika by previous administrations, the country's growing cases of coronavirus were a result of mixed messages from President Bolsonaro's administration regarding the severity of the outbreak (Urban & Saad-Diniz, 2020), alongside failure to coordinate a nationwide protocol in line with WHO recommendations (Londoño, Andreoni, & Casado, 2020). Instead, disease control efforts were largely localized and varied immensely among subregions (Leite et al., 2020), a clear indicator of a mixed response by officials in the nation as some cooperated and others defected on COVID-19 mitigation actions. A similar mixed response is found in the nation's efforts toward climate change readiness. Ranked 96th out of 181 nations, Brazil has received the lowest ND-GAIN (2018) ranking of the seven nations assessed here, having implemented few policies and possessing inadequate infrastructure to counter the dangers posed by climate change, making the nation's response mixed-cooperative at best and wholly uncooperative at worst. The 2018 election of far-right President Bolsonaro has since resulted in policies that incentivize economic development at the cost of climate change readiness, leading to unprecedented and unsustainable levels of forest destruction for artisanal gold mining (Cannon, 2020), timber harvesting (Spring, 2020), and livestock grazing (Ferrante & Fearnside, 2019). ND-GAIN suggests that while the nation faces pressing challenges, there is still a window of time (albeit rapidly closing) to redirect Brazil's course and improve its climate change readiness. If Brazil is to contain the spread of a pandemic or slow the effects of climate change long term, it will have to overcome its largely uncooperative tendencies that value current financial gain over the recommendations of WHO, IPCC, and other entities to foster cooperation and overcome these challenges.

United States

Despite several months' notice of COVID-19 outbreaks in nations like China and Italy, the United States was underprepared to contain the imminent outbreak. Similar to other failed nations' strategies, the approach of the United States was characterized by a delayed and irregularly implemented response that cost the nation both human lives and economic returns (Carter & May, 2020; Khanna et al., 2020). Politicization of the pandemic (Baker, 2020), a general disregard for evidence-based approaches (Cohen, 2017), and a prioritization of economic growth (Tankersly, Haberman, & Rabin, 2020) under President Trump resulted in over five million confirmed cases and over 150,000 deaths by August 2020 (CDC, 2020). At both the collective and individual levels, Americans exhibited an extremely mixed response to COVID-19 containment measures like social distancing, self-quarantining, and wearing adequate face coverings (Tabari et al., 2020). The same variation toward cooperative strategies can be seen in America's response to climate change mitigation. ND-GAIN (2018) ranked the United States 19th out of 181 nations in terms of climate readiness, suggesting that the nation has decently positioned infrastructure to adapt to and mitigate climate-related challenges, but noting that it lacks a comprehensive climate policy. At the federal level, although the United States has continued to invest heavily in the development of renewable energy sources (UNEP, 2020), the Trump administration struck all "evidence-based" language from materials and censored scientifically oriented government agencies such as the Environmental Protection Agency (EPA) and the Centers for Disease

Control (CDC), effectively delegating climate mitigation policy to the state level (Cohen, 2017). States like California and New Mexico are passing ambitious policies to reduce carbon emissions and invest in renewable energy, while Delaware, Maine, and New York have banned the use of plastic bags. Even conservative-majority states like Florida and Louisiana have put taxpayer dollars toward the construction of climate adaptation structures like seawalls and levees, but the vast majority of states have done little in the way of legislation, again lending support to the mixed-cooperation scenario of the Prisoner's Dilemma. These discrepancies in action, risk perception, and values may be attributed in large part to the nation's increasingly bipartisan way of life, such that shared threats like climate change and pandemics have become a sort of party-loyalty litmus test that prevents a fully cooperative strategy.

China

Home to the initial outbreak, China has received immense criticism over its handling of COVID-19. Claims of silencing whistleblower Dr. Wenliang (who died of COVID-19; Xiong & Gan, 2020), faulty reporting of true COVID-19 numbers, and production of faulty COVID-19 detection tests (which were sold to the United Kingdom for a staggering US\$20 million; Manning, 2020) plague the nation, even in the wake of its recovery from the pandemic. Despite these early setbacks, China's strong, centralized government has uniquely positioned it to implement sweeping changes including strict lockdown procedures, aggressive contact tracing, and enforcement of face coverings (Tabari et al., 2020). China averaged fewer than 100 cases per day in August 2020, whereas its peak infection of nearly 20,000 people in a single day was back in mid-February 2020, suggesting that the nation reversed its strategy of not cooperating to fully cooperating to contain COVID-19 in a matter of months (Manikandan, 2020). The decisive cooperation that characterizes the latter, more successful coronavirus response is also seen in how the nation handles the long-term threat of climate change. Ranked 61st out of 181 nations by ND-GAIN (2018), China was noted to be vulnerable to insufficient water as well as shortages in medical staff, the latter becoming particularly relevant in China's COVID-19 response only one year later, in late 2019. China emits more than a quarter of the world's carbon dioxide and approximately one-third of its greenhouse gases (World Bank, 2022). The amount of greenhouse gases produced by the nation, coupled with the fact that China has also been the world's primary investor in renewable energy alternatives (UNEP, 2020), suggests that the nation operates with a mixed-cooperation approach. In some ways, China is positioning itself to become a global leader in the fight against climate change by becoming a leader in renewable energy products, which will support its own economic development, yet it is still heavily dependent on coal, suggesting that it prefers a mixed-cooperation strategy.

Prison Break: Learning from the Prisoner's Dilemma to Foster Cooperation

The Prisoner's Dilemma provides a useful framework by which to classify and better understand how and why nations all facing the same stimuli can react in such different ways. When rational actors are faced with a problem greater than themselves, each actor is free to choose whether to cooperate to overcome that problem. However, irrespective of each party's choice, neither actor is free from the consequences of his or her own actions, or those of the other actor. This interconnectedness of decision-making, whether at the individual level or aggregated into the international level, suggests something perhaps intuitive to the human spirit—we all need each other. In examining a small subset of all the national responses possible to both the COVID-19 pandemic and climate change, we discerned a few powerful lessons and noted some likely trends about the relationship between response to a short-term cooperative challenge like COVID-19 and a long-term cooperative challenge like climate change.

Given the parallels between the COVID-19 outbreak and climate change, we hypothesized that response to the former, a relatively short-term challenge, would be predictive of response to the latter, a long-term challenge relying on the same principles of global cooperation. We anticipated that nations with successful containment of the COVID-19 pandemic would be more likely to have passed legislation to potentially mitigate climate change successfully. We also anticipated the antithesis to be true: nations with a poor response to

COVID-19 would also have a poor response to climate change, likely passing few or ineffective policies toward successful mitigation. Of the seven nations we analyzed, we found that for the most part, each nation responded similarly to both threats, suggesting that COVID-19 response may indeed be a good proxy by which to predict how a nation may respond to a more diffuse, global threat on a long-term scale, like climate change. This may be because the mechanisms and rationale for combating both events remain the same, even if the relevant timescales differ (Kaushik, 2020). Countries that successfully responded to COVID-19 were characterized by a rapid response time, evidence-based strategies recommended by medical professionals, and direct, transparent communication of aims and goals by government officials. These traits led to successful cooperation by individual constituents by clearly defining the challenge at hand—the goal—as well as the directives to achieve that goal and the risks associated with not meeting that goal. By utilizing evidence-based strategies published by research entities to inform policy and by providing individual actors with both knowledge and skills to overcome COVID-19, these successful nations empowered their citizens to fully cooperate to combat a problem while preventing interactor conflict (Beaubien, 2020). Contrast this approach with some of the hallmarks of nations with failed responses to COVID-19: delayed and inconsistent responses, skepticism toward evidence-based techniques to reduce spread, and conflicting communications between government officials and their constituents. When individual actors observe a mixed response by government officials and policymakers, it undermines the legitimacy of the danger posed by pandemics and, by extension, the legitimacy of containment measures, encouraging at best a mixed response by individuals, or at worst a wholly uncooperative response wherein no one partakes in vital containment measures like social distancing, quarantining, and so on. Instead, across the four nations with poor or inconsistent responses to COVID-19, we see that leadership in those nations was often slow to react and often propagated misinformed or contradictory messages (Davis, 2020).

At the heart of the three potential outcomes hypothesized by the Prisoner's Dilemma is the underlying question of how to ensure that all actors have a shared base of knowledge and values. When all actors align in knowledge and values, it is possible, easy even, to foster coop-eration because the group interest now readily matches the individual interest (Ostrom, 1990; Ostrom et al., 1999). In countries with poorer responses to COVID-19, it may be worthwhile to note that such failed responses, when responses have even occurred, are driven by disparate information and values. It is difficult, if not impossible, to foster coop-erative sacrifice of individual freedoms to solve a problem that is con-sidered a hoax or whose threat level is considered exaggerated by any sizable number of a nation's constituents. Where disparate knowledge or conflicting values exist, it becomes the responsibility of the govern-ing body to equalize those factors by providing clear facts and unify-ing, national aims that overcome lesser divisions such that cooperation at every tier of organization becomes possible. In times of trial, people turn to their leaders for guidance, so when an administration is char-acterized by mixed cooperation, it is only reasonable to expect that its constituents will emulate such an example. It is increasingly clear that the threshold between one Prisoner's Dilemma scenario and another is leadership style (Somvichian-Clausen, 2020).

Effective leadership is a tool, but ineffective leadership is a weapon. The Prisoner's Dilemma has shown that the decisions of every actor, whether effective or ineffective, good or bad, all have a universal impact, but that impact is weighted considerably more when the actor is the leader of a nation. In coordinating global responses, it would be reckless to underestimate the personal power and sway of political fig-ures in influencing the perception, narrative, and response protocols surrounding challenges like pandemics or climate change. Countless examples demonstrate how national politics have shaped and even interfered with the response to an otherwise nonpartisan threat for purposes of individual gain. When we consider the harrowing circum-stances and grim prospects offered by the challenges of a pandemic or climate change, however, there is no such thing as an individual gain or loss. Nature cares not for human delineations—natural disasters and diseases transcend politics and national boundaries and will continue to do so with increasing frequency and intensity. There may be short-term winners and losers, but when it comes to widespread, globalized challenges, the effects will diffuse such that net benefits and losses will be universally and evenly distributed.

The intent of this work is neither to condemn nor to laud the advent of globalization, but rather to point out that it has already happened and that the future of all meaningful and effective policy must be developed and enacted in this global framework (Collins, 2015; West, 2017). Successful leaders should recognize the inherent linkages between every nation's decision-making and work to cooperate so as to generate diffuse but universal benefits for all of humanity. As it stands, the world at large remains locked in a mixed-response scenario from the Prisoner's Dilemma. We hold the key but must turn it together— only by fostering cooperation can we attempt a successful prison break.

References

Ackerman, F., & Stanton, E. A. (2008). *The cost of climate change: What we'll pay if global warming continues unchecked.* Report commissioned by the Natural Resources Defense Council. https://www.nrdc.org/sites/default/files/cost.pdf

Andreoni, M. (2020, August 20). Coronavirus in Brazil: What you need to know. *New York Times.* Accessed August 20, 2020. https://www.nytimes.com/article/brazil-coronavirus-cases.html?auth=linked-google

Baker, G. (2020, March 13). The politicization of a pandemic. *Wall Street Journal.* Accessed August 15, 2020. https://www.wsj.com/articles/the-politicization -of-a-pandemic-11584115592

Beaubien, J. (2020, May 27). Some countries have brought new cases down to nearly zero. How did they do it? National Public Radio (NPR). Accessed August 12, 2020. https://www.npr.org/sections/goatsandsoda/2020/05/23/861577367/ messaging-from-leaders-who-have-tamed-their-countrys-coronavirus-outbreaks

Beck, J. (2011, June 12). Sweden, UK and Germany rank most active on climate. *Deutsche Welle.* Accessed August 13, 2020. https://www.dw.com/en/sweden -uk-and-germany-rank-most-active-on-climate/a-15582525

Cannon, J. C. (2020, April 8). Gold mining threatens indigenous forests in the Brazilian Amazon. *Mongabay.* Accessed August 18, 2020. https://news .mongabay.com/2020/04/gold-mining-threatens-indigenous-forests-in -the-brazilian-amazon/

Carter, D. P., & May, P. J. (2020). Making sense of the U.S. COVID-19 pandemic response: A policy regime perspective. *Administrative Theory and Praxis*, 42(2), 265–77. https://doi.org/10.1080/10841806.2020.1758991

CCC (Climate Change Commission). (2020). *Statement of intent: July 2020–June 2024.* Climate Change Commission of New Zealand. https://ccc-production -media.s3.ap-southeast-2.amazonaws.com/public/documents/Corporate -publications-/CCC-SOI-July-2020-June-2024.pdf

CDC (Centers for Disease Control and Prevention). (2020, August 13). Cases in the U.S. Accessed August 13, 2020. https://www.cdc.gov/coronavirus/2019-ncov/ cases-updates/cases-in-us.html

Chen, C., Noble, I., Hellmann, J., Coffee, J., Murillo, M., & Chawla, N. (2015). *University of Notre Dame Global Adaptation Index: Country Index technical report*. Notre Dame, IN: University of Notre Dame Global Adaptation Index (ND-GAIN).

Chen, L. (2020, July 10). The US has a lot to learn from Taiwan's Covid fight. CNN. Accessed August 1, 2020. https://www.cnn.com/2020/07/10/opinions/taiwan-covid-19-lesson-united-states-chen/index.html

Cohen, J. (2017, December 18). CDC word ban? The fight over seven health-related words in the president's next budget. *Science*, 1–5. https://doi.org/10.1126/science.aar7959

Collins, M. (2015, May 6). The pros and cons of globalization. *Forbes*, 1–5.

Contini, C., Di Nuzzo, M., Barp, N., Bonazza, A., de Giorgio, R., Tognon, M., & Rubino, S. (2020). The novel zoonotic COVID-19 pandemic: An expected global health concern. *Journal of Infection in Developing Countries*, 14(3), 254–64. https://doi.org/10.3855/jidc.12671

Davis, W. (2020, August 6). The unravelling of America. *Rolling Stone*. Accessed August 14, 2020. https://www.rollingstone.com/politics/political-commentary/covid-19-end-of-american-era-wade-davis-1038206/?jwsource=cl&fbclid=IwAR25omECignvH2QHhhO30C5OMgRNX2CrkGrXjGxuIABCVdYISX6SWV3y-EE

DeCanio, S. J., & Fremstad, A. (2013). Game theory and climate diplomacy. *Ecological Economics*, 85, 177–87. doi:10.1016/j.ecolecon.2011.04.016

DeFries, R., Rudel, T., Uriarte, M., & Hansen, M. (2010). Deforestation driven by urban population growth and agricultural trade in the twenty-first century. *Nature Geoscience*, 3, 178–81. https://doi.org/10.1038/ngeo756

Emanuel, E. J., Zhang, C., & Glickman, A. (2020, June 30). Learning from Taiwan about responding to Covid-19—and using electronic health records. *STAT News*. Accessed August 12, 2020. https://www.statnews.com/2020/06/30/taiwan-lessons-fighting-covid-19-using-electronic-health-records/

EM-DAT. (2020). EM-DAT public: Natural disasters in 2019–2020. EM-DAT: The International Disasters Database. https://public.emdat.be/

Fauci, A. S., Lane, H. C., & Redfield, R. R. (2020). Covid-19—Navigating the uncharted. *New England Journal of Medicine*, 382(13), 1268–69. https://doi.org/10.1056/NEJMe2002387

Ferrante, L., and Fearnside, P. M. (2019). Brazil's new president and "ruralists" threaten Amazonia's environment, traditional peoples and the global climate. *Environmental Conservation*, 46, 261–63. doi:10.1017/ S0376892919000213

Fischer, F. (2019). Knowledge politics and post-truth in climate denial: On the social construction of alternative facts. *Critical Policy Studies*, 13(2), 133–52. https://doi.org/10.1080/19460171.2019.1602067

Goudarzi, S. (2020, April 29). How a warming climate could affect the spread of diseases similar to COVID-19. *Scientific American*, 1–7.

IPCC (Intergovernmental Panel on Climate Change). 2014. *Climate Change 2014: Synthesis Report. Contribution of Working Groups I, II, and III to the Fifth Assessment Report of the Intergovernmental Panel on Climate Change*, R. K. Pachauri & L. A. Meyer (Eds.). Geneva, Switzerland: IPCC.

Johns Hopkins University. (2022, April 5). COVID-19 Dashboard. https://coronavirus
.jhu.edu/map.html.

Kaushik, P. (2020, March 17). Covid-19 and the Prisoner's Dilemma. *Asia Times*, 1–6.

Keating, D. (2017, June 16). Sweden to end net carbon emissions by 2045. *Deutsche
Welle*. Accessed August 15, 2020. https://www.dw.com/en/sweden-to-end-net
-carbon-emissions-by-2045/a-39280147

Khanna, R. C., Cicinelli, M. V., Gilbert, S. S., Honavar, S. G., & Murthy, G. V. S. (2020).
COVID19 pandemic: Lessons learned and future directions. *Indian Journal of
Ophthalmology*, *68*(5), 703–10. https://doi.org/10.4103/ijo.IJO_843_20

Klare, M. (2019, November 12). If the US military is facing up to the climate crisis,
shouldn't we all? *The Guardian*. Accessed August 8, 2020. https://www
.theguardian.com/commentisfree/2019/nov/12/us-military-pentagon
-climate-crisis-breakdown-

Leite, J., Preissler Iglesias, S., Viotti Beck, M., & Bronner, E. (2020, June 24). The
pandemic's worst-case scenario is unfolding in Brazil. *Bloomberg Businessweek*.
Accessed August 15, 2020. https://www.bloomberg.com/news/features/2020
-06-24/coronavirus-pandemic-brazil-faces-worst-case-scenario

Levy, B. S., & Patz, J. A. (2015). Climate change, human rights, and social justice.
Annals of Global Health, *81*, 310–22.

Li, Q., Guan, X., Wu, P., Wang, X, Zhou, L., Tong, Y., . . . Feng, M. (2020). Early transmission dynamics in Wuhan, China, of novel coronavirus–infected pneumonia.
New England Journal of Medicine, *382*, 1199–207.

Liu, H., Liu, J., & You, X. (2021, December 3). Q&A: What does China's 14th "five year
plan" mean for climate change? Carbon Brief. https://www.carbonbrief.org/
qa-what-does-chinas-14th-five-year-plan-mean-for-climate-change

Londoño, E., Andreoni, M., & Casado, L. (2020, June 18). Brazil, once a leader,
struggles to contain virus amid political turmoil. *New York Times*. Accessed
August 18, 2020. https://www.nytimes.com/2020/05/16/world/americas/virus
-brazil-deaths.html

Manikandan N. (2020). Are social distancing, hand washing and wearing masks
appropriate measures to mitigate transmission of COVID-19? [¿Son el distan-
ciamiento social, lavado de manos y uso de mascarilla medidas apropiadas para
mitigar la transmisión de la COVID-19?]. *Vacunas* (English Edition), *21*(2),
136–37. https://doi.org/10.1016/j.vacune.2020.10.010

Manning, R. A. (2020, April 21). Why China will be the biggest COVID-19 loser.
The Hill. Accessed August 14, 2020. https://thehill.com/opinion/international/
493876-why-china-will-be-the-biggest-covid-19-loser

Masola, J. (2020, August 14). New Zealand is "going hard and going early" after learning from Australia's outbreak. *Sydney Morning Herald*. Accessed August 16,
2020. https://www.smh.com.au/world/oceania/new-zealand-is-going-hard-and
-going-early-after-learning-from-australia-s-outbreak-20200814-p55lv3.html

Mehran, A., AghaKouchak, A., Nakhjiri, N., Stewardson, M. J., Peel, M. C.,
Phillips, T. J., Wada, Y., & Ravalico, J. K. (2017). Compounding impacts
of human-induced water stress and climate change on water availability.
Scientific Reports, *7*(6282). https://doi.org/10.1038/s41598-017-06765-0

Menon, P. (2020, July 26). New Zealand PM Ardern's ratings sky high ahead of election. Reuters. Accessed November 14, 2020. https://www.reuters.com/ article/us-newzealand-election-ardern/new-zealand-pm-arderns-ratings-sky -high-ahead-of-election-idUSKCN24R0UI

Mongelli, I., Tassielli, G., & Notarnicola, B. (2009). Carbon tax and its short-term effects in Italy: An evaluation through the input-output model. In S. Suh (Ed.), *Handbook of input-output economics in industrial ecology: Eco-efficiency in industry and science* (vol. 23, pp. 357–77). Dordrecht, Netherlands: Springer. https://doi.org/10.1007/978-1-4020-5737-3_18

Mulaney, A. (2020, June 21). A COVID-19 prisoner's dilemma. *Stanford Daily*, 1–3.

Muno, M. (2020, April 30). Coronavirus lockdowns lose support in Germany. *Deutsche Welle*. Accessed August 15, 2020: https://www.dw.com/en/opinion -coronavirus-lockdowns-lose-support-in-germany/a-53297044

ND-GAIN (Notre Dame Global Adaptation Initiative). (2018). ND-GAIN Country Index. Accessed August 1, 2020. https://gain.nd.edu/our-work/country-index/

Odell, S. D., Bebbington, A., & Frey, K. E. (2018). Mining and climate change: A review and framework for analysis. *Extractive Industries and Society*, 5(1), 201–14. doi:10.1016/j.exis.2017.12.004.

Ostrom, E. (1990). *Governing the commons: The evolution of institutions for collective action*. Cambridge: Cambridge University Press.

Ostrom, E., Burger, J., Field, C. B., Norgaard, R. B., & Policansky, D. (1999). Revisiting the commons: Local lessons, global challenges. *Science*, 248(5412), 278–82. doi:10.1126/science.284.5412.278

Pittel, K., & Rübbelke, D. T. (2010). Transitions in the negotiations on climate change: From prisoner's dilemma to chicken and beyond. *International Environmental Agreements: Politics, Law and Economics*, 12(1), 23–39. doi:10.1007/s10784-010 -9126-6

Regan, P. M. (2016). *The politics of global climate change*. London: Routledge.

Reynolds, E. (2020, July 17). Coronavirus and animals: From farmed mink to your pet cat, here's what we know. CNN. https://www.cnn.com/2020/07/17/health/ animals-coronavirus-infection-explained-intl/index.html.

Somvichian-Clausen, A. (2020, August 21). New study confirms that female-led countries fared better against coronavirus. *The Hill*. Accessed August 24, 2020. https://thehill.com/changing-america/respect/equality/513163-new-study -confirms-that-female-led-countries-fared-better?fbclid=IwAR3Gxfx7qtp1 TU5TYcoSX5zEmtVgn74cn8MPS3M8UoaG_cy5GFfvCy23fSk

Spring, J. (2020, March 4). Brazil exported thousands of shipments of unauthorized wood from Amazon port. Reuters. Accessed August 20, 2020. https://www .reuters.com/article/us-brazil-environment-lumber-exclusive/exclusive-brazil -exported-thousands-of-shipments-of-unauthorized-wood-from-amazon -port-idUSKBN20R15X

Tabari, P., Amini, M., Moghadami, M., & Moosavi, M. (2020). International public health responses to COVID-19 outbreak: A rapid review. *Iranian Journal of Medical Sciences*, 45(3), 157–69. https://doi.org/10.30476/ijms.2020.85810.1537

Tankersley, J., Haberman, M., & Rabin, R. C. (2020, March 23). Trump considers reopening economy, over health experts' objections. *New York Times*. Accessed August 15, 2020. https://www.nytimes.com/2020/03/23/business/trump-coronavirus-economy.html

Thompson, M. (2019, September 20). Germany unveils $60 billion plan to fight the climate crisis. CNN. Accessed August 15, 2020. https://www.cnn.com/2019/09/20/economy/germany-climate-crisis-package/index.html.

UNEP (United Nations Environment Programme). (2020). Frankfurt School—UNEP Collaborating Centre for Climate and Sustainable Energy Finance. Accessed August 20, 2020. http://www.fs-unep-centre.org

Urban, M., & Saad-Diniz, E. (2020, June 22). Why Brazil's COVID-19 response is failing. *Regulatory Review*. Accessed August 20, 2020. https://www.theregreview.org/2020/06/22/urban-saad-diniz-brazil-covid-19-response-failing/

West, G. B. (2017). *Scale: The universal laws of growth, innovation, sustainability, and the pace of life in organisms, cities, economies, and companies*. New York: Penguin Press.

World Bank (2022, October 12). China's transition to a low-carbon economy and climate resilience needs shift in resources and technologies. https://www.world-bank.org/en/news/press-release/2022/10/12/china-s-transition-to-a-low-carbon-economy-and-climate-resilience-needs-shifts-in-resources-and-technologies#:~:text=China%20emits%2027%20percent%20of,of%20the%20world's%20greenhouse%20gases

Xiong, Y., & Gan, N. (2020, February 4). This Chinese doctor tried to save lives, but was silenced. Now he has coronavirus. CNN. Accessed August 1, 2020. https://www.cnn.com/2020/02/03/asia/coronavirus-doctor-whistle-blower-intl-hnk/index.html

CHAPTER 4

Operation Warp Speed and COVID-19 Vaccines in the United States

GERALD W. PARKER

Background

The World Health Organization (WHO) was notified on December 31, 2019, about an unusual pneumonia cluster in Wuhan, China. The Shanghai Public Health Center received clinical samples on January 3, 2020, and generated the first genomic sequence two days later for a novel coronavirus, subsequently named Severe Respiratory Coronavirus 2 (SARS-CoV-2), which was found to cause Coronavirus Disease-19 (COVID-19). The sequence was uploaded to a public database by the University of Sydney in Australia on January 11, 2020. By that time, 41 patients had been diagnosed with COVID-19 and one death had been reported in Wuhan. Scientists and public health authorities realized a public health crisis was unfolding, and the race was on to develop vaccines based on the genomic sequence.

Exactly eleven months later, on December 11, 2020, the Food and Drug Administration (FDA) granted the first emergency use authorization (EUA) for the Pfizer-BioNTech vaccine to prevent COVID-19 illness in individuals 16 years old and older (FDA, 2020d). One week later, on December 18, 2020, the FDA granted the second EUA for the Moderna COVID-19 vaccine for use in individuals 18 years old and older (FDA, 2020e).

These first two EUAs marked a significant milestone in the fight against COVID-19 and came at a time when severe disease was accelerating, deaths were mounting, hospitals were overwhelmed, and crisis standards of care were being implemented in communities across the United States. The pace at which the vaccine was developed was unprecedented in vaccine development history and an extraordinary public health achievement. Vaccine development and approval is estimated in most cases to take 10 years or longer, and most vaccine candidates fail to attain full FDA approval. The acceleration of safe and effective COVID-19 vaccines was the equivalent of a vaccine moonshot that came at the right time, and this achievement would not have been possible without prior investments in biodefense and public health preparedness; vaccine research, development, manufacturing; and regulatory science over the last 20 years—and the hard lessons learned over that 20-year journey.

A key early decision that enabled accelerated development was to proceed through the development pipeline in parallel rather than in series, as is normally done in the financially risk-averse environment of the vaccine industry. The architects of Operation Warp Speed (OWS) established checks that prevented cutting corners to avoid jeopardizing vaccine quality, safety, and efficacy. Finally, it took extraordinary leadership, focus, discipline, and resources from OWS and the vaccine industry.

Past Lessons Learned from Anthrax to Ebola (2001–2018)

A series of events and crises, as well as 20 years of public health preparedness policy evolution, set the stage for the COVID-19 vaccine development response. Along that journey, progress was not always apparent, but with two decades of successes and failures along the way, the medical countermeasures (MCM) enterprise was poised to respond to COVID-19.

The Anthrax Letter Attacks

Letters containing dried anthrax spores were mailed in the aftermath of the terrorist attacks of September 11, 2001. The first batch of anthrax letters were postmarked on September 11 and sent to major media addresses in New York City and Florida. The second batch of letters were postmarked on October 12 and sent to the Hart Senate Office Building in Washington, DC. These letters constituted the first significant act of bioterrorism in the United States and highlighted our vulnerability to biological threats, whether intentional, accidental, or natural in origin. Lessons learned revealed a lack of vaccines and other potentially lifesaving treatments, as well as a lack of logistical plans needed for the rapid distribution and administration of antibiotics or vaccines, had they been available. In the aftermath, the Bush administration and Congress established new biodefense and infectious disease research programs, allocated funding for new high-containment laboratory construction, and established new partnerships with the private sector for vaccine research, development, and planning for mass prophylaxis of therapeutics and vaccines.

Severe Acute Respiratory Syndrome (SARS)

SARS was a previously unknown viral respiratory illness caused by a coronavirus. The disease was first reported in China in November 2002, and over the next few months it spread to 26 countries before the outbreak was contained. There were over 8,000 cases and 774 deaths reported worldwide, and the outbreak caused significant economic consequences in affected countries.

Lessons learned were like those of the anthrax attacks, but in an international context. The National Institutes of Health (NIH) and scientists worldwide initiated vaccine research projects, and several candidates made it to preclinical trials. Only a few made it to phase 1 clinical trials to evaluate safety and immune response to the SARS coronavirus spike protein, and this commenced only after the SARS epidemic ended. NIH redirected funding to other priorities, and SARS vaccine development stopped soon thereafter. However, the experience provided valuable insights about the SARS-CoV-2 immunogenic targets needed for COVID-19 vaccine development 15 years later.

Project BioShield

Project BioShield was enacted by Congress in 2004 to accelerate research, development, purchase, and availability of biodefense vaccines, therapeutics, and diagnostics (US Department of Health and

Human Services, Administration for Strategic Preparedness and Response, 2004). Project BioShield had three components: (1) funding authorized and appropriated for MCMs in a Special Reserve Fund ($5.6 billion over 10 years); (2) new authorities at NIH to expedite and simplify biodefense and emerging infectious disease research grants; and (3) the use of MCMs in an emergency.

A 10-year extended appropriation and an advance purchase agreement were intended to incentivize and stimulate industry innovation and public-private partnerships. Unfortunately, the initial high-profile BioShield contract for a recombinant anthrax vaccine, still in early R&D phases, failed miserably (Miller, 2006). Over time, both the government and the vaccine industry learned from early mistakes. For example, a subsequent Project BioShield advance purchase agreement led to the successful development of a new smallpox vaccine that could be administered to immune-compromised individuals (Bavarian Nordic, 2010).

OWS succeeded in using advance purchase agreements thanks to early BioShield lessons learned. Pfizer-BioNTech did not take R&D funding from OWS but utilized the advance purchase agreement business model consistent with experienced pharmaceutical manufacturers.

The third BioShield component, the EUA, provided FDA legal authority for the distribution and use of Pfizer-BioNTech, Moderna, and Johnson & Johnson COVID-19 vaccines.

When enacted as a component of Project BioShield, the EUA was intended to provide the best available MCMs to the public following a declaration of a public health emergency by the secretary of Health and Human Services (HHS). An EUA is an evidence-based mechanism to facilitate the availability and use of MCMs, including vaccines, during public health emergencies. Under an EUA, the FDA may allow the use of unapproved medical products, or unapproved uses of approved medical products in an emergency to diagnose, treat, or prevent serious or life-threatening diseases or conditions. Certain statutory criteria must be met, including that there are no adequate, approved, and available alternatives. EUAs have been used in past public health emergencies, such as the 2009 H1N1 pandemic and the MERS, Ebola virus, and Zika virus outbreaks.

Lessons learned from past EUAs provided industry and the FDA with the demonstrated ability and confidence to utilize the authorization for COVID-19 vaccines, treatments, and diagnostics, and on a scale never used prior to COVID-19 (FDA, 2020c). Never has an EUA been used knowing that a vaccine would be administered to more than 300 million people of all ages before granting a full biological license agreement (BLA).

The Public Readiness and Emergency Preparedness (PREP) Act

The PREP Act, which passed in 2005, allows the secretary of HHS to issue declarations of immunity from liability, except for willful misconduct, for the following claims: (1) loss resulting from the administration or use of MCMs for diseases or threat conditions; (2) a situation determined by the secretary to constitute present or credible risk of a future public health emergency; and (3) claims by entities involved in the development, manufacture, testing, distribution, administration, and use of covered MCMs (ASPR, 2021).

PREP Act declarations have been used during at least seven public health crises since the act's authorization. The secretary of HHS utilized the act to cover COVID-19 MCMs beginning in March 2020. This power was essential for providing liability protection for all entities and individuals involved in the manufacturing and vaccination campaign for COVID-19, including the hundreds of thousands of volunteers administering vaccinations on the front line (US Department of Health and Human Services, 2020).

The Pandemic and All-Hazards Preparedness Act (PAHPA)

PAHPA legislation was originally authorized in 2006 and reauthorized in 2013 and 2019 (ASPR, 2006, 2013, 2019). The act provided HHS with new authorities, new organizations, and new programs for public health preparedness and response. The most notable new entities with implications for COVID-19 vaccines were the Administration for Strategic Preparedness and Response (ASPR) and the Biomedical Advanced Research and Development Authority (BARDA), which leads and oversees advanced development, manufacture, and federal acquisition of pandemic and biodefense MCMs.

The Public Health Emergency Medical Countermeasures
Enterprise (PHEMCE)

In 2006, ASPR established the PHEMCE to coordinate across HHS and with other federal departments for MCM research, development, and procurement for the Strategic National Stockpile (SNS) (ASPR, 2021). Led by ASPR, the PHEMCE includes partners from BARDA, NIH, FDA, Centers for Disease Control and Prevention (CDC), Department of Defense (DOD), Department of Homeland Security (DHS), Veterans Administration (VA), and Department of Agriculture (USDA). The PHEMCE was the first attempt to organize, coordinate, and integrate decision-making for all MCM preparedness programs across the federal government. It was upon this ecosystem that OWS began to build in the spring of 2020, albeit avoiding and shedding the PHEMCE's bureaucratic inertia that had evolved between 2006 and 2020.

The Joint Program Executive Office for Chemical, Biological, Radiological,
and Nuclear Defense (JPEO-CBRND)

The JPEO-CBRND was established to manage DOD's investments in advanced development, manufacture, and acquisition of chemical, biological, radiological, and nuclear (CBRN) defense equipment and MCMs (JPEO-CBRND, 2021) in the early 2000s. In recent years, the JPEO-CBRND's acquisition programs have adopted innovative and agile contracting mechanisms, such as Other Transaction Authorities (OTA) (DAU, 2021). Lessons were learned on how best to utilize agile contracting tools for MCMs that were in the best interest of DOD and biotechnology industry partners.

OWS utilized the project management and contracting infrastructure and expertise available in both BARDA and JPEO-CBRND for many contractual agreements. These agreements enabled COVID-19 vaccine advanced development and procurement. The application of JPEO-CBRND's OTA lessons learned and business tools were essential to OWS and industry success.

The H5N1 Pandemic Influenza National Strategy
and Implementation Plan

The pandemic strategy and implementation plan were initiated in 2005 and 2006, respectively (Homeland Security Council, 2005, 2006). The national strategy guided preparedness and response to an influenza pandemic, with the intent of (1) slowing the spread of a pandemic to the United States to provide time to take preparedness actions, like surge vaccine manufacturing; (2) limiting the domestic spread of a novel influenza viral strain once it arrived, and mitigating disease, suffering, and death; and (3) sustaining infrastructure and mitigating economic and societal impact. The Bush administration requested and Congress approved about $6 billion in emergency supplemental appropriations for pandemic preparedness in 2006, the first time an appropriation was made for preparation ahead of a pandemic.

A key pillar of both documents was pandemic vaccine advanced development, surge manufacturing, stockpiling, and distribution planning (Homeland Security Council, 2006). The goal was to establish domestic production capacity and countermeasure stockpiles to ensure sufficient H5N1 influenza vaccines for all front-line personnel and at-risk populations, including military personnel; sufficient manufacturing surge capacity to vaccinate the entire US population within six months of the emergence of a virus with pandemic potential; and advancement in regulatory science and the removal of other legal barriers to the expansion of our domestic vaccine production capacity.

To achieve surge manufacturing capacity goals for pandemic readiness, the influenza vaccine industry needed to move away from its decades-old approach of culturing influenza viruses in large-scale egg production facilities and instead move toward modern cell-based technology. Unfortunately, this proved more technically and financially difficult than anticipated. Today, nearly 15 years later, most FDA-approved influenza vaccines still use egg-based manufacturing technology. Pandemic vaccine readiness funding resulted in FDA approval of only one cell-based and one recombinant subunit protein-based vaccine in 2012 and 2013, respectively (GEN, 2012; Ledford, 2013).

Preparedness efforts during that era pushed the vaccine industry toward understanding the need to modernize vaccine technology platforms for both seasonal and pandemic influenza readiness. One of the six COVID-19 vaccine candidates supported by OWS used the recombinant subunit vaccine technology platform approved in 2013.

The Defense Production Act (DPA)

The DPA and its potential application to public health preparedness and crisis response were initiated as an action of the National Strategy for Pandemic Influenza Implementation plan in the 2006–2008 time frame (Homeland Security Council, 2006). Vaccine surge planning revealed that extraordinary measures were needed to mobilize industry during a pandemic crisis. To address this challenge, innovative contracting and public-private business models were explored, including the utilization of the DPA, which had rarely been used beyond DOD and military requirements prior to that time.

Modeled on the War Powers Acts of 1941 and 1942, the DPA was originally passed during the Korean War. The current version of the law gives the executive branch substantial powers to direct private companies to prioritize orders from the federal government to allocate materiel, services, and facilities for national defense. It also includes the power to restrict hoarding of essential supplies. Additionally, companies can be authorized to coordinate with each other in ways that might otherwise violate antitrust laws (Tucker, 2020).

OWS application of the DPA was a key enabler that focused essential supply chains for priority COVID-19 vaccine development, manufacturing, and distribution, including many ancillary supplies like bioreactor supplies, glass vials, stoppers, needles, syringes, and other items (GAO, 2020).

2009 H1N1 Influenza Pandemic

In April 2009, a new influenza virus subtype was identified that was radically different from other circulating seasonal influenza viruses. Within just a few weeks, this virus spread globally, and WHO declared it a pandemic in June 2009.

Numerous 2009 H1N1 after-action reports revealed some success in tackling the pandemic, but many shortcomings were identified that would have had serious, if not catastrophic, ramifications during an outbreak of a more virulent influenza virus. For example, an H1N1 influenza monovalent vaccine was rapidly developed and manufactured. However, the vaccine was not available before the pandemic peaked in the Northern Hemisphere, and ultimately it had little impact on slowing the trajectory of viral spread and disease.

The HHS after action review of the pandemic concluded that the United States must have "nimble and flexible capabilities to produce medical countermeasures rapidly in the face of any attack or threat, whether known or unknown, novel or reemerging or intentional" (US Department of Health and Human Services, Administration for Strategic Preparedness and Response, 2010). Various technology platforms were proposed by the report, but adaptable and flexible manufacturing innovation was deemed essential.

That recommendation led to the construction and establishment of the Centers for Innovation in Advanced Development and Manufacturing (CIADMs) at the Texas A&M University System (TAMUS) and Emergent BioSolutions. The TAMUS CIADM and its subcontractor, Fujifilm Diosynth Biotechnologies, are supporting advanced development and manufacture of Novavax's COVID-19 vaccine candidate. Emergent BioSolutions is supporting the manufacture of Johnson & Johnson's COVID-19 vaccine.

Inadequate domestic manufacturing capacity and supply chains for specialized vaccine equipment and supplies were the most difficult challenges faced by OWS. The CIADMs were available and tasked to provide their manufacturing capacity for OWS, which alleviated some of these obstacles.

A final lesson learned from the 2009 pandemic was that inadequate access to global influenza pandemic vaccine became a major diplomatic problem for the United States and other high-income nations. It was never solved in the 2009 pandemic, and global COVID-19 vaccine access is still a significant gap today.

Ebola, 2014–2016 and 2018

The West African Ebola virus epidemic was a tragic public health emergency and humanitarian crisis. It was by far the largest Ebola outbreak on record and caused significant morbidity and mortality, accompanied by major socioeconomic consequences for the region, mainly in Guinea, Liberia, and Sierra Leone. There were 28,646 reported cases and 11,323 deaths worldwide, with isolated travel-related and/or health care provider cases occurring in Europe and the United States.

An Ebola vaccine, which had been developed by the Public Health Agency of Canada years earlier based on a live, attenuated vaccine platform technology and had been put on hold for lack of funding, was transferred to Merck in 2014 and rushed into advanced development, clinical trials, and manufacture with funding provided by the United States. When the Ebola outbreak was contained in 2016, funding was paused again and development stopped. Johnson & Johnson also developed an Ebola vaccine candidate based on a nonreplicating adenovirus vector vaccine platform technology, and like Merck, it paused clinical development when the outbreak ended. This was a noble public service by both Merck and Johnson & Johnson, but the experience also left the companies with significant financial losses and some uncertainty regarding future opportunities through public-private partnerships.

Another Ebola outbreak occurred in the Democratic Republic of the Congo (DRC) starting in 2018. Because of past financial losses and uncertainty regarding federal commitment, Merck was reluctant at first but was quickly persuaded to restart clinical trials and potential manufacture of its investigational Ebola vaccine candidate at financial risk. Merck's Ebola vaccine received conditional European Commission and FDA approval in 2019 (Branswell, 2019; FDA, 2019). Merck's live, attenuated vaccine platform technology was subsequently used to develop a COVID-19 vaccine candidate but did not meet OWS technology readiness levels, as discussed in more detail later.

Johnson & Johnson also moved its Ebola vaccine candidate back into clinical development and achieved European authorization in 2020. The Johnson & Johnson nonreplicating viral vector technology platform was used to develop a COVID-19 vaccine candidate and has achieved FDA EUA status.

However, the financial losses, government contract uncertainty, and difficult federal acquisition regulations experienced by Merck and Johnson & Johnson rippled through the vaccine industry. Concerns remained that the federal government did not fully recognize the commitment and funding needed for vaccine development and manufacturing for emergency response.

Vaccine development and manufacturing cannot simply be turned on and off repeatedly. These concerns impacted initial negotiations with industry in the early days of the COVID-19 response. Industry understandably needed to see demonstrated commitment by the US government to support accelerated development of a COVID vaccine.

Vaccine Platform Technology Research

Both the NIH and the Coalition for Epidemic Preparedness Innovations (CEPI, established after Ebola in 2014–2016) made focused investments in vaccine platform technologies and tested platforms against prototype pathogens from viral families thought to have pandemic potential (Martson, Paules, & Fauci, 2017; CEPI, 2017). This moved platform technologies from basic science to potential real-world application.

Although basic research on vaccine platforms started well over 20 years ago, many, including the author, considered it the holy grail of biodefense and public health preparedness because threats are constantly emerging and changing. Traditional vaccine development is a lengthy, expensive process with no guarantee of success. Project BioShield envisioned innovative platform technologies needed to move away from the "one-drug-for-one-bug" paradigm as early as 2004, but platform technology was still at only a basic readiness level.

The ideal goal is to have a pathogen-agnostic platform technology for a disease X, or capability to respond rapidly in a matter of weeks to an unknown disease. Although pathogen-agnostic platforms have not yet been demonstrated, the focus on platform technologies after Ebola in 2014–2016 helped facilitate the application of mRNA, nonreplicating viral vector, live attenuated viral vector, and subunit protein vaccine platform technologies pursued by OWS, which will be covered in more detail later.

Clinical Trials during an Outbreak Response

Regulatory approval to distribute and use vaccines requires randomized, double-blind, placebo-controlled clinical trials to support safety and efficacy demonstration for FDA EUA and BLA approvals. This is a challenge during an epidemic or a pandemic. The Merck and Johnson & Johnson Ebola vaccines were the first in the modern era to successfully complete necessary phase 1, phase 2, and phase 3 clinical trials during an outbreak while also having an impact on containing and preventing further Ebola disease and achieving regulatory approvals.

Outbreak clinical trial experience and lessons learned informed the FDA and industry in the design of COVID-19 clinical trials.

Defense Advanced Research Projects Agency (DARPA)
Grand Challenges
DARPA first established biodefense programs in 1998, and early investments included basic research for platform technologies and manufacturing innovation.

The COVID-19 mRNA vaccine platform will likely be one of the greatest success stories of the COVID-19 vaccine response. But like other technologies previously discussed, mRNA vaccine technology has its roots in the 1990s. Fortunately, a few dedicated scientists had the resilience to continue researching the technology and finally discovered how to drive the mRNA into a cell so that the cell's machinery could produce the immunogen from the encoded ribonucleic acid message (Kolata, 2021). Several biotechnology venture capital funding organizations soon grasped the potential of this new technology and made significant investments to move it forward.

DARPA, known to drive innovation through grand challenges, also picked up on the potential of mRNA for biodefense applications starting in 2012. DARPA's grand challenges pushed the biotechnology and pharmaceutical industry to think outside the box to accelerate the response to all biological threats, whether intentional, accidental, or natural. In 2017, DARPA established the Pandemic Prevention Platform with the goal of creating MCMs within 60 days of a viral outbreak. DNA and RNA technology platforms were the foundation of this new grand challenge. The innovations spurred by DARPA were extensively leveraged by OWS for vaccines and monoclonal antibody therapeutics (Duke Human Vaccine Institute, 2017; Dolgin, 2021).

Summary of Past Lessons Learned
Over a two-decade journey in biodefense and public health preparedness, lessons learned were not always apparent through different crises, policy changes, and boom-and-bust funding cycles. There were successes and failures along the way, but the MCM enterprise in the government and private sector made steady long-term progress that enabled accelerated vaccine development, manufacture, and access

that otherwise would not have been possible. COVID-19 vaccines were developed and authorized in 11 months, but the research, development, and acquisition foundations were over 20 years in the making.

Some of the more notable tools leveraged to success by OWS, industry, and the FDA include EUA, OTA, the PREP Act, DPA, FDA regulatory science and reforms, clinical trials during an outbreak, advanced development and agile manufacturing capacity, and advance purchase agreements. Key coordinating and integrating structures established in the last 20 years were also vital, including ASPR, BARDA, JPEO-CBRND, PHEMCE, and DARPA.

But the most important component when COVID-19 hit was a willing and able biotechnology and pharmaceutical industry, or *bio-economy*, that answered the call to pivot resources aggressively and work closely with OWS in a focused public-private partnership.

Operation Warp Speed
Operation Warp Speed Stand-Up and Strategy
After the publication of the SARS-CoV-2 genetic sequence on January 11, 2020, scientists and biotechnology companies around the world began to unravel the genetic code to develop candidate vaccine strategies. On March 16, 2020, Moderna began its NIH-funded phase 1 clinical trial, only 45 days after the sequence went public, a record time from sequence to first human vaccination.

US philanthropic organizations, CEPI (headquartered in Europe), NIH, BARDA, and DOD rushed into action to establish vaccine development contracts domestically and internationally.

ASPR and BARDA established an interagency MCM task force in late January 2020, even before the secretary of HHS declared a public health emergency on January 31. The task force included ASPR, BARDA, CDC, NIH, and DOD. Under task force guidance, NIH, BARDA, and DOD began to independently explore modifying existing contracts and initiating new contracts for vaccine development that included outreach to industry stakeholders in a manner that encouraged a broad portfolio of vaccine platform technology approaches. They also initiated what would become one of the greatest early challenges: securing vaccine manufacturing capacity and supply chains.

BARDA modified existing Johnson & Johnson and Sanofi vaccine development contracts by mid-February 2020 and redirected their adenoviral vector and recombinant subunit vaccine platforms, respectively, for COVID-19 vaccine advanced development. On March 21, 2020, BARDA awarded Moderna a contract to bridge from NIH's preclinical and phase 1 clinical development to phase 2 advanced development and beyond.

Although the MCM task force made early progress, it was essentially an extension of the PHEMCE model, which had become overburdened by bureaucratic inertia and lacked timely decision-making ability and authority. Pandemic crisis response requires strong leadership and an organizational culture that enables effective leaders to drive collaboration, cooperation, innovation, and communication with a sense of urgency. The PHEMCE is a long-standing and established interagency coordination ecosystem that works in peacetime, but not in crisis response. Also, HHS secretaries going back to the original 2006 PAHPA never empowered the ASPR with the full authority of that legislation. Unfortunately, that meant that a sense of urgency, innovation, and quick decision-making ability were not the strengths and the culture of the PHEMCE, or of supporting components BARDA, NIH, CDC, FDA, and DOD, even with effective top-level leadership. It was also clear that DOD would need to provide significant contracting and logistics support that was not available in HHS to the degree,

Figure 4.1. Traditional vaccine development timelines.

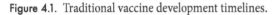
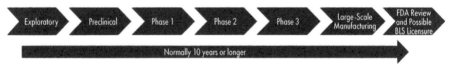

Phase 1 clinical trials test the initial safety profile in human volunteers with increasing doses.

Phase 2 clinical trials are designed to evaluate the ability of vaccine candidates to elicit immune responses indicating potential for efficacy and common short-term safety side effects.

Phase 3 clinical studies determine preliminary evidence of efficacy in large field studies and additional safety information.

Commercial large-scale manufacturing normally does not occur until after Phase 3 clinical trials and are subject to rigorous FDA quality control good manufacturing standards.

speed, and sophistication needed. Finally, the HHS MCM task force was starting to suffer counterproductive influence by the White House COVID-19 Task Force, which itself was not compatible with established incident command discipline under the National Response Plan.

By late March 2020, HHS leadership from ASPR up to the secretary recognized that a new leadership paradigm was needed to accelerate and innovate vaccine development and manufacture with a new public-private business model in what was becoming a very serious unfolding pandemic. ASPR and the FDA director of the Center for Biologics Evaluation and Research analyzed options and proposed recommendations for a new approach. From the start, the two established a bold goal to develop COVID-19 vaccines and achieve FDA EUA in less than a year. Vaccine development normally takes years to progress from preclinical development through phase 1, phase 2, and phase 3 clinical trials, plus the associated small-scale clinical manufacturing, manufacturing scale-up, commercial-scale validation, and large-scale manufacturing under good manufacturing quality standards. Development normally proceeds through the phases in order after established checkpoints, moving from one phase to the next based on analysis of the data from the last phase. Large-scale manufacturing normally starts after completion of phase 3 clinical trials (fig. 4.1). OWS sought to change the vaccine development timeline to address the needs of the crisis (fig. 4.2).

Figure 4.2. Operation Warp Speed vaccine development.

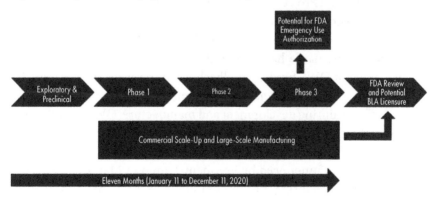

On the surface, the innovative concept and strategy that evolved was simple. Eliminate the dead space, or time, between normal development milestones that occur in series and, where possible, proceed with development steps in parallel. This strategy allowed all development steps and phases to proceed without shortcuts during the manufacturing development and clinical trials needed to demonstrate safety and efficacy. Actual implementation was extraordinarily complex and had never been tried before, largely for financial reasons. The biomedical research enterprise in peacetime is risk averse and operates far below "warp speed."

Because of the gravity of the pandemic, the full power of the federal government—financial and other authorities—was needed to mitigate financial risks for industry and to drive an innovative business model to leverage vaccine platform technologies, other technological advances, and federal authorities such as the DPA, OTA, PREP Act, FDA EUA, and others that had been honed over the last 20 years for the strategy to have a chance of success.

The strategy was initially called Manhattan Project 2, after the first Manhattan Project during World War II, which similarly achieved what many considered impossible at the project's inception. The Manhattan Project during World War II integrated the nation's best scientists and military might to develop the first atomic weapon to end the war. In a similar fashion, Manhattan Project 2 paired the best vaccine scientists from government and industry with military program and logistics disciplines in pursuit of vaccines to end the pandemic.

Manhattan Project 2 was later rebranded "Operation Warp Speed," since the effort was to create a vaccine as fast as possible to end the pandemic, not a bomb (Robert Kadlec, ASPR, pers. comm., 2020). Although the name had and continues to have critics, there is no denying that OWS fundamentally changed the speed of the biomedical research enterprise without compromising vaccine quality, safety, and efficacy during development and manufacture. OWS took the biomedical research enterprise and vaccine industry where it had never gone before.

OWS was announced by President Trump in May 2020, with the goal of manufacturing 300 million doses by mid-2021 and starting delivery of FDA-authorized COVID-19 vaccines by December 31, 2020.

This was an audacious goal. Leveraging past lessons learned and relying on the expertise of BARDA, NIH, FDA, CDC, DOD, and industry were essential, but the MCM enterprise needed a fundamental restructuring to manage and support the vaccine industry for an accelerated COVID-19 vaccine response. OWS was a leadership paradigm shift for government and industry that combined the best capabilities of DOD and HHS with their private-sector partners in the vaccine industry.

Leadership was essential, and the HHS and DOD secretaries took charge, established a strict chain of command, and put in place procedures that would protect the integrity of OWS from undue influence, including counterproductive political pressure from the White House COVID-19 Task Force.

The most important first decision was selecting the chief operations officer and chief scientist to drive day-to-day, hour-to-hour, and minute-to-minute operations and decisions in what became a vast public-private enterprise that included thousands of people involved in research, development, manufacture, and distribution. General Gustave Perna, former commanding general of the US Army Materiel Command, and Moncef Slaoui, a vaccine industry specialist and former head of vaccines at GlaxoSmithKline, were selected to serve as the chief operations officer and chief scientist, respectively. General Perna brought DOD logistics, materiel supply chain, program management, and leadership discipline not characteristic of a health agency like HHS. Moncef Slaoui brought decades of industry leadership and vaccine science experience. As a government outsider, Dr. Slaoui was also not burdened with historical bureaucratic tendencies, which allowed him to cut through long-standing government silos.

From May 2020 to February 2, 2021 (which was my last day of direct involvement in and observation of OWS as a senior adviser to the ASPR), OWS practiced very disciplined program management through a "battle rhythm" to drive operations, milestone deliverables, and timelines.

Product development teams were established for each vaccine candidate in the portfolio that focused on the most minuscule of details. Government program managers and scientists worked closely with their private sector counterparts, whether vaccine industry primary contractors or one of the myriad supply chain subcontractors.

Problems were rapidly elevated to government and industry leadership for resolution or alternative plans as quickly as possible.

But before this battle rhythm could get started in earnest, key decisions loomed—specifically, the base OWS vaccine candidate portfolio. Success or failure hinged on these decisions. OWS leadership established criteria and key principles that guided selection of vaccine candidates for the portfolio.

OWS's strategy included several key principles that enhanced its chance of success. The first was establishing a diverse portfolio that included two vaccine candidates for each of the three vaccine platform technologies: the mRNA vaccine platform; the recombinant-subunit adjuvanted protein vaccine platform; and the replication-defective live-vector vaccine platform. The four vaccine platform technologies were selected to permit fast and effective manufacturing potential. Vaccine candidates had to demonstrate a technology readiness level that would allow the scalability and consistency necessary to reliably produce 100 million doses by mid-2021, with preclinical or early clinical data to indicate the potential for clinical safety, efficacy, and potential to enter phase 3 clinical studies by July to November 2020. This timeline was necessary to deliver clinical safety and efficacy outcomes by the end of 2020 to mid-2021, aligned to overarching goals (Slaoui & Hepburn, 2020).

The second key principle was accelerating advanced development without compromising vaccine safety, efficacy, and product quality. Acceleration potential was predicated on running all development streams fully resourced in parallel rather than in series. Phase 3 clinical trials proceeded under time-tested randomized, double-blind, placebo-controlled research protocols, after phase 1 and phase 2 clinical studies showed that vaccine candidates were well tolerated and elicited an immune response in adult volunteers. The number of patients and trial site locations for phase 3 clinical trials were increased and guided by COVID-19 disease forecasting models to optimize safety and efficacy signals. Volunteer patient enrollment in clinical trials sought diversity that was representative of the US population.

The third key principle was providing financial resources and technical assistance to companies supporting OWS to commence process development and scale up manufacturing while vaccine candidates were in preclinical through clinical safety and efficacy testing. This included facility construction or renovations, equipment fitting, staff hiring and training, raw material sourcing, and technology transfer as well as acquisition of vials, syringes, needles, and ancillary supplies for each vaccine candidate.

The overall strategy was to support a diverse but focused vaccine candidate portfolio with the highest potential for moving through the development pipeline, and to accelerate vaccine development without curtailing quality processes and checkpoints required for objective program management and regulatory science standards. The ability to move through the development timeline in parallel was aided by early and unambiguous guidance to manufacturers from the FDA on how and when, based on required data, to seek EUA to allow vaccine administration before all BLA procedures were completed.

Operation Warp Speed Vaccine Development Portfolio

As previously stated, OWS ended up supporting six vaccine candidates. Vaccine candidates based on attenuated live-viral vector vaccine platform technology, like Merck's COVID-19 vaccine candidate, did not meet the technology readiness criteria of OWS and were not included in the base portfolio. Below is a brief overview of each platform.

MRNA VACCINE PLATFORM

The mRNA platform delivers the genetic sequence of the SARS-CoV-2 spike protein directly into cells. The mRNA molecule contains the code that causes host cells to make the spike protein. The host immune system recognizes the spike protein and elicits a protective immune response. The mRNA does not enter the nucleus of the cell, only the cytoplasm, and the molecule needs to be encased in a lipid nanoparticle to enter cells.

The two mRNA vaccines supported by OWS were those of Pfizer-BioNTech and Moderna. Pfizer-BioNTech's mRNA vaccine candidate, BNT162b2, consists of mRNA that encodes the viral spike protein of SARS-CoV-2, transported inside lipid nanoparticles that allow the mRNA to enter cells. Two doses are required, with the second dose administered no sooner than 21 days after the first dose. The vaccine must be kept frozen and stored in an ultra-low-temperature freezer between -80 and -60 degrees centigrade, and protected from light until ready to use. The vaccine remains shelf stable for up to five days at standard refrigerator temperatures (between 2 and 8 degrees centigrade).

Moderna's mRNA-1273 vaccine candidate consists of mRNA encoding the viral spike protein of SARS-CoV-2, transported in lipid nanoparticles, and also requires two doses, with the second dose administered no sooner than 28 days after the first dose. The Moderna vaccine is stable for six months during shipping and storage at freezer temperatures of -20 degrees centigrade. The vaccine is shelf stable at refrigerator temperatures (between 2 and 8 degrees centigrade) for 30 days.

REPLICATION-DEFECTIVE LIVE-VECTOR VACCINE PLATFORM

The two vaccine candidates based on the replication-defective live-vector platform use a weakened adenovirus that cannot reproduce or cause disease. The adenovirus serves as a viral vector to carry a DNA molecule coding for the SARS-CoV-2 spike protein to the nucleus of host cells. The cell then generates the spike protein immunogen, which is recognized by the immune system and elicits an immune response. The two replication-defective live-vector vaccines supported by OWS were the Johnson & Johnson and the AstraZeneca–University of Oxford vaccine.

The Johnson & Johnson vaccine candidate uses a nonreplicating adenovirus 26 vector platform, the same platform it used in its Ebola vaccine. The vaccine requires one dose and can be stored at refrigerator temperatures (between 2 and 8 degrees centigrade) for at least three months. The AstraZeneca–Oxford AZD1222 vaccine candidate consists of nonreplicating chimpanzee adenovirus, ChAdOx1, which is a weakened virus that causes infections in nonhuman primates. The vaccine requires two doses and can be stored at refrigerator temperatures (between 2 and 8 degrees centigrade).

RECOMBINANT-SUBUNIT ADJUVANTED PROTEIN PLATFORM

The two vaccine candidates based on this platform utilize purified SARS-CoV-2 spike protein subunits to stimulate an immune response. An adjuvant is required to help boost the immune response. This is a more traditional vaccine approach. Vaccines using this platform include those for hepatitis B, human papillomavirus, and tetanus. The two recombinant-subunit adjuvanted protein vaccines supported by OWS were Novavax and Sanofi-GSK. Novavax's NVX-CoV2373 vaccine candidate is a recombinant nanoparticle spike protein that includes a proprietary adjuvant to increase the immune response. The vaccine requires two doses and can be stored at refrigerator temperatures (between 2 and 8 degrees centigrade). Sanofi-GSK's vaccine candidate uses the same recombinant protein-based technology as one of Sanofi's seasonal influenza vaccines along with GSK's established pandemic vaccine adjuvant technology. The vaccine will require two doses if authorized for use in the United States and can be stored at refrigerator temperatures (between 2 and 8 degrees centigrade).

The total value of OWS-supported vaccine candidates, manufacturing capacity expansion, and ancillary supplies as of March 1, 2021, was over $23 billion, as summarized in tables 4.1 and 4.2 (CRS, 2021).

COVID-19 VACCINE EFFICACY AND EFFECTIVENESS IN REDUCING RISK OF SARS-COV-2 SEVERE CLINICAL OUTCOMES

The phase 3 clinical trial results for the Pfizer-BioNTech and Moderna vaccines showed 95 percent and 94 percent efficacy against symptomatic COVID-19 illness caused by the original SARS-CoV-2 strains in circulation during the fall of 2020. Johnson & Johnson's vaccine showed 66 percent efficacy against moderate COVID-19 illness and 85 percent efficacy against severe illness.

Table 4.1. Contract value for OWS-supported vaccines as of March 1, 2021.

COMPANY	CONTRACT VALUE	SPECIFICATIONS
Pfizer-BioNTech	$5.97 billion	300 million doses
Moderna	$4.94 billion	300 million doses
AstraZeneca	$1.2 billion	300 million doses
Johnson & Johnson	$1.5 billion	100 million doses
Novavax	$1.6 billion	100 million doses
Sanofi-GSK	$2.3 billion	100 million doses

Table 4.2. Contract value for other COVID-19 vaccine supplies as of March 1, 2021.

COMPANY	CONTRACT VALUE	PURPOSE OR SPECIFICATIONS
Emergent BioSolutions	$628 million	Manufacturing support
Texas A&M University with Fujifilm Diosynth Biotechnologies	$265 million	Manufacturing support for Novavax
ApiJect Systems America	$138 million	100 million prefilled syringes by the end of 2020
Corning Pharmaceutical Technologies	$204 million	Manufacturing capacity expansion to produce an additional 164 million glass vials per year if needed
SiO2 Materials Science	$143 million	Manufacturing capacity expansion to produce 120 million glass-coated containers
Becton Dickinson and Co.	$42.3 million	Manufacturing capacity expansion to produce needles and syringes
Smiths Medical, Inc.	$20.6 million	Manufacturing capacity expansion to produce needles and syringes
Goldbelt Security, LLC	$125 million	530 million needles and syringes
Retractable Technologies, Inc.	$53.6 million	Manufacturing capacity expansion to produce safety needles and syringes
Retractable Technologies, Inc.	$93.8 million	530 million safety needles and syringes
Marathon Medical	$27.5 million	N/A

Table 4.2. *continued*

COMPANY	CONTRACT VALUE	PURPOSE OR SPECIFICATIONS
DuoProSS Meditech Corp.	$48 million	134 million safety syringes by the end of 2020
Cardinal Health, Inc.	$15 million	500 million safety syringes over a 12-month period (August 2020 to August 2021)
Gold Coast Medical Supply, LP	$14 million	N/A
HTL-STREFA, Inc.	$12 million	N/A
Quality Impact, Inc.	$9 million	N/A
Medline Industries	$6 million	N/A

However, the phase 3 clinical trials were conducted at the same time as nonpharmaceutical interventions were being widely used to help mitigate viral community transmission, which could have impacted vaccine efficacy estimates against mild to moderate clinical illness. The clinical trials did not measure protection against asymptomatic infection or potential to transmit SARS-CoV-2 after vaccination. Nonetheless, the phase 3 clinical trial results were extraordinary, far exceeding the FDA efficacy threshold of 50 percent.

Vaccine distribution began within 24 hours of the FDA granting the EUA, and the largest and most complex vaccination campaign in US public health history was underway. The campaign was bumpy until vaccine production stabilized, health care systems vaccinated frontline health care providers at highest risk of exposure, and state and local authorities geared up mass vaccination sites in urban centers and other means to reach underserved communities and rural areas across the United States. As vaccine coverage increased from January to June 2021, new daily COVID-19 cases, hospitalizations, and deaths dropped precipitously from their January 2021 highs.

Real-world data have continued to accrue since phase 3 clinical trial results were first reported in November and December 2020.

Since then, COVID-19 vaccines have stood the test of time, but SARS-CoV-2 continues to move through the population worldwide, adapting new variants to favor its own survival and continued transmission to vulnerable individuals. For example, the Delta variant emerged in India in March 2021 and rapidly spread globally. This highly contagious variant started its ascent to become the predominant viral strain in the United States in the summer of 2021, at a time when vaccinations had slowed significantly, with only 50 percent of the population fully vaccinated. During July and August 2021, new COVID-19 cases and hospitalizations surged in the United States and reports of vaccination breakthrough infections increased.

The Delta variant demonstrated that emerging variants will challenge all nations. Public health and national leaders must continuously monitor vaccine effectiveness through population studies, maintain vigilance, and take appropriate actions to protect the most vulnerable populations. This will include updating vaccine booster recommendations to account for changing immunogenic targets and waning immunity following the initial vaccination series. Continued deployment of nonpharmaceutical interventions for unvaccinated and vaccinated individuals may be necessary in communities experiencing high community viral transmission.

Israel's Ministry of Health conducted what was arguably the most comprehensive population-based, real-world study on the effectiveness of the Pfizer-BioNTech vaccine. Results of this study from January 24 through April 3, 2021, demonstrated remarkable vaccine effectiveness in preventing asymptomatic and symptomatic cases, hospitalization, critical disease, and death caused by SARS-CoV-2, even against the B.1.1.7 variant, which became the dominant variant in Israel during the study period. The incidence of SARS-CoV-2 infections and severe COVID-19 disease outcomes decreased as vaccine coverage increased, even after nonpharmaceutical interventions were relaxed, indicating that vaccinations were mitigating severe outcomes of the pandemic.

However, Israeli health authorities subsequently reported potential for waning immunity with the Pfizer-BioNTech vaccine during the summer of 2021 (unpublished). Preliminary findings from Israel's Ministry of Health suggest the Pfizer-BioNTech vaccine was only 40 percent effective at reducing the risk of symptomatic disease from

June through July 2021, when the Delta variant was becoming the predominant strain (Lovelace, 2021). This compared unfavorably to the more than 95 percent effectiveness against symptomatic illness reported from January 24 through April 3, 2021 (Haas et al., 2021). However, the vaccine remained 91 percent effective at preventing hospitalization, critical disease, and death against the Delta variant through July 2021 (Lovelace, 2021).

It was unclear whether reduced effectiveness against mild to moderate infection was the result of waning immunity from the vaccine, Delta's increased contagiousness, or both. Israeli authorities decided not to make any changes and authorized a third booster dose for people over 60 years of age and immunocompromised individuals starting August 1, 2021 (BBC, 2021).

By the end of July 2021, more than 163 million people in the United States were fully vaccinated. There were 6,239 reported hospitalizations in vaccinated people diagnosed with SARS-CoV-2 infection, compared to over 35 million confirmed COVID-19 cases. In about 25 percent of the reported vaccine breakthrough cases, patients were asymptomatic, or their diagnosis appeared secondary to the primary cause of hospitalization. This indicates what we knew when the vaccination campaign started and what we know now, that vaccine breakthrough infections are expected.

COVID-19 vaccines are not 100 percent effective. No vaccine is perfect, but to date, COVID-19 vaccines authorized for use in the United States remain effective in reducing the risk of severe disease and death. Table 4.3 shows the risk of infection, hospitalization, and death in unvaccinated compared to vaccinated people through July 2021. According to the CDC, COVID-19 vaccines provide 8-, 25-, and 25-fold reductions in symptomatic disease incidence, hospitalization incidence, and death, respectively (CDC, 2021a).

But the CDC's data have limitations because they depend on passive reporting from states on vaccine breakthroughs that led to hospitalization or death. The CDC did not require reporting of asymptomatic or symptomatic mild-to-moderate infections of individuals partially or fully vaccinated, and few states reported COVID-19 cases by vaccination status. The Virginia Department of Health did report COVID-19 cases by vaccination status, and it showed that 98.5 percent of total cases,

Table **4.3.** US weekly COVID-19 incidence per 100,000 in unvaccinated and vaccinated.

	UNVACCINATED	VACCINATED	REDUCTION DUE TO VACCINATION
Cases per 100K	178.6	21.4	8-fold reduction
Hospitalized per 100K	2.52	0.1	25-fold reduction
Deaths per 100K	0.96	0.04	25-fold reduction

Source: CDC (2021a).

97.3 percent of hospitalizations, and 98.2 percent of deaths occurred in people not fully vaccinated through July (VDH, 2021). Additionally, the Delta and Omicron variants demonstrated that vaccinated people can become infected and transmit the virus to others (Ledger, 2021).

More population-based studies like the one done in Israel, and better reporting are needed to gain an understanding of estimated rates of breakthrough cases of mild-to-moderate infection, vaccine effectiveness against new variants, and durability of immunity.

Real-world studies during the earliest phase of the Delta variant–driven outbreak reported from the United Kingdom indicated that the Pfizer-BioNTech COVID vaccine remained about 88 percent effective against symptomatic illness and 96 percent effective at preventing hospitalization and death against the Delta variant in June to July 2021 (Bernal et al., 2021; Stowe et al., 2021).

In the United States, the Mayo Clinic published data in August 2021 that showed similar findings from patients in the Mayo Clinic health care system in Minnesota compared to patients in Israel. The Mayo Clinic study included data on both the Moderna and Pfizer-BioNTech vaccines from January through July 2021. Both vaccines were highly effective against mild-to-moderate infection with SARS-CoV-2: Moderna, 86 percent; and Pfizer-BioNTech, 76 percent. Vaccine effectiveness was also estimated against hospitalization: Moderna, 91.6 percent; and Pfizer-BioNTech, 85 percent. However, during July 2021, as the Delta variant was becoming the predominant strain, vaccine effectiveness against mild-to-moderate infection dropped for both vaccines: Moderna to 76 percent; and Pfizer-BioNTech to 42 percent. Estimated effectiveness against hospitalization remained above 75 percent for both vaccines. No deaths were reported from either vaccine cohort in Minnesota from January through July 2021.

Despite increasing vaccination breakthrough infections with newly emerging variants, COVID-19 vaccines remain effective and our best tool to reduce risk of severe disease and death from COVID-19. Public health authorities and medical professionals must continually monitor vaccine effectiveness and enhance surveillance efforts to detect new variants. Near-real-time genomic sequence surveillance data are essential to guide vaccine manufacturers to anticipate new vaccine candidates specific to emerging variants.

Fortunately, OWS and industry successfully generated mRNA and adenoviral vector vaccine platform technologies that can rapidly adapt to changing requirements. Pfizer, Moderna, and Johnson & Johnson are conducting new clinical trials with vaccine candidates designed to combat new variants and are prepared to pivot to manufacturing boosters against specific new variants, as we do every year for seasonal influenza. National public health authorities must likewise be prepared to make timely and decisive decisions for the pivot to be effective.

COVID-19 Vaccine Distribution and Administration in the United States
OWS coordinated distribution planning with the CDC starting in the summer of 2020. Vaccine distribution rollout began 24 hours after the FDA issued the first EUA on December 11, 2020. The CDC and state public health authorities have lead responsibilities for implementing distribution and administration once a vaccine is shipped from federal control to state and local authorities.

There have been many criticisms of OWS, the CDC, and state authorities regarding vaccine distribution, which were especially acute during the first two months when vaccines were scarce and in high demand. Some criticisms are well founded. This chapter will not discuss in detail the many aspects of distribution and administration, but a few observations are offered from the inside to provide a big-picture perspective.

The COVID-19 vaccination campaign was and continues to be the largest and most complex mass prophylaxis campaign ever attempted by the public health system in the United States. A logistics platform to distribute and administer vaccines under an EUA to everyone in the United States over the course of a few months did not exist.

But as vaccine manufacturing stabilized and became more predictable, the vaccine distribution system evolved in concert across a vast enterprise that spanned from vaccine manufacturers, distributors, and shippers to hospitals, long-term care facilities, state and local authorities, and pharmacies, which similarly had to develop capacities to administer vaccines in their communities.

Preparedness plans since the anthrax attacks in 2001 required mass prophylaxis plans per CDC public health preparedness grant funding. Some states and local communities understood that requirement and exercised their plans, while others apparently did not take the CDC grant funding requirement seriously. However, no one, from the federal to the local level, regardless of past planning experience, could have been fully prepared for the enormity of the task at hand. This required keeping pace with the evolving lessons learned during the rollout to improve the efficiency of vaccine distribution, logistics, and administration as the rollout progressed.

Unfortunately, the CDC's initial vaccine allocation guidance was logistically complex and did not focus on the most vulnerable populations at risk of severe COVID-19 disease, hospitalization, and death. Every state prioritized the first vaccine allocations to frontline health care providers, who were clearly at high risk of exposure. After that, many different allocation priorities were tried with varying levels of success. Some states, like Texas, once health care providers had an opportunity to get vaccinated, provided the next priority allocation to all people over 65 years of age plus all people with medical comorbidities who were at highest risk of hospitalization and death. States that took this approach were generally able to establish more effective distribution systems more quickly. This allowed them to start to mitigate severe disease outcomes from COVID-19 in the most vulnerable populations sooner.

Global COVID-19 Vaccine Development and Access

It was estimated that 11 billion COVID-19 vaccine doses had been administered and 66.4 percent of the global population had received at least one dose as of April 2022 (Holder, 2022). However, large vaccine incquitics remain, as less than 10 percent of the population in many low-income countries is fully vaccinated. On the African continent specifically, the vaccination rate is only 20 percent (Holder, 2022).

The United States is contributing to the improvement of global vaccine access in terms of monetary donations, vaccine doses, and manufacturing capacity needed to manufacture donated doses. For example, the United States committed $4 billion to COVAX and has donated AstraZeneca vaccine originally manufactured for the United States but not yet approved here. Doses of Moderna and Johnson & Johnson vaccines have been donated, and the administration announced in June 2021 that 500 million doses of Pfizer-BioNTech would be made available for global distribution to low- and middle-income nations. The United States is also supporting vaccine administration efforts through the US Agency for International Development (USAID) and GAVI (US Department of State, 2021; White House, 2021). Despite these efforts, the United States can do better and should take a leadership role with other high-income nations to establish an international vaccine strategy to accelerate global vaccine access that goes beyond the current piecemeal approach.

Operation Warp Speed Lessons Learned

The number of federal pandemic response critics continues to flourish into the third year of the pandemic. Many criticisms are deserved. There have been many failures, but there are successes too. Despite many setbacks, the United States was better prepared for SARS-CoV-2 because of past investments in biodefense, public health preparedness, and health security vaccine research and development. This came with hard and sometimes painful lessons learned, but steady progress was made over a 20-year journey built on the backs of many dedicated professionals in government at all levels as well as in industry, academia, and other NGOs.

The accelerated development of safe and effective COVID-19 vaccines through OWS is one of the bright spots among many response failures. OWS, however, would not have been possible without public support, which came with new congressional authorities and appropriations after the anthrax letter attacks in the fall of 2001. This allowed the executive branch to establish new and evolving programs in health security vaccine and therapeutics research, development, manufacturing, and regulatory science over the last 20 years. OWS was also successful in the crisis because HHS and DOD leaders took charge, each assuming ownership and accountability while they established a strict chain of command, empowered their subordinates, and put in place procedures to protect the integrity of OWS. The FDA provided a defined regulatory pathway without ambiguity, industry stepped up to the challenge, and Congress provided appropriations. Together, a sort of symphony was established with countless moving parts, diverse expertise, and a clear conductor bringing the pieces together.

Despite the extraordinary success of OWS, lessons learned are apparent. The Biden administration and Congress need to understand the leadership lessons learned, and how to institutionalize the effective leadership paradigm of OWS to continue fighting COVID-19 now and to prepare for future regional epidemics and pandemics. Federal program managers and acquisition authorities will likewise need to assess reforms needed at the operational level to maintain effective public-private partnerships. Effective business models for vaccine R&D preparedness are elusive, especially for vaccine manufacturing, which needs to scale up rapidly in a crisis. There are no easy solutions.

Key Enablers of Success

Several key factors allowed OWS to be successful. These included leadership, commitment, governance, regulatory science, contracting business models and resources, judicial use of the power of the federal government, a diverse portfolio to reduce technology risk, and industry best practices. Regarding leadership, there was an unprecedented reduction of government silos, which enabled rapid decision-making by the best government and industry scientists, focused on a common and clearly articulated end goal. Regarding commitment, committed leaders at all levels of government and industry drove day-to-day operations under a strict battle rhythm that also promoted open communication so problems could be elevated quickly for resolution. Regarding governance, there was a whole-government approach with an industry structure that was flat organizationally and took a task-force approach.

Each portfolio had single points of contact between government product coordination teams and industry counterparts to facilitate communication. Regarding regulatory science, there was early, rapid, and regular input from the FDA while a regulatory firewall and independence were maintained. Unambiguous regulatory pathways were established early and had minimal changes so that vaccine developers knew the steps to reach FDA authorization. For judicial use of the power of the federal government, there was targeted use of the DPA ratings, and the DOD was mobilized along with other government resources. These resources included contracting that prioritized supply chains and other resources for manufacturing and clinical trials.

The establishment of a diversified portfolio to reduce technology risk, as discussed earlier, allowed focus on the vaccine candidates with the highest potential for success. These were selected from a wide range of acceptable platforms. Finally, OWS maintained industry best practices for independence, oversight, and safety standards. These included maintaining political independence in day-to-day operations.

Key Challenges

While OWS had significant successes, it also faced key challenges during vaccine development. The first was the limited vaccine manufacturing capacity in the United States and worldwide. The second key challenge was the disruptions to manufacturing supply chains. The third key challenge was the lack of a ready and available trained workforce. The fourth and final challenge was finding a way to distribute and administer vaccines from the federal to the local level throughout the United States.

Risks and Challenges That Require Continued Leadership and Management for Pandemic Medical Countermeasures Preparedness

Many aspects of vaccine development and distribution required continued leadership and management. These areas included the urgency of pandemic vaccine research, development, manufacturing, and regulatory science innovation for preparedness, preparing for the last pandemic, leveraging innovation in academia and industry, vaccine hesitancy and messaging, global access to COVID-19 vaccines, and the lack of a global vaccine manufacturing and distribution capacity.

After past infectious disease crises, the public, Congress, and the administration's interest in biodefense and the health security medical countermeasures enterprise waned, and preparedness suffered. Preparedness during interpandemic periods requires sustained urgency and investments. The successful OWS public-private partnership lessons learned during the crisis response must be applied to preparedness.

PREPARING FOR THE LAST PANDEMIC

After the 2009 H1N1 influenza pandemic, the HHS adopted several new initiatives to address lessons learned. One of the primary initiatives was the establishment of Centers for Innovation in Advanced Development and Manufacturing (CIADMs). Each CIADM was intended to provide flexible, surge vaccine manufacturing capacity that could respond to novel influenza viruses with pandemic potential. Unfortunately, the program investments and goals of all administrations fell short of what was required to maintain operational readiness for a crisis. That was apparent during the COVID-19 response. The original goal of these public-private partnerships was to create vaccine manufacturing facilities with the capacity to produce 50 million dose-equivalents of influenza vaccine drug substance within four months of a declared pandemic. Those capacities were established. But facility and capacity expansion were only the first step. To establish and maintain a state of readiness, continued investments are essential. The government maintained that it would provide the CIADMs with investments and vaccine advanced development work to build, sustain, and exercise those capacities, but that did not happen.

As we build the systems needed to prepare for future pandemics, we should assume that the next pandemic will not be like COVID-19. The government's business model for the CIADM program after the 2009 pandemic was built on influenza. We fought the last pandemic rather than looking sufficiently to the future with an expansive view of potential pandemic threats. Because the business model was built on influenza, it was doomed to fail. Physical facility and workforce capacities are still needed, but next time we must put more emphasis on effective business models with flexible contracting processes that will sustain such facilities and the workforce.

As with the first point above, we need to approach vaccine manufacturing preparedness with a military readiness mindset and exercise those capabilities. Proactively producing a variety of vaccine drug substances will allow the United States to perfect the processes, technologies, and workforce expertise needed to scale up manufacturing to face new threats and defeat the next pandemic. Workforce training and expertise are essential. The CIADM programs included a workforce training element, but that needs to be expanded. A university federally funded R&D center (FFRDC) network could be an essential component of a future vaccine pandemic preparedness and response ecosystem.

LEVERAGE INNOVATION IN ACADEMIA AND INDUSTRY

Many government vaccine R&D programs have not effectively leveraged innovation in academia and industry during preparedness. Universities are uniquely positioned to help overcome barriers confronted by the biotechnology industry through their research and service core missions, which could be better leveraged to support government requirements in partnership with the biotechnology industry. For vaccine manufacturing, this could be provided through advanced development solutions with platform technologies and innovative manufacturing strategies. Commercial vaccine manufacturers could then quickly adapt those platforms for surge production at a commercial scale. Universities also have international biomedical research collaborators to assist US global health security and diplomatic efforts to promote international vaccine advanced development and manufacturing networks. Universities also bring innovative vaccine technology platforms and manufacturing into the mix for technology transfer into industry as well. HHS and DOD should take stock of the CIADM lessons learned. The concept can work, and similar models have proven successful in other national security domains. The federal government should establish a network of FFRDCs for vaccine advanced development and manufacturing research, like the Department of

Energy's National Laboratory Network. A focused network of university FFRDCs in this mission space could also serve as a neutral "smart scientific buyer or adviser" for the federal government.

Vaccine availability does not equate to vaccinations. Vaccine hesitancy was a concern that was anticipated early on and remains an issue as of this writing. Unfortunately, initial scare-tactic public health messaging around the emergence of the Delta variant and reports of vaccination breakthroughs were confusing and inconsistent and derailed the importance of COVID-19 vaccines. Public health messaging should use a reasoned tone to emphasize the reassuring data on vaccine safety and efficacy in preventing severe disease and death in vaccinated people compared to unvaccinated people. The ensuing federal mandates and harsh tone that continued through the fall of 2021 eroded public trust in institutions and vaccines. Good leaders use the power of persuasion with a reasoned tone. COVID-19 vaccine safety and efficacy data are reassuring and almost tell their own story if explained properly. Public messaging from trusted voices will be more successful in future vaccination campaigns. Public policy leaders need to heed this advice.

GLOBAL ACCESS TO COVID-19 VACCINES

Approximately 68 percent of the US population was fully vaccinated and 65 percent of the global population was fully vaccinated as of November 2022. In many low-income countries, particularly those in Africa, less 10 percent of the population is fully vaccinated. Global vaccine access is essential. The longer we take to provide worldwide vaccine access, the more likely a vaccine-resistant variant will emerge that will prolong the pandemic.

Global vaccine manufacturing capacity for all other licensed vaccines prior to COVID-19 was about 6 billion doses annually. The global COVID-19 vaccine requirement, assuming 90 percent population vaccination with an initial two-dose regimen, is 14.2 billion doses. We have a long way to go to establish sustainable global vaccine manufacturing capacity and distribution systems to finish the fight against COVID-19 and be prepared for the next inevitable pandemic.

COORDINATED GLOBAL VACCINE MANUFACTURING CAPACITY AND
DISTRIBUTION ECOSYSTEMS DO NOT EXIST

When the COVID-19 vaccine was under development, many obstacles hindered our ability to manufacture and distribute the candidates worldwide. And despite advances, a number of obstacles still need to be overcome. The development of a coordinated global vaccine manufacturing capacity and distribution ecosystem requires a global development and manufacturing network consisting of regional, decentralized capacity in low- and middle-income countries and large, centralized manufacturing capacity in middle- and high-income countries. It also requires sustained financing, flexible business models, investment in design, construction of manufacturing innovations, and efficient mechanisms to facilitate and sustain technology transfer. It requires equitable vaccine allocation priorities and distribution system innovations. Finally, it requires a system of global coordination of phase 4, postmarket research to document near-real-time ongoing safety and efficacy vaccine data in populations, and to overcome vaccine misinformation and build trust across many different cultures and norms.

Final Thoughts: COVID-19 Vaccines and Vaccinations in the United States

The pace of OWS was unprecedented and groundbreaking, and it was an extraordinary public health achievement. It would not have been possible without prior investments in biodefense and pandemic preparedness vaccine research, development, manufacturing, regulatory science, and mass prophylaxis planning over the last 20 years, and the hard essons learned over that journey.

It took leadership, focus, discipline, and resources from OWS and a strong bioeconomy to capitalize on past lessons learned. This was followed by extraordinary leadership by public health and emergency management at state, county, and local levels, and hundreds of thousands of health care workers, logisticians, volunteers, and others to administer the shots in every community across the United States.

As of November 2022, more than 224 million people in the United States were fully vaccinated against COVID-19. While that is remarkable, it is only 68 percent of the US population, and vaccine is plentiful for those who wish to get vaccinated. Worldwide, estimates show that about 65 percent are fully vaccinated, with less than 10 percent of the population fully vaccinated in several low-income countries. Action is needed to accelerate global vaccine access.

The emergence of new variants, waning vaccine immunity, and surges of new cases require continued vigilance. Despite increasing vaccine breakthroughs in the United States and elsewhere, nearly all hospitalizations, severe disease, and deaths have occurred in unvaccinated people.

SARS-CoV-2 and the coming new variants will become endemic for the foreseeable future. We must learn how to live safely with SARS-CoV-2, as we have with other risks associated with daily life. Vaccines are the most effective tool for individuals to reduce their risk of hospitalization, severe disease, and death.

References

ASPR (Administration for Strategic Preparedness and Response, Department of Health and Human Services). (2006, December). Pandemic and All-Hazards Preparedness Act (PAHPA). https://www.phe.gov/Preparedness/legal/pahpa/Pages/default.aspx

ASPR (Administration for Strategic Preparedness and Response, Department of Health and Human Services). (2013, March). Pandemic and All-Hazards Preparedness Reauthorization Act (PAHPRA). Administration for Strategic Preparedness and Response, Department of Health and Human Services. https://www.phe.gov/Preparedness/legal/pahpa/Pages/pahpra.aspx

ASPR (Administration for Strategic Preparedness and Response, Department of Health and Human Services). (2019, June 24). Pandemic and All-Hazards Preparedness and Advancing Innovation Act (PAHPAIA). Administration for Strategic Preparedness and Response, Department of Health and Human Services. https://www.phe.gov/Preparedness/legal/pahpa/Pages/pahpaia.aspx

ASPR (Administration for Strategic Preparedness and Response, Department of Health and Human Services). (2021, March 26). Public Health Emergency Medical Countermeasures Enterprise. Administration for Strategic Preparedness and Response, Department of Health and Human Services. https://www.phe.gov/Preparedness/mcm/phemce/Pages/default.aspx

ASPR (Administration for Strategic Preparedness and Response, Department of Health and Human Services). (2021, August 6). Public Readiness and Emergency Preparedness (PREP) Act. Administration for Strategic Preparedness and Response, Department of Health and Human Services. https://www.phe.gov/Preparedness/legal/prepact/Pages/default.aspx

Bavarian Nordic. (2010, July 13). Bavarian Nordic delivers 1 million doses of first vaccine developed under US. biopreparedness program to the Strategic National Stockpile. https://www.bavarian-nordic.com/investor/news/news .aspx?news=2041

Bernal, J. L, Andrews, N., Gower, C., Gallagher, E., Simmons, R., Thelwall, S., . . . Ramsay, M. (2021, July 21). Effectiveness of Covid-19 vaccines against the B.1.617.2 (Delta) variant. *New England Journal of Medicine, 385*, 585–94. https:// www.nejm.org/doi/full/10.1056/NEJMoa2108891

BBC (British Broadcasting Corporation). (2021, July 29). Coronavirus: Israel to give third jab to people aged over 60. https://www.bbc.com/news/world-middle-east -58021386

Branswell, H. (2019, November 11). Ebola vaccine approved in Europe in landmark moment in fight against a deadly disease. STAT. https://www.statnews.com/ 2019/11/11/ebola-vaccine-approved-in-europe-in-landmark-moment-in-fight -against-a-deadly-disease/

CDC (Centers for Disease Control and Prevention). (2021a, July 26). COVID-19 vaccine breakthrough case investigation and reporting. https://www.cdc.gov/ vaccines/covid-19/health-departments/breakthrough-cases.html

CDC (Centers for Disease Control and Prevention). (2021b, August 1). COVID vaccinations in the United States. https://covid.cdc.gov/covid-data-tracker/ #vaccinations_vacc-total-admin-rate-total

CEPI (Coalition for Epidemic Preparedness Innovations). (2017, September). Platform technologies. Accessed July 12, 2021. https://cepi.net/research _dev/technology/

CRS (Congressional Research Service). (2021, March 1). Operation Warp Speed contracts for COVID-19 vaccines and ancillary vaccination materials. https:// crsreports.congress.gov/product/pdf/IN/IN11560

DAU (Defense Acquisition University). (2021, August 6). Other transactions. https:// aaf.dau.edu/aaf/contracting-cone/ot/

Dolgin, E. (2021, January 12). How COVID unlocked the power of mRNA vaccines. *Nature*. Accessed July 26, 2021. https://www.nature.com/articles/d41586-021 -00019-w

Duke Human Vaccine Institute. (2017). Duke DARPA pandemic prevention platform. Accessed July 26, 2021. https://dhvi.duke.edu/programs-and -centers/pandemic-preparedness/duke-darpa-pandemic-prevention -platform-p3

FDA (US Food and Drug Administration). (2019, December 19). First FDA-approved vaccine for the prevention of Ebola virus disease, marking a critical milestone in public health preparedness and response. https://www.fda.gov/news-events/ press-announcements/first-fda-approved-vaccine-prevention-ebola-virus -disease-marking-critical-milestone-public-health

FDA (US Food and Drug Administration). (2020a, February 27). FDA issues emergency use authorization for third COVID vaccine. https://www.fda.gov/news -events/press-announcements/fda-issues-emergency-use-authorization-third -covid-19-vaccine

FDA (US Food and Drug Administration). (2020b, May 27). Coronavirus
(COVID-19) update: FDA authorizes Pfizer-BioNTech COVID-19 vaccine
for emergency use in adolescents in another important action in fight
against pandemic. https://www.fda.gov/news-events/press-announcements/
coronavirus-covid-19-update-fda-authorizes-pfizer-biontech-covid-19
-vaccine-emergency-use

FDA (US Food and Drug Administration). (2020c, November 20). Emergency use
authorization for vaccines explained. https://www.fda.gov/vaccines-blood
-biologics/vaccines/emergency-use-authorization-vaccines-explained

FDA (US Food and Drug Administration). (2020d, December 11). FDA takes key
action in fight against COVID-19 by issuing emergency use authorization for
first COVID-19 vaccine. Accessed July 6, 2021. https://www.fda.gov/news
-events/press-announcements/fda-takes-key-action-fight-against-covid-19
-issuing-emergency-use-authorization-first-covid-19

FDA (US Food and Drug Administration). (2020e, December 18). FDA takes additional action in fight against COVID-19 by issuing emergency use authorization
for second COVID-19 vaccine. Accessed August 6, 2021. https://www.fda.gov/
news-events/press-announcements/fda-takes-additional-action-fight-against
-covid-19-issuing-emergency-use-authorization-second-covid

FDA (US Food and Drug Administration). (2021a, April 23). FDA and CDC lift
recommended pause on Johnson & Johnson (Janssen) COVID-19 vaccine use
following thorough safety review. https://www.fda.gov/news-events/press
-announcements/fda-and-cdc-lift-recommended-pause-johnson-johnson
-janssen-covid-19-vaccine-use-following-thorough

FDA (US Food and Drug Administration). (2021b, June 25). Coronavirus
(COVID-19) update: June 25, 2021. https://www.fda.gov/news-events/press
-announcements/coronavirus-covid-19-update-june-25-2021

GAO (Government Accountability Office). (2020, November). *Defense Production
Act: Opportunities exist to increase transparency and identify future actions to
mitigate medical supply chain issues.* GAO-21-108. https://www.gao.gov/assets/
gao-21-108.pdf

GEN (Genetic Engineering and Biotechnology News). (2012, November 21). FDA
approves Novartis' Flucelvax. https://www.genengnews.com/topics/drug
-discovery/fda-approves-novartis-flucelvax/

Haas, E. J., Angulo, F. J., McLaughlin, J. M., Anis, E., Singer, S. R., Khan, F., . . . Alroy-
Preis, S. (2021, May 15). Impact and effectiveness of mRNA BNT162b2 vaccine
against SARS-CoV-2 infections and COVID-19 cases, hospitalisations, and
deaths following a nationwide vaccination campaign in Israel: An observational
study using national surveillance data. *Lancet.* https://www.thelancet.com/
journals/lancet/article/PIIS0140-6736(21)00947-8/fulltext#sec1

Holder, J. (2022, April 7). Tracking coronavirus vaccinations around the world.
New York Times. https://www.nytimes.com/interactive/2021/world/covid
-vaccinations-tracker.html

Homeland Security Council. (2005, November). *National Strategy for Pandemic
Influenza.* https://www.cdc.gov/flu/pandemic-resources/pdf/pandemic
-influenza-strategy-2005.pdf

Homeland Security Council. (2006, May). *National Strategy for Pandemic Influenza: Implementation Plan* https://www.cdc.gov/flu/pandemic-resources/pdf/pandemic-influenza-implementation.pdf

JPEO-CBRND (Joint Program Executive Office for Chemical, Biological, Radiological, and Nuclear Defense). (2021, August 6). We are JPEO. https://www.jpeocbrnd.osd.mil/

Kolata, G. (2021, April 8). Kati Kariko helped shield the world from the coronavirus. *New York Times*. https://www.nytimes.com/2021/04/08/health/coronavirus-mrna-kariko.html

Ledford, H. (2013, January 22). FDA approves recombinant flu vaccine. *Scientific American*. https://www.scientificamerican.com/article/fda-approves-recombinant-flu-vaccine/

Ledger, J. (2021, August 11). You've had a COVID "breakthrough infection"—can you really spread it to others? YaleMedicine. https://www.yalemedicine.org/news/covid-breakthrough-infection-transmission

Lovelace, B., Jr. (2021, July 23). Israel says Pfizer Covid vaccine is just 39% effective as delta spreads, but still prevents severe illness. CNBC. https://www.cnbc.com/2021/07/23/delta-variant-pfizer-covid-vaccine-39percent-effective-in-israel-prevents-severe-illness.html

Martson, H. D., Paules, C. I., & Fauci, A. S. (2017). The critical role of biomedical research in pandemic preparedness. *JAMA, 318*(18), 1757–58.

Miller, J. D. (2006, December 20). US cancels anthrax vaccine contract. *The Scientist*. https://www.the-scientist.com/daily-news/us-cancels-anthrax-vaccine-contract-46942

Our World in Data. (2021, August 6). Coronavirus (COVID-19) vaccinations. https://ourworldindata.org/covid-vaccinations

Slaoui, M., & Hepburn, M. (2020, October 29). Developing safe and effective COVID vaccines—Operation Warp Speed's strategy and approach. *New England Journal of Medicine, 383*, 1701–3. https://www.nejm.org/doi/full/10.1056/NEJMp2027405

Stowe, J., Andrews, N., Gower, C., Gallagher, E., Utsi, L., Simmons, R., . . . Bernal, J. L. (2021, July). Effectiveness of COVID vaccines against hospital admission with the Delta (B.1.617.2) variant. UK Health Security Agency. https://khub.net/web/phe-national/public-library/-/document_library/v2WsRK3ZlEig/view_file/479607329?_com_liferay_document_library_web_portlet_DLPortlet_INSTANCE_v2WsRK3ZlEig_redirect=https%3A%2F%2Fkhub.net%3A443%2Fweb%2Fphe-national%2Fpublic-library%2F-%

Tucker, E. (2020, March 19). What exactly is the Defense Production Act? *Military Times*. https://www.militarytimes.com/news/your-military/2020/03/19/what-exactly-is-the-defense-production-act/

US Department of Health and Human Services. (2020, March 17). Declaration under the Public Readiness and Emergency Preparedness Act for medical countermeasures against COVID-19. Accessed July 12, 2021. https://www.federalregister.gov/documents/2020/03/17/2020-05484/declaration-under-the-public-readiness-and-emergency-preparedness-act-for-medical-countermeasures

US Department of Health and Human Services, Administration for Strategic Preparedness and Response. (2004, July 24). Project BioShield overview. Medical Countermeasures.gov. https://www.medicalcountermeasures.gov/barda/cbrn/project-bioshield-overview/

US Department of Health and Human Services, Administration for Strategic Preparedness and Response. (2010, August). *The Public Health Emergency Medical Countermeasures Enterprise review: Transforming the enterprise to meet long-range national needs.* https://www.medicalcountermeasures.gov/media/1138/mcmreviewfinalcover-508.pdf

US Department of State. (2021, July 21). Digital press briefing on the U.S. donations of COVID-19 vaccines to the African union. https://www.state.gov/digital-press-briefing-on-the-u-s-donations-of-covid-19-vaccines-to-the-african-union/

US Embassy in Barbados, the Eastern Caribbean, and the OECS. (2021, February 18). The United States announces a US$4 billion contribution to a global vaccine initiative. https://bb.usembassy.gov/the-united-states-announces-a-us4-billion-contribution-to-a-global-vaccine-initiative/

VDH (Virginia Department of Health). (2021, August 16). COVID-19 cases by vaccination status. https://www.vdh.virginia.gov/coronavirus/covid-19-in-virginia/covid-19-cases-by-vaccination-status/

White House. (2021, June 10). FACT SHEET: President Biden announces historic vaccine donation: Half a billion Pfizer vaccines to the world's lowest-income nations. https://www.whitehouse.gov/briefing-room/statements-releases/2021/06/10/fact-sheet-president-biden-announces-historic-vaccine-donation-half-a-billion-pfizer-vaccines-to-the-worlds-lowest-income-nations/#:~:text=Today%2C%20President%20Biden%20will%20announ

PART 3

ECONOMIC IMPACTS OF COVID-19

CHAPTER 5

Economic Consequences of the COVID-19 Crisis

RAYMOND ROBERTSON, HUYEN PHAM,
ERNESTO AMARAL, AND SOUJIN WANG

Introduction: The Economic Magnitude of the Crisis

AS THE HIGHLY INFECTIOUS SARS-COV-2 (COVID-19) VIRUS SPREAD quickly through the world, different countries imposed different policies to control its spread. Figure 5.1 shows the spread of the virus by tracking monthly new cases in the United States, China, Germany, Sweden, and the world from the beginning of the crisis through the beginning of August 2020. The contrast between the US experience and that of the other countries (and the world) is striking. China, the first to be infected, quickly controlled the domestic spread of the virus through very aggressive (some have said draconian) policies that may not have worked in a free society. Germany and the United States experienced similar rises in cases in the middle of March 2020, but around the beginning of April, the trends sharply diverged. Germany's aggressive stay-in-place orders, testing, and tracking helped bring the spread under control. In the United States, the trend continued to rise through the beginning of April 2020 before it seemed to reverse in the second quarter. In the middle of June 2020, however, the number of new cases began to rise sharply. The increase in new cases continued into the beginning of July and then stabilized at a relatively high level. Sweden's model, discussed in more detail later, resulted in a path similar to that of the United States, but with important deviations in July 2020 and again in early 2021.

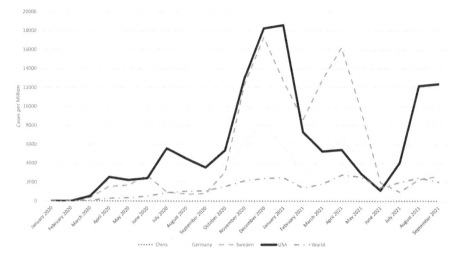

Figure 5.1. The United States stands out.

Nearly all sectors of the economy contracted because of this crisis. Stock prices fell sharply but recovered later in the summer. Various estimates put the economic contraction of gross domestic product in double digits. Global supply chains were significantly disrupted, spreading the problem across borders and into low-income countries that depend on exports for jobs and income. Possibly the most salient aspect of the situation, however, was in US labor markets. In particular, the effects fell unevenly across the US population. We document how the COVID-19 economic impact affected different groups and segments of the US population by presenting an original analysis and drawing on the explosion of academic analyses.

Academics and policymakers debate the degree to which the crisis was the result of policy (such as stay-in-place orders). We review the literature that seeks to estimate the degree to which the policy response contributed to the economic contraction. While it is probably too soon to claim that a consensus has emerged in the literature, the preponderance of evidence suggests that the policy response to the crisis explains less than half of its economic consequences.

A pandemic, by definition, sweeps across many countries. Economic integration through trade and global value chains contributes to the spread of economic effects across countries. Policy debate about disruptions in global value chains will have important implications for the structure of international trade and, we argue, for economic development in the world's poor countries. In this chapter, we review this debate and present recent research that explores the long-run implications of the economic crisis for global economic development.

Finally, zooming in on the United States, we address some of the less-discussed long-run concerns of the pandemic, including how it affected low-wage workers. To do this, we focus on the restaurant industry because restaurant-related occupations are the third largest occupational group in the US economy and have the lowest average wages. Finally, we offer some concluding thoughts and policy lessons.

Not a Typical Crisis

From a macroeconomic perspective, the COVID-19 crisis was very different from any of the four previous recessions. Reinhart and Reinhart (2020) described the "pandemic depression" and noted that the World Bank predicted that global output would fall 5.2 percent in 2020. The International Monetary Fund (IMF) reported that world output actually fell by 3.27 percent in 2020 (IMF, 2021). Baker et al. (2020a) argued that the reaction of the US stock market was stronger than in all previous disease outbreaks (including the 1918 flu). Alfaro et al. (2020b) found that the stock market reaction was oddly divergent from labor market indicators. Figure 5.2 shows the peaks and troughs of the unemployment rate during the last four recessions, demonstrating three key differences between the COVID-19 crisis and these four recessions. The most obvious is the striking increase in unemployment. The recession began with the sharpest increase in unemployment seen in the United States over the last 40 years.

The second key difference is the peak level of unemployment, which reached 14.7 percent in April 2020. Some economists such as Fairlie, Couch, and Xu (2020) adjusted for measurement concerns expressed by the US Bureau of Labor Statistics and estimated that the US unemployment rate could have been closer to 26.5 percent. Cajner et al. (2020)

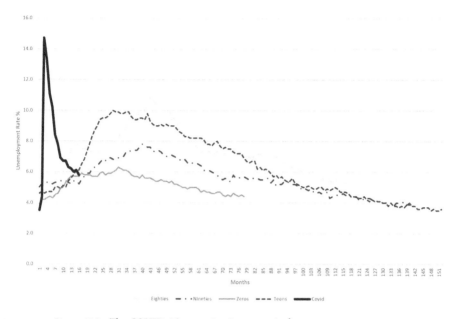

Figure 5.2. The COVID-19 recession is not typical.

used weekly payroll data to show that aggregate employment fell by 21 percent from February to near the end of April 2020 and that employers cut wages for nearly seven million workers. Figure 5.2 also shows that the previous post-Depression record of 10.8 percent unemployment was in November and December 1982. The global financial crisis had the next highest maximum unemployment rate, 10 percent, in September 2009. High unemployment is an important indicator of loss in economic output. Studies such as that by Ludvigson, Ma, and Ng (2020) have estimated that the loss of industrial production was as high as 20 percent.

The third key feature is that the unemployment rate began to fall much more quickly than in previous recessions. The sharp increase and fall seem more similar to unemployment rates observed after natural disasters like hurricanes or earthquakes, which come and go quickly (Ludvigson, Ma, and Ng 2020). The length of the line for each time span represents the number of months in which unemployment fell—in other words, the length of the economic expansion as measured by falling unemployment rates. Note that the longest expansion (by several months) was the 2009–2020 expansion, which lasted for over

100 months. The second longest expansion in the last 50 years was during the 1990s, which started from a peak unemployment of 7.8 percent in June 1992.

Unemployment across Demographic Groups

Differences in unemployment rates across demographic groups have been relatively stable across the last four business cycles. Figure 5.3 shows the average US monthly unemployment rates for white people, Black people, males, and females (patterns for Hispanics and Asian Americans are similar). In general, recessions result in higher unemployment rates for men. Unemployment rates of Black people are consistently higher than those of other groups. The changes in unemployment during the COVID-19 crisis are very hard to see in figure 5.3, which is a problem because these changes are very different from the changes in previous recessions.

To illustrate these changes more clearly, figure 5.4 shows the change in unemployment for several US demographic groups between March and April 2020. These changes are different from those of previous

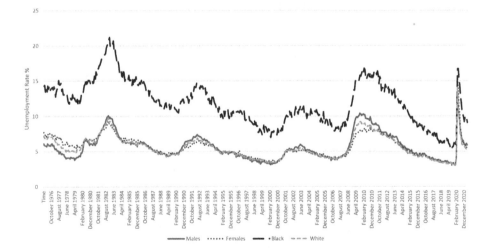

Figure 5.3. Unemployment rates by demographic group.

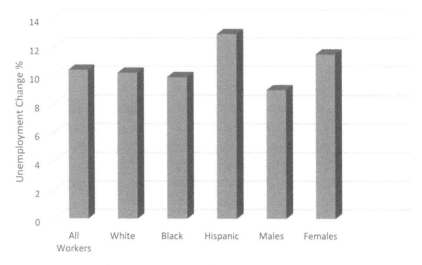

Figure 5.4. Unemployment change, March to April 2020.

recessions in several ways. For example, Fairlie, Couch, and Xu (2020) pointed out that unemployment for Black people increased less than expected based on previous recessions.

The change in unemployment rates hides the "churning" in the labor market, or the combination of hiring patterns and layoffs that generate the aggregate unemployment rate. Barrero, Bloom, and Davis (2020) found that there were just 3 new hires for every 10 layoffs in the first months of the pandemic. Using real-time data on job vacancies, which measure the number of jobs available for workers looking for jobs, Forsythe et al. (2020) estimated that between early March and late April 2020, job vacancies fell by over 40 percent and that almost all occupations and industries experienced a drop in job vacancies, but vacancies in the leisure and hospitality sectors fell the most. In particular, restaurant-related occupations help explain some of the different changes in unemployment rates across demographic and income groups. Analyzing weekly administrative payroll data, Cajner et al. (2020) found that worker recall explained much of the rebound, but nevertheless they agreed with studies using other datasets that found that losses were largest among low-wage workers.

On the other hand, Campello, Kankanhalli, and Muthukrishnan (2020) found that high-skilled job postings fell much more than low-skilled jobs within firms and that small firms were more affected than larger firms. In fact, they showed that small firms reduced job postings to nearly zero. Fairlie (2020) found that the number of business owners in the United States fell nearly 22 percent between February and April 2020. The loss of small, independent businesses (which are generally understood to be the engine of job growth) implied by Fairlie's (2020) results suggests that economic recovery will both be slow and require financing for business owners to restart. In a survey of more than 5,800 small businesses, Bartik et al. (2020a) found that nearly 43 percent of these businesses temporarily closed, and they reduced their workforce by 40 percent on average. Bartik et al. (2020b) showed that many of the small businesses that shed workers—especially those that were already unhealthy—closed entirely. Barrero, Bloom, and Davis (2020) estimated that 42 percent of the layoffs would result in permanent job loss.

To provide a sense of how the recovery began, figure 5.5 shows the change in unemployment rates after April 2020, when unemployment rates started to come down. The sharp decline in unemployment rates was not evenly shared across demographic groups. The rates for Hispanics, who had the highest increases in figure 5.4, fell the most, but African American unemployment rates fell the least between June and July 2020. The unemployment rate for women, which had risen the most between March and April, fell about twice as much as the unemployment rate for men. These differences may mask changes that happened at home during the crisis. Costoya et al. (2022) and Del Boca et al. (2020) found that women allocated more time toward unpaid ("home") activities during the pandemic. Thus, while the recovery was rapid for women, the situation laid bare some of the persistent underlying differences in the total work burden (paid and unpaid) between genders.

Figures 5.4 and 5.5 suggest that the labor market after COVID-19 might look very different in the future. Cheng et al. (2020) echoed this view, reporting that groups that had the highest April 2020 unemployment rates had the lowest reemployment rates during the months after April 2020. They also found that reemployment rates fell with the amount of time away from work. This finding has two implications. First, unemployment for some people may be long lasting. Second,

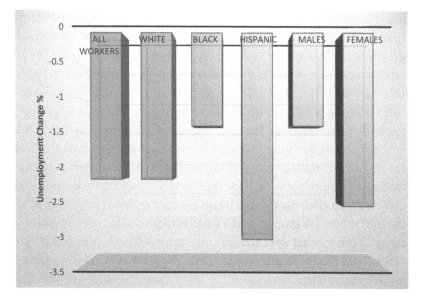

Figure 5.5. Unemployment change, April to June/July 2020.

many workers responded by simply dropping out of the labor force (i.e., increased the "discouraged worker" population). Cowan (2020), for example, documented a decline in labor force participation for workers who lost their jobs. Coibion, Gorodnichenko, and Weber (2020a) estimated that labor force participation fell by 7 percent, which was more than twice the decline observed between 2008 and 2016.

Additionally, older workers and immigrants seem to have been hit harder in 2020 than in 2009. Bui, Button, and Picciotti (2020) found that the effects of COVID-19 fell disproportionately on older workers, whose April unemployment rates reached 15.4 percent. Borjas and Cassidy (2020) found that COVID-19 reversed the pattern of employment differences between immigrants and natives. Prior to COVID-19, immigrant men in the United States had higher employment rates than native men, but this reversed in April 2020. Borjas and Cassidy also noted that undocumented workers experienced much higher rates of job loss than legal migrants.

Several papers about the economic impacts of COVID-19 focus on women. As figures 5.4 and 5.5 show, the effects of COVID-19 were different from those of the previous four business cycles because women's unemployment increased more than men's. Alon et al. (2020a) showed that women were particularly affected because they tend to work in restaurants, and school and day care closings increased the demand for childcare, which tends to fall on women. Alon et al. (2020b) optimistically argued, however, that changes in work flexibility and the increasing role of fathers in childcare (possibly spurred by COVID-19) might ultimately help increase gender equality in the labor market. It is also possible that the crisis simply cast into sharper relief the unequal burden of total work that women bear around the world.

One of the main themes of many 2020 COVID-19 studies is that job loss fell more heavily on workers who were not able to work remotely, and those workers, either voluntarily or because of available opportunities, tended to sort between jobs that did and did not allow remote work (Montenovo et al. 2020). Papanikolaou and Schmidt (2020) found that sectors with workers who were less able to work remotely were more likely to contract in employment, revenue, and stock performance. Dingel and Neiman (2020) estimated that only 37 percent of US jobs can be performed entirely at home, but these jobs pay more than other jobs and account for 46 percent of all US wages. In other words, jobs that can be performed at home tend to be higher-wage jobs. Studies that track movement, such as that of Mongey, Pilossoph, and Weinberg (2020), found that workers whose jobs were not conducive to working at home were less likely to actually stay home, and they experienced higher rates of job loss. Given that higher-income workers are more likely to have internet access, it becomes clear that low-wage workers bore a larger share of the economic burden of COVID-19.

Unemployment by Industry: US Restaurants Hit Especially Hard

US restaurants were especially affected by the pandemic. The effects on restaurant workers are important because they are the third largest occupational group in the United States, constituting 13.5 million workers in 2019 (BLS 2019). Restaurant workers have the lowest median and mean hourly wages and the lowest annual earnings of all major occupational groups. With its low barriers to entry, the industry attracts marginalized or vulnerable workers: the young, the low skilled, and immigrants.* Immigrants in particular are overrepresented in the restaurant industry, making up 17 percent of the total workforce but 21 percent of the restaurant industry workforce (Gelatt, 2020). In 2020, the restaurant industry lost $240 billion in sales and 3.1 million jobs, compared with 2019 (National Restaurant Association, n.d.).

Starting in the spring of 2021, our team conducted 19 in-depth interviews with restaurant owners and managers to help shape a nationally representative survey. The interviews focused on the implications of drastically reduced employment. As restaurants have reopened, employment structures and practices have shifted unexpectedly. The interviews suggest that the country experienced a "negative labor supply shock": fewer workers are applying for the available restaurant jobs, and even when applications are numerous, few workers accept jobs when offered. We also observed rising hourly wages, increased cross-training of employees (to do multiple jobs), steady employment of immigrant workers (even as employment of native-born workers dropped), and the increased use of delivery, "ghost kitchens," and technology, which require fewer front-of-house workers.

Results from our novel, yet preliminary, survey suggest that the record levels of unemployment in the restaurant industry were not shared equally across different occupations and differed between native and immigrant workers. We found that COVID-19 may have contributed to a hollowing out or job polarization within the restaurant industry, increasing the need for low-wage, back-of-house workers and for managers to supervise their work. The middle group of waitstaff, bartenders, and similar workers were most likely to have been laid off or furloughed. Because marginal workers, such as immigrants, are overrepresented in the restaurant industry and in those back-of-house jobs in particular, our preliminary study suggests that the demand for immigrant workers may have increased during this pandemic relative to native workers, even as the sector as a whole contracted.

---

* In contrast to native-born workers, immigrants have less access to safety-net programs (e.g., unemployment benefits, health care, and the $3 trillion in federal stimulus aid). Driven by economic necessity and lacking access to safety-net programs, immigrant workers tend to work in more dangerous settings (Orrenius & Zavodny, 2009) and for lower wages than native-born workers (Wright & Clibborn, 2019).

Among restaurants interviewed, one of the most common pandemic struggles was difficulty adapting to safety guidelines. These included local mandates such as restricted occupancy, mask requirements, and sanitation protocols, among others. Several restaurants interviewed reported that getting both staff and customers to adhere to mask requirements was challenging. Staff at one Texas location indicated that many men who entered the restaurant did not want to put on a mask, which the workers attributed to "cowboy culture," similar to a show of masculinity. Those at another location described difficulty in getting their chefs to wear masks, as they spent a lot of time in front of hot ovens or open flames, which made wearing a mask cumbersome.

Many restaurants interviewed complained about unemployment benefits, which were higher than their current employee wages. One reason for this phenomenon is that tips make up a significant portion of a restaurant worker's income, and tip income fell dramatically during the crisis and the early months of recovery. Several locations stated that they thought things "going back to normal" after the pandemic would bring in potential hires looking for work. Our survey results, however, suggest that restaurants continued to struggle to hire despite the rollbacks of safety guidelines in early 2021. Some suggested that workers may have realized that they were not getting paid enough at these restaurant jobs (especially without tip income), and that unemployment benefits may have been greater than wages without tips.

Changes in low-wage jobs following COVID-19 have at least four significant policy implications. First, the crisis cast into sharp relief the differences in time dedicated to non-labor-market activities ("home" activities) between men and women. The labor force implications of this reveal persistent differences that were exacerbated during the pandemic. Second, understanding the demand for low-income workers is important for anyone concerned about income inequality. The loss of restaurants and the shifts in employment across occupations affect the design of support programs for the unemployed. Third, understanding the shifts in demand for occupations and firms in which immigrants work helps shape our immigration policy, which has become increasingly restrictive. Fourth, understanding the changing demand that arises from a preference for natives—or the lack of this preference—is important for the national immigration debate. Our findings also raise questions about the unintended consequences of government COVID-19 relief funds; by excluding most immigrants, these funds may also be affecting labor markets by increasing the risk-taking behavior of immigrant workers and increasing their employability in pandemic times.

Was the Economic Impact a Result of Policy?

Was the economic contraction we saw during the pandemic, within the restaurant industry and other industries, caused by government stay-at-home policies? Within popular and policy debates, there seems to be an implicit belief that there has to be a trade-off between an adverse economic impact and lives saved. The same implicit belief can be found in academic studies as well (see, for example, Hall, Jones, and Klenow, 2020). In fact, one of the key questions debated among recent studies of the economic impact of COVID-19 is how much of it was the result of policies implemented to control the crisis. On the surface, such policies—including stay-at-home orders and the closure of "non-essential" businesses—seemed to be directly causing the economic contraction. Some studies that did not differentiate policies from the incidence of the virus alone (without lockdown policies) have concluded that lockdown policies greatly increased poverty. For example, Lustig et al. (2020) simulated the effects of lockdown in four Latin American countries and predicted large increases in poverty. When analyzing the stock market, Baker et al. (2020d) grouped government policies with other aspects of COVID-19. The question for policymakers, however, is how much of the economic contraction was a result of these policies and how much was a result of the virus itself. The emerging evidence from empirical economic studies may surprise most readers.

To answer this question, economists have taken several approaches. The central factor in identifying the role of policy, as in most contemporary economics, is the ability of researchers to find the kind of variation in the data that will allow them to identify a relationship between policy and outcomes that is not plausibly affected by other variables. To try to establish the link between policies and the economic impact of COVID-19, researchers have turned to differences both across and within countries and have tried to take advantage of differences in policy implementation across time and space.

One of the first questions asked to address this issue is, which policies reduce mobility? That is, how effective are government policies at reducing local travel? Governments implemented several policies aimed at reducing movement, including declaring a state of emergency, stay-at-home orders, school closings, and restrictions on social gatherings (including restaurants and entertainment). By tracking mobility with cell phone records, Cronin and Evans (2020) found that stay-in-place orders explained only a small part of the reduction in mobility but declaring a state of emergency had a large effect. Industry-specific restrictions, such as those on restaurants, also had a large effect on observed mobility, but private, self-regulating behavior explained more than three-fourths of traffic reductions for most businesses.

Most studies have found that government policies do not explain the rise in unemployment. Using differences across US states that implemented stay-at-home policies and those that did not, Lin and Meissner (2020) found that job losses were not higher in the states with stay-at-home policies. Rojas et al. (2020) showed that unemployment claims increased in all states and did not vary significantly in states that had different policies. Bartik et al. (2020b) analyzed employment data at the firm level and concluded that shelter-in-place orders contributed to only a small share of total job losses, at most. Using cell phone records that reflected visits to more than 2.25 million businesses in 110 different industries, Goolsbee and Syverson (2020) also concluded that government policies explained only 7 percent of the 60-percentage-point decline in overall consumer traffic because the decline in traffic started before the legal restrictions were put in place and consumers shifted from larger, busier stores to smaller stores. Forsythe et al. (2020) also concluded that the economic contraction was not the result of stay-at-home orders because these orders were not correlated with the contraction, and unemployment claims increased across both "essential" and other industries.

Of course, a consensus has not yet emerged. Baker et al. (2020c) found that contractions in consumer spending were associated with greater levels of social distancing, which were in turn linked to shelter-in-place orders that had been established by the end of March. Gupta et al. (2020) estimated that about 60 percent of the drop in employment was the result of state-mandated stay-in-place orders, and the remaining 40 percent was the result of the nationwide shock, but they admitted that they could not rule out the potential role of voluntary reductions in mobility that are described in other studies.

Evidence from other countries also suggests that stay-in-place orders may not have been driving the rise in unemployment. Korea, for example, did not have stay-in-place orders, but the emergence of COVID-19 cases was still associated with a drop in local employment of nearly 3 percent (Aum, Lee, and Shin 2020a). For Colombia, Alfaro, Becerra, and Eslava (2020a) suggested that the initial stages of the COVID-19 crisis put 50 percent of jobs at risk.

While not unanimous, these studies suggest that it was fear of the virus, more than government policies, that reduced mobility and contributed to rising unemployment. Would lifting these policies have contributed more to reducing unemployment? To answer this question, other studies have focused on the symmetry of the "reopening" policies. The simple answer is "no" because the policy effect of closing seems to be about the same in magnitude as that of opening (although reversed in sign). For example, using granular activity data, Chettey et al. (2020) found that when governments lifted the stay-in-place orders and other measures, local employment did not change very much.

Did Stay-in-Place Orders Reduce COVID-19 Cases?

Lin and Meissner (2020) found that stay-at-home policies were, at most, weakly related to local COVID-19 cases. Part of the reason the United States had more cases than many other countries and struggled to control the virus was that many people would not or could not accept the recommendations of health experts in particular or the scientific community more generally. Fan, Yeşim, and Turjeman (2020), in an original survey of 5,500 US adults, found significant heterogeneity across different groups (including along partisan lines) that correlated to mobility and other behaviors related to COVID-19. Pulejo and Querubín (2020) showed that incumbents who were likely to be running for reelection were less likely to vote for more stringent restrictions that they perceived would have a stronger economic impact. Comparing South Korea and the United Kingdom, however, Aum, Lee, and Shin (2020b) found that a longer lockdown would have reduced infections significantly. They suggested that if the United Kingdom had adopted South Korea's approach, it would have had a smaller outbreak. In the United States, Brown and Ravallion (2020) found that infection rates were higher in poor and unequal counties but suggested that these results may have been driven by racial composition and greater gains from social distancing in wealthier counties.

What About the Stimulus Policies?

The US government implemented both fiscal and monetary policies in response to the COVID-19 pandemic. Fiscal policies included the $483 billion Paycheck Protection Program (PPP) and Health Care Enhancement Act, the $2.3 trillion Coronavirus Aid, Relief, and Economic Security (CARES) Act, the $8.3 billion Coronavirus Preparedness and Response Supplemental Appropriations Act, and the $192 billion Families First Coronavirus Response Act. Monetary policies included a reduction of the federal funds rate to 0–0.25 basis points in March 2020, facilities to support credit flow, and other regulatory actions. The effects of these programs as a whole on the macroeconomy are still being estimated (and therefore were unknown at the time this chapter was written), but the sharp decrease in the unemployment rate suggests that these policies as a group may have cushioned the fall.

Various studies have estimated the effects of specific programs. Both Chetty et al. (2020) and Neilson, Humphries, and Ulyssea (2020) analyzed the effects of the Paycheck Protection Program loans. Chetty et al. (2020) found that these had, at most, small effects on small-business employment. Neilson, Humphries, and Ulyssea (2020) suggested that one possible reason for the relatively small observed effect was that the smallest businesses were not aware of the program and/or did not know how to apply. The smaller businesses that did apply faced longer processing times and had higher rejection rates. Furthermore, Granja et al. (2020) found very little evidence to suggest that funds flowed to higher-need areas. Instead, funds seemed to flow to the less-affected areas. The authors of all three of these studies agreed that the PPP, at least in the early stages, did very little to improve local economic outcomes. Guerrieri et al. (2020) took a step back and considered macroeconomic stimulus policies, such as Keynesian fiscal policies broadly, and monetary policy. They concluded that both were somewhat limited by the extent to which underlying consumer behavior was driven by the presence of the virus. As a result, the direct payments to households seem to have been effective in mitigating the adverse consequences of the crisis (Bachas et al. 2020), but the real solution rests in containing the virus. We discuss these policies and other options that show promise later in this chapter.

If Not Policy, Then What?

Figure 5.3 shows that the United States had been experiencing the longest expansion in over 40 years, but it also shows that business cycles are a regular feature of the US economy. Together, these points suggest that a recession of some form was imminent. The COVID-19 shock may have been the spark, rather than the lockdown policies. But what was it about COVID-19 that induced the rise in unemployment? Hassan et al. (2020) pointed to three specific links between the virus and economic contraction: falling consumer demand, rising uncertainty, and supply chain disruption. We will discuss each of these in turn.

The first link between the virus and the economic contraction was that consumers stopped spending in stores and chose to stay at home in the early stages of the spread of the virus. Analysis of US household-level bank account data shows that consumers significantly reallocated and reduced spending during the early weeks of the pandemic (Bachas et al. 2020). Coibion, Gorodnichenko, and Weber (2020b) showed that aggregate consumer spending dropped by about 31 percent. Baker et al. (2020c) also documented a strong contraction in overall consumer spending, using household financial data. Falling demand was closely linked to consumer perception of the infectiousness of the disease (Akesson et al. 2020), which implies that accurate information is critical for shaping the most appropriate behavioral responses.

The second link between the virus and economic contraction was rising uncertainty. Rising uncertainty affects both consumers and firms, but risk is often a dominating factor that firms consider when making investment decisions. It is very difficult to overstate the importance of mitigating risk to businesses, but risk is often difficult to measure. By combining stock market volatility, newspaper analysis, and business surveys, Altig et al. (2020) found that COVID-19 dramatically increased common measures of risk. Others, such as Baker et al. (2020b), carried out a similar exercise and estimated that about half of the expected contraction in US economic output was a result of the increased risk from COVID-19. COVID-19 is also likely to increase the perception of risk far into the future. Even with accurate current information, the large shock that the world suffered has increased consumer perceptions that another large shock is possible (Kozlowski, Veldkamp, and Venkateswaran, 2020). By definition, this increases the perception of risk.

The third link listed by Hassan et al. (2020) was supply chain disruption. Supply chains linking the US economy to the rest of the world and the global economic system after the pandemic are different than they were during 2000–2009. Trade conflicts between the United States and its main trading partners had begun to reshape global trade patterns prior to the COVID-19 crisis (Datamyne 2020). After the onset of the pandemic, protectionist sentiment grew worldwide, and there seems to be a great deal of sympathy for further restrictions on globalization (Razin, Sadka, and Schwemmer, 2020).

Since the 1990s, low-income countries have increased their exports of goods manufactured from parts and materials produced elsewhere in the world. The new production relationships resulting from these changes are now known as global supply chains (when focused on specific products) or global value chains (when the complete production chain is considered). The growth in supply chains increased US interdependence with its trading partners around the world. The 2020 *World Development Report* (World Bank, 2020) describes how value chains shape global trade and contribute to economic development—in low- and middle-income as well as high-income countries.

COVID-19 has complicated global value chains in three important ways. First, the reduction in demand in high-income countries has disrupted production in countries producing final goods. As the COVID-19 crisis hit the United States in March 2020, US retail sales fell 8.7 percent, the largest decline since 1992. Closing retail stores in the United States caused many sectors to contract, and apparel (clothing) was one of the hardest hit. Some (e.g., Perez & Devnath, 2020) described how the contraction in the apparel sector put millions of garment workers, already some of the lowest-wage manufacturing workers in the world, at risk of falling into abject poverty. Additionally, the World Bank predicted that COVID-19 could plunge as many as 60 million people into poverty (Reinhart & Reinhart, 2020).

Some countries bore more of the economic impact than others. In Bangladesh, for example, 89 percent of the country's exports are garments. These exports create opportunities for women in the formal sector, and the increased demand for women in this sector has been shown to be linked to rising wages for women throughout the country—not just in apparel (Robertson et al., 2020). Since women are key for economic development (ILO, 2017), the loss of these jobs puts economic development of some of the world's poorest countries at risk. During recovery, women came back to work, but the pandemic revealed that women on the margins of the workforce are both especially vulnerable and yet critical to many sectors of the economy.

In addition to the indirect development effects implied by the adverse effects on women, Ray and Subramanian (2020) argued that the economic cost in India of a lockdown policy put lives at risk because of the prevalence of extreme poverty (the Asian Development Bank estimated that in 2019, 10.7 percent of India's 400 million employed workers earned less than $1.90 per day in purchasing power parity). Bonadio et al. (2020) estimated that lifting lockdowns in the largest economies could increase GDP in smaller trade partners as much as 2.5 percent. Studies from other countries have highlighted the importance of international linkages. For example, Çakmaklı et al. (2020) showed that in Turkey, sectors with stronger input-output connections had larger losses from COVID-19.

The second way that COVID-19 complicates global value chains is by disrupting the supply of inputs. Bonadio et al. (2020) found that as much as 25 percent of the reduction in GDP expected from the crisis could be attributed to disruptions in that input supply. Ding et al. (2020) surveyed more than 6,000 firms across 56 countries and found that countries that were less exposed to the supply chain disruptions of COVID-19 had smaller drops in stock prices. Interestingly, they also noted that companies with more corporate social responsibility (CSR) programs were more likely to have smaller reductions in stock prices as well. CSR programs help companies engage with their in-country suppliers and may improve resilience through cooperative activities.

Balla-Elliott et al. (2020) surveyed US small businesses in 2020 and found that a large minority expected to delay their opening, mainly because of access to inputs (i.e., supply chain issues).

The third way that COVID-19 complicates global supply chains is in the subsequent policy response. COVID-19 cast the vulnerabilities of global economic integration into sharp relief. As a result, many nations, especially the United States, are actively exploring "reshoring" policies for sensitive and defense-related industries. Some researchers, including Campello, Kankanhalli, and Muthukrishnan (2020) and Bonadio et al. (2020), are skeptical of the increase in GDP that might come from reshoring because producing inputs domestically increases the risk of a domestic shock. As a result, policymakers and private sector actors will have to carefully evaluate the costs and benefits of reshoring.

So, What Does Work?

As noted earlier, the adverse economic impact of COVID-19 was driven by three key factors: falling consumer demand, a sharp increase in uncertainty, and disruptions of global supply chains. Some might question whether there is a role for government in this situation. Mainstream economic theory teaches us that government intervention is justified when externalities exist. That is, if the actions of individuals impose costs on others that are not easily measured or paid, then some coordination is necessary to help reduce these costs. COVID-19, in particular, is a clear example of a situation with negative externalities. Individuals who are, or may be, infectious impose costs on others by spreading the disease. As a result, the estimated private costs (the perceived costs to healthy individuals of getting sick themselves) are much lower than the costs to society of those same individuals infecting others. Bethune and Korinek (2020) applied this reasoning to estimate the difference in the private and public costs of COVID-19 infection and estimated that the private cost was about $80,000. In contrast, they estimated that the social cost was around $286,000. This large difference suggests that government coordination is justified. Eichenbaum, Rebelo, and Trabandt (2020) agreed, noting that the failure of individuals to consider the costs they impose on others justified government-led containment policies.

Of course, we have already discussed government policies that did not work. Several policy options other than PPP and local stay-in-place orders (broadly defined) have been evaluated in the academic literature. The main message from these studies is that the chief objective must be to contain the spread of the virus. Krueger, Uhlig, and Xie (2020) argued for the "Swedish solution," which allowed individuals to modify their behavior in ways that would both contain the crisis and minimize the adverse economic impact. Unfortunately, the previously discussed study by Fan, Yeşim, and Turjeman (2020) showed that in the United States this option would have come with significant loss of life.

As suggested earlier, direct payments to workers would help mitigate the drop in demand. The 2020 CARES Act did exactly that. Predictably, Baker et al. (2020d) found that lower-income houses responded most strongly to CARES Act payments, and much of this spending went to food rather than consumer durables.

The other key policy that seemed to work best was direct containment of the virus because this addressed falling consumer demand as well as the rise in uncertainty that was driving economic contraction. Berger, Herkenhoff, and Mongey (2020) demonstrated the effectiveness of testing, tracing, and targeted quarantine policies with a Susceptible-Exposed-Infectious-Recovered (SEIR) model. This model suggests that the economic costs in the United States could have been greatly mitigated with clear national leadership and targeted virus control.

Conclusion

The COVID-19 crisis has been unprecedented in terms of both lives lost and economic cost. The United States has not done as well as other countries. The range of policies implemented by federal and state governments have had mixed success because of a combination of factors. The preponderance of the literature suggests that the economic cost in the United States was not entirely, or even mostly, a result of the policies implemented. Instead, the virus changed spending behavior, increased uncertainty, and disrupted supply chains in wages to amplify the economic cost. The solution implied by the more than 80 studies reviewed in this chapter depends critically on controlling the spread of the virus. Masks, testing, and targeted quarantine policies seem to be especially effective. Although the United States continues to focus on the short-term costs of the crisis, the long-run implications may significantly affect how we work and the financial viability of the federal government.

Acknowledgments

The authors thank Brian Nakamura, Sharon Nakamura, Mark Robertson, Justin Bullock, Maija Robertson, and Christine Blackburn for helpful comments and support, and Ashley Beaudreau, Mary Jane Vickers, Areala Mendoza, Angelique Maes, Patricia Partida, Fizza Raza, and Laila Alvi for outstanding research assistance.

References

Akesson, J., Ashworth-Hayes, S., Hahn, R., Metcalfe, R., & Rasooly, I. (2020). Fatalism, beliefs, and behaviors during the COVID-19 pandemic. National Bureau of Economic Research Working Paper No. 27245. http://www.nber.org/papers/w27245

Alfaro, L., Becerra, O., & Eslava, M. (2020a). EMEs and COVID-19: Shutting down in a world of informal and tiny firms. National Bureau of Economic Research Working Paper No. 27360. http://www.nber.org/papers/w27360

Alfaro, L., Chari, A., Greenland, A., & Schott, P. (2020b). Aggregate and firm-level stock returns during pandemics, in real time. National Bureau of Economic Research Working Paper No. 26950. http://www.nber.org/papers/w26950

Alon, T., Doepke, M., Olmstead-Rumsey, J., & Tertilt, M. (2020a). This time it's different: The role of women's employment in a pandemic recession. National Bureau of Economic Research Working Paper No. 27660. http://www.nber.org/papers/w27660

Alon, T., Doepke, M., Olmstead-Rumsey, J., & Tertilt, M. (2020b). The impact of COVID-19 on gender equality. National Bureau of Economic Research Working Paper No. 26947. http://www.nber.org/papers/w26947

Altig, D., Baker, S., Barrero, J., Bloom, N., Bunn, P., Chen, S., . . . Thwaites, G. (2020). Economic uncertainty before and during the COVID-19 pandemic. National Bureau of Economic Research Working Paper No. 27418. http://www.nber.org/papers/w27418

Arellano, C., Bai, Y., & Mihalache, G. (2020). Deadly debt crises: COVID-19 in emerging markets. National Bureau of Economic Research Working Paper No. 27275. http://www.nber.org/papers/w27275

Aucejo, E., French, J., Araya, M., & Zafar, B. (2020). The impact of COVID-19 on student experiences and expectations: Evidence from a survey. National Bureau of Economic Research Working Paper No. 27392. http://www.nber.org/papers/w27392

Aum, S., Lee, S., & Shin, Y. (2020a). COVID-19 doesn't need lockdowns to destroy jobs: The effect of local outbreaks in Korea. National Bureau of Economic Research Working Paper No. 27264. http://www.nber.org/papers/w27264

Aum, S., Lee, S., & Shin, Y. (2020b). Inequality of fear and self-quarantine: Is there a trade-off between GDP and public health? National Bureau of Economic Research Working Paper No. 27100. http://www.nber.org/papers/w27100

Bachas, N., Ganong, P., Noel, P., Vavra, J., Wong, A., Farrell, D., & Greig, F. (2020). Initial impacts of the pandemic on consumer behavior: Evidence from linked income, spending, and savings data. National Bureau of Economic Research Working Paper No. 27617. http://www.nber.org/papers/w27617

Bacher-Hicks, A., Goodman, J., & Mulhern, C. (2020). Inequality in household adaptation to schooling shocks: Covid-induced online learning engagement in real time. National Bureau of Economic Research Working Paper No. 27555. http://www.nber.org/papers/w27555

Baker, S., Bloom, N., Davis, S., Kost, K., Sammon, M., & Viratyosin, T. (2020a). The unprecedented stock market impact of COVID-19. National Bureau of Economic Research Working Paper No. 26945. http://www.nber.org/papers/w26945

Baker, S., Bloom, N., Davis, S., & Terry, S. (2020b). COVID-induced economic uncertainty. National Bureau of Economic Research Working Paper No. 26983. http://www.nber.org/papers/w26983

Baker, S., Farrokhnia, R. A., Meyer, S., Pagel, M., & Yannelis, C. (2020c). How does household spending respond to an epidemic? Consumption during the 2020 COVID-19 pandemic. National Bureau of Economic Research Working Paper No. 26949. http://www.nber.org/papers/w26949

Baker, S., Farrokhnia, R. A., Meyer, S., Pagel, M., & Yannelis, C. (2020d). Income, liquidity, and the consumption response to the 2020 economic stimulus payments. National Bureau of Economic Research Working Paper No. 27097. http://www.nber.org/papers/w27097

Balla-Elliott, D., Cullen, Z., Glaeser, E., Luca, M., & Stanton, C. (2020). Business reopening decisions and demand forecasts during the COVID-19 pandemic. National Bureau of Economic Research Working Paper No. 27362. http://www.nber.org/papers/w27362

Barrero, J., Bloom, N., & Davis, S. (2020). COVID-19 is also a reallocation shock. National Bureau of Economic Research Working Paper No. 27137. http://www.nber.org/papers/w27137

Bartik, A., Bertrand, M., Cullen, Z., Glaeser, E., Luca, M., & Stanton, C. (2020a). How are small businesses adjusting to COVID-19? Early evidence from a survey. National Bureau of Economic Research Working Paper No. 26989. http://www.nber.org/papers/w26989

Bartik, A., Bertrand, M., Lin, F., Rothstein, J., & Unrath, M. (2020b). Measuring the labor market at the onset of the COVID-19 crisis. National Bureau of Economic Research Working Paper No. 27613. http://www.nber.org/papers/w27613

Berger, D., Herkenhoff, K., & Mongey, S. (2020). An SEIR infectious disease model with testing and conditional quarantine. National Bureau of Economic Research Working Paper No. 26901. http://www.nber.org/papers/w26901

Bethune, Z., & Korinek, A. (2020). Covid-19 infection externalities: Trading off lives vs. livelihoods. National Bureau of Economic Research Working Paper No. 27009. http://www.nber.org/papers/w27009

BLS (US Bureau of Labor Statistics). (2019) Occupational employment and wage statistics. https://www.bls.gov/oes/current/oes_nat.htm

Bonadio, B., Huo, Z., Levchenko, A., & Pandalai-Nayar, N. (2020). Global supply chains in the pandemic. National Bureau of Economic Research Working Paper No. 27224. http://www.nber.org/papers/w27224

Borjas, G., & Cassidy, H. (2020). The adverse effect of the COVID-19 labor market shock on immigrant employment. National Bureau of Economic Research Working Paper No. 27243. http://www.nber.org/papers/w27243

Brown, C., & Ravallion, M. (2020). Inequality and the coronavirus: Socioeconomic covariates of behavioral responses and viral outcomes across US counties. National Bureau of Economic Research Working Paper No. 27549. http://www.nber.org/papers/w27549

Bui, T., Button, P., & Picciotti, E. (2020). Early evidence on the impact of COVID-19 and the recession on older workers. National Bureau of Economic Research Working Paper No. 27448. http://www.nber.org/papers/w27448

Cajner, T., Crane, L., Decker, R., Grigsby, J., Hamins-Puertolas, A., Hurst, E., Kurz, C., & Yildirmaz, A. (2020). The U.S. labor market during the beginning of the pandemic recession. National Bureau of Economic Research Working Paper No. 27159. http://www.nber.org/papers/w27159

Çakmaklı, C., Demiralp, S., Kalemli-Özcan, S., Yesiltas, S., & Yildirim, M. (2020). COVID-19 and emerging markets: An epidemiological model with international production networks and capital flows. National Bureau of Economic Research Working Paper No. 27191. http://www.nber.org/papers/w27191

Campello, M., Kankanhalli, G., & Muthukrishnan, P. (2020). Corporate hiring under COVID-19: Labor market concentration, downskilling, and income inequality. National Bureau of Economic Research Working Paper No. 27208. http://www.nber.org/papers/w27208

Cheng, W., Carlin, P., Carroll, J., Gupta, S., Rojas, F., Montenovo, L., . . . Weinberg, B. (2020). Back to business and (re)employing workers? Labor market activity during state COVID-19 reopenings. National Bureau of Economic Research Working Paper No. 27419. http://www.nber.org/papers/w27419

Chernoff, A., & Warman, C. (2020). COVID-19 and implications for automation. National Bureau of Economic Research Working Paper No. 27249. http://www.nber.org/papers/w27249

Chetty, R., Friedman, J., Hendren, N., Stepner, M., & the Opportunity Insights Team (2020). How did COVID-19 and stabilization policies affect spending and employment? A new real-time economic tracker based on private sector data. National Bureau of Economic Research Working Paper No. 27431. http://www.nber.org/papers/w27431

Chiou, L., & Tucker, C. (2020). Social distancing, internet access, and inequality. National Bureau of Economic Research Working Paper No. 26982. http://www.nber.org/papers/w26982

Clemens, J., & Veuger, S. (2020). Implications of the Covid-19 pandemic for state government tax revenues. National Bureau of Economic Research Working Paper No. 27426. http://www.nber.org/papers/w27426

Coibion, O., Gorodnichenko, Y., & Weber, M. (2020a). Labor markets during the COVID-19 crisis: A preliminary view. National Bureau of Economic Research Working Paper No. 27017. http://www.nber.org/papers/w27017

Coibion, O., Gorodnichenko, Y., & Weber, M. (2020b). The cost of the Covid-19 crisis: Lockdowns, macroeconomic expectations, and consumer spending. National Bureau of Economic Research Working Paper No. 27141. http://www.nber.org/papers/w27141

Congressional Budget Office. (2018). Options for reducing the deficit: 2019 to 2028. https://www.cbo.gov/publication/54667

Costoya, V., Echeverría, L., & Edo, M. (2022). Gender gaps within couples: Evidence of time re-allocations during COVID-19 in Argentina. *Journal of Family and Economic Issues*, *43*, 213–26. https://doi.org/10.1007/s10834-021-09770-8

Cowan, B. (2020). Short-run effects of COVID-19 on U.S. worker transitions. National Bureau of Economic Research Working Paper No. 27315. http://www.nber.org/papers/w27315

Cronin, C., & Evans, W. (2020). Private precaution and public restrictions: What drives social distancing and industry foot traffic in the COVID-19 era? National Bureau of Economic Research Working Paper No. 27531. http://www.nber.org/papers/w27531

Datamyne. (2020, April 7). Covid-19: Global trade braces for epochal change. Descartes Datamyne blog. https://www.datamyne.com/blog/markets/covid-19-global-trade-braces-for-epochal-change/

Del Boca, D., Oggero, N., Profeta, P., and Rossi, M. (2020). Women's and men's work, housework and childcare, before and during COVID-19. *Review of Economics of the Household*, *18*, 1001–17. https://doi.org/10.1007/s11150-020-09502-1

Ding, W., Levine, R., Lin, C., & Xie, W. (2020). Corporate immunity to the COVID-19 pandemic. National Bureau of Economic Research Working Paper No. 27055. http://www.nber.org/papers/w27055

Dingel, J., & Neiman, B. (2020). How many jobs can be done at home? National Bureau of Economic Research Working Paper No. 26948. http://www.nber.org/papers/w26948

Eichenbaum, M., Rebelo, S., & Trabandt, M. (2020). The macroeconomics of epidemics. National Bureau of Economic Research Working Paper No. 26882. http://www.nber.org/papers/w26882

Fairlie, R. W. (2020). The impact of COVID-19 on small business owners: The first three months after social-distancing restrictions. National Bureau of Economic Research Working Paper No. 27462. http://www.nber.org/papers/w27462

Fairlie, R. W., Couch, K., & Xu, H. (2020). The impacts of COVID-19 on minority unemployment: First evidence from April 2020 CPS microdata. National Bureau of Economic Research Working Paper No. 27246. http://www.nber.org/papers/w27246

Fan, Y., Yeşim, A. Y., & Turjeman, D. (2020). Heterogeneous actions, beliefs, constraints and risk tolerance during the COVID-19 pandemic. National Bureau of Economic Research Working Paper No. 27211. http://www.nber.org/papers/w27211

Forsythe, E., Kahn, L., Lange, F., & Wiczer, D. (2020). Labor demand in the time of COVID-19: Evidence from vacancy postings and UI claims. National Bureau of Economic Research Working Paper No. 27061. http://www.nber.org/papers/w27061

Fukuyama, F. (2020, September/October). The pandemic and political order. *Foreign Affairs*. https://www.foreignaffairs.com/articles/world/2020-06-09/pandemic-and-political-order

Gelatt, Julia. (2020). Immigrant workers: Vital to the U.S. COVID-19 response, disproportionately vulnerable. Migration Policy Institute fact sheet. https://www.migrationpolicy.org/research/immigrant-workers-us-covid-19-response

Goolsbee, A., & Syverson, C. (2020). Fear, lockdown, and diversion: Comparing drivers of pandemic economic decline 2020. National Bureau of Economic Research Working Paper No. 27432. http://www.nber.org/papers/w27432

Granja, J., Makridis, C., Yannelis, C., & Zwick, E. (2020). Did the Paycheck Protection Program hit the target? National Bureau of Economic Research Working Paper No. 27095. http://www.nber.org/papers/w27095

Guerrieri, V., Lorenzoni, G., Straub, L., & Werning, I. (2020). Macroeconomic implications of COVID-19: Can negative supply shocks cause demand shortages? National Bureau of Economic Research Working Paper No. 26918. http://www.nber.org/papers/w26918

Gupta, S., Montenovo, L., Nguyen, T., Rojas, F., Schmutte, I., Simon, K., Weinberg, B., & Wing, C. (2020). Effects of social distancing policy on labor market outcomes. National Bureau of Economic Research Working Paper No. 27280. http://www.nber.org/papers/w27280

Hall, R., Jones, C., & Klenow, P. (2020). Trading off consumption and COVID-19 deaths. National Bureau of Economic Research Working Paper No. 27340. http://www.nber.org/papers/w27340

Hassan, T., Hollander, S., van Lent, L., & Tahoun, A. (2020). Firm-level exposure to epidemic diseases: Covid-19, SARS, and H1N1. National Bureau of Economic Research Working Paper No. 26971. http://www.nber.org/papers/w26971

Howell, S., Lerner, J., Nanda, R., & Townsend, R. (2020). Financial distancing: How venture capital follows the economy down and curtails innovation. National Bureau of Economic Research Working Paper No. 27150. http://www.nber.org/papers/w27150

ILO (International Labour Organization). (2017). *World Employment and Social Outlook: Trends for Women 2017*. https://www.ilo.org/global/research/global-reports/weso/trends-for-women2017/lang--en/index.htm

IMF (International Monetary Fund). (2021, April). World Economic Outlook Database. https://www.imf.org/en/Publications/WEO/weo-database/2021/April

Jorda, O., Singh, S., & Taylor, A. (2020). Longer-run economic consequences of pandemics. National Bureau of Economic Research Working Paper No. 26934. http://www.nber.org/papers/w26934

Kozlowski, J., Veldkamp, L., & Venkateswaran, V. (2020). Scarring body and mind: The long-term belief-scarring effects of COVID-19. National Bureau of Economic Research Working Paper No. 27439. http://www.nber.org/papers/w27439

Krueger, D., Uhlig, H., & Xie, T. (2020). Macroeconomic dynamics and reallocation in an epidemic. National Bureau of Economic Research Working Paper
No. 27047. http://www.nber.org/papers/w27047

Lin, Z., & Meissner, C. (2020). Health vs. wealth? Public health policies and the economy during Covid-19. National Bureau of Economic Research Working Paper
No. 27099. http://www.nber.org/papers/w27099

Ludvigson, S. C., Ma, S., & Ng, S. (2020). COVID-19 and the macroeconomic effects
of costly disasters. National Bureau of Economic Research Working Paper
No. 26987. http://www.nber.org/papers/w26987

Lustig, N., Martinez Pabon, V., Sanz, F., & Younger, S. D. (2020). The impact of
COVID-19 lockdowns and expanded social assistance on inequality, poverty
and mobility in Argentina, Brazil, Colombia and Mexico. ECINEQ, Society
for the Study of Economic Inequality Working Paper 2020 558. https://www
.cgdev.org/publication/impact-covid-19-lockdowns-and-expanded-social
-assistance-inequality-poverty-and-mobility

Mongey, S., Pilossoph, L., & Weinberg, A. (2020). Which workers bear the burden
of social distancing? National Bureau of Economic Research Working Paper
No. 27085. http://www.nber.org/papers/w27085

Montenovo, L., Jiang, X., Rojas, F., Schmutte, I., Simon, K., Weinberg, B., & Wing,
C. (2020). Determinant of disparities in Covid-19 job losses. National Bureau
of Economic Research Working Paper No. 27132. http://www.nber.org/papers/
w27132

Mulligan, C. (2020). Economic activity and the value of medical innovation during
a pandemic. National Bureau of Economic Research Working Paper No. 27060.
http://www.nber.org/papers/w27060

National Restaurant Association. (n.d.). Coronavirus information. Accessed
February 3, 2021. https://restaurant.org/research/restaurant-statistics/
restaurant-industry-facts-at-a-glance

Neilson, C., Humphries, J., & Ulyssea, G. (2020). Information frictions and access
to the Paycheck Protection Program. National Bureau of Economic Research
Working Paper No. 27624. http://www.nber.org/papers/w27624

Orrenius, P. M., & Zavodny, M. (2009). Tied to the business cycle: How immigrants
fare in good and bad economic times. Migration Policy Institute. https://www
.migrationpolicy.org/pubs/orrenius-Nov09.pdf

Papanikolaou, D., & Schmidt, L. (2020). Working remotely and the supply-side
impact of Covid-19. National Bureau of Economic Research Working Paper
No. 27330. http://www.nber.org/papers/w27330

Perez, M., & Devnath, A. (2020) Workers who make the world's clothes are facing
abject poverty. Bloomberg Business. https://www.bloomberg.com/news/articles/
2020-04-20/faded-desire-for-fashion-leaves-global-garment-workers-destitute

Pindyck, R. S. (2020). COVID-19 and the welfare effects of reducing contagion.
National Bureau of Economic Research Working Paper No. 27121. http://www
.nber.org/papers/w27121

Pulejo, M., & Querubín, P. (2020). Electoral concerns reduce restrictive measures
during the COVID-19 pandemic. National Bureau of Economic Research
Working Paper No. 27498. http://www.nber.org/papers/w27498

Ray, D., & Subramanian, S. (2020). India's lockdown: An interim report. National Bureau of Economic Research Working Paper No. 27282. http://www.nber.org/papers/w27282

Razin, A., Sadka, E., & Schwemmer, A. (2020). Deglobalization and social safety nets in post-Covid-19 era: Textbook macroeconomic analysis. National Bureau of Economic Research Working Paper No. 27239. http://www.nber.org/papers/w27239

Reinhart, C., & Reinhart, V. (2020, September/October). The pandemic depression. *Foreign Affairs*. https://www.foreignaffairs.com/articles/united-states/2020-08-06/coronavirus-depression-global-economy

Robertson, R., Kokas, D., Cardozo, D., & Lopez-Acevedo, G. (2020). Short and long-run labor market effects of developing country exports: Evidence from Bangladesh. Policy Research Working Paper WPS 9176. Washington, DC: World Bank Group. http://documents.worldbank.org/curated/en/545471583761343054/Short-and-Long-Run-Labor-Market-Effects-of-Developing-Country-Exports-Evidence-from-Bangladesh

Rojas, F., Jiang, X., Montenovo, L., Simon, K., Weiberg, B., & Wing, C. (2020). Is the cure worse than the problem itself? Immediate labor market effects of COVID-19 case rates and school closures in the U.S. National Bureau of Economic Research Working Paper No. 27127. http://www.nber.org/papers/w27127

World Bank (2020). *World Development Report 2020: Trading for Development in the Age of Global Value Chains*. Washington, DC: World Bank. https://www.worldbank.org/en/publication/wdr2020

Wright, C. F., and Clibborn, S. (2019). Migrant labour and low-quality work: A persistent relationship. *Journal of Industrial Relations*, 61(2), 157–75. https://doi.org/10.1177/0022185618824137

CHAPTER 6

COVID-19 Approach, Challenges, and Lessons Learned

The ExxonMobil Experience

MALICK DIARA, SUSAN NGUNJIRI,
CANDACE MCALESTER, DAMOLA ADESAKIN,
MOE FAZAIL, RICHARD GELATT, AND VICKI WELDON

Summary

PANDEMICS AND OTHER LARGE-SCALE GLOBAL HEALTH THREATS have the ability to significantly impact individuals, communities, public services, and country economies, as well as multinational corporations such as ExxonMobil. The human coronavirus disease 2019, or COVID-19, has affected people all over the world and was declared a public health emergency of international concern (PHEIC) by the World Health Organization (WHO) in January 2020 (WHO, 2020c). COVID-19 has the potential to affect the health, safety, and productivity of workers, in addition to a company's operations and reputation (Garrett, 2007). Considering the magnitude of these risks while knowing that no one sector can do it all, ExxonMobil committed to the early detection of such health threats, with adequate preparedness and swift responses triggered in coordination with stakeholders at the global and local levels.

The primordial responsibility of business leadership during a pandemic is to guide workers in maintaining good health while limiting the severity of business disruption. The optimal approach is built across and within public and private sectors in coordination with communities and other stakeholders for effective global pandemic preparedness and response, with local solutions (Diara et al., 2019, 2016,

2014, 2013). This approach should align with International Health Regulations (WHO, 2005) and country-level aspects assessed by joint external evaluations (JEEs) (GHSA, n.d.) where available in the context of the Global Health Security Agenda (White House, Office of the Press Secretary, 2015). The approach includes both preventive and mitigation measures established to minimize the impact of the disease on workers and company business. These measures should be based on the company's business continuity plans (BCPs) and infectious disease outbreak management program elements, with their implementation guided by emergency support groups (ESGs) established, as appropriate, at the global, regional, and country levels (Diara et al., 2019, 2016, 2014, 2013).

At ExxonMobil, experiences from past pandemics and outbreaks of severe acute respiratory syndrome (SARS), Middle East respiratory syndrome (MERS), and Ebola were instrumental in modeling a framework of preparedness and response (Diara et al., 2019, 2016, 2014, 2013). This framework is built on the safety culture of the company, structured as a "bow-tie safety" approach, using ESG concepts and tools.

Because COVID-19 was a novel disease, unprecedented challenges emerged. We applied safeguards used in prior coronavirus epidemics initially, while developing more knowledge about the nuances of SARS-CoV-2. Areas for clarification included determining the infectivity period, mechanisms of transmission, and viability of the virus in different environments. Safeguards such as social distancing and the use of masks arose as the science emerged for these important factors. In addition to disease prevention, the clinical aspects of COVID-19 were rapidly evolving, including improved understanding of the clinical manifestations, diagnosis, vaccination, and treatment. Given the knowledge gaps, the rapid pace of emerging science, and inconsistent health authority guidance across countries—and even within countries—effective information management and coordinated communication were critical to a successful response.

As the pandemic evolved, with disease waves occurring at different times within countries and across regions, we learned more about its transmission, and which measures to adopt for prevention and mitigation. The swift development and progressive rollout of vaccines further contributed to flattening the pandemic curve where implemented, with a progressive return to normal in areas with extensive vaccine coverage. As long as all people are not protected everywhere, however, the persistence of the pandemic and the emergence of variant viruses will remain a potential threat to the laboriously achieved results in the fight against COVID-19.

The four areas of focus for lessons learned are leadership, communication, medical-clinical capacity, and incident management. Among these aspects, the most critical are leadership and the ability to introduce new, effective, preventive pharmaceutical measures such as vaccines. At ExxonMobil, early and continued engagement between company executives and health and safety experts, combined with a collaborative framework for engaging public, private, and community stakeholders, continues to drive effective pandemic preparedness and response and successful mitigation, including the promotion and use of vaccines.

The Evolution of the COVID-19 Pandemic and ExxonMobil's Early Response

ExxonMobil's Early Response: A Timeline

ExxonMobil operates in more than 45 countries, and an important stance of the company is the health and safety of all personnel regardless of location, as well as those living in the communities where the company operates. ExxonMobil implemented incremental disease prevention and transmission risk mitigation to workers as soon as the first cases were reported in China. The company applied and globally communicated these preventive and mitigation safeguards in alignment with country health requirements. At the onset of cases in China, ExxonMobil's medical lead overseeing local operations liaised with the company's Infectious Disease Control unit to mount a swift and adapted response for personnel and business travelers in the region.

Because COVID-19 was a novel disease, significant knowledge gaps existed, but after daily reviews of scientific publications and meetings with external health experts at the headquarters and country levels, ExxonMobil initiated practical site guidance on infectious disease outbreak management at its sites in China (International Association of Oil & Gas Producers, 2016). A global travel health platform informed travelers about the features of COVID-19 and related restrictions. As the risk became better characterized and presented the potential for large-scale impact in the region, the company leveraged its pandemic flu framework to support business continuity planning in China and countries in the Asia-Pacific region. In the second half of January 2020, ExxonMobil established ESGs to implement the BCP.

By the end of January 2020, with close to 10,000 cases in China and just over 106 cases detected in 16 other countries (WHO, 2020a), ExxonMobil assembled regional representatives from each affiliate in the Asia-Pacific region for a coordinated response and established a corporate working group for global guidance. On February 29, 2020, the company activated its Europe, Africa, and Middle East ESGs, although country mechanisms were already in place (initiated by Italy, which was reporting over 800 cumulative cases by then).

On March 31, 2020, as the disease peaked in China and spread to Europe (400,000-plus cases) and the United States (180,000-plus cases, more than in any other single country), ExxonMobil activated the Americas ESG, in addition to business-line ESGs in manufacturing and upstream oil and gas, which have very specific operational needs. The timeline in figure 6.1 illustrates the progression of COVID-19 and the establishment of company ESGs in the first quarter of 2020.

As the pandemic continued, with expectations that it would prevail, ExxonMobil established a corporate data analytics team, which consolidated internal and external COVID-19 data collection, analysis, and reporting efforts to better understand, anticipate, adapt to, and communicate information company-wide. Related initiatives conducted by this team included using predictive modeling for community disease progression, immunity aspects, vaccine introduction, and the determination of quarantine duration before deployment to congregate settings with testing, among other key aspects of pandemic preventive and mitigation safeguards.

Support from the Medicine and Occupational Health (MOH) group to the data analytics team (beyond allocated members) included establishing strategic technical teams for continued surveillance and reporting, with internal or external interfaces as appropriate on specific COVID-19 health topics. Topics tracked by MOH included disease evolution, disease transmission, biological diagnostics and testing, vaccines, treatment, and workplace case management. As the

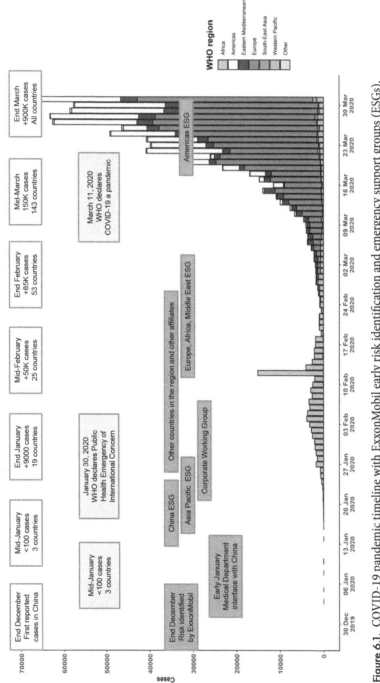

Figure 6.1. COVID-19 pandemic timeline with ExxonMobil early risk identification and emergency support groups (ESGs).

situation evolved, the MOH department continued to closely monitor such topics in order to anticipate and adapt recommendations to protect employees and the business, and to support surrounding communities where appropriate. Recommendations and guidance continued to align with those from the US Centers for Disease Control and Prevention, WHO, European Centre for Disease Prevention and Control, and other reputable authorities. Where health authorities had divergent opinions, we reviewed the science to help make an informed decision based on the evidence available at the time.

ExxonMobil's Approach to Pandemic Risk
Global Health Perspectives

During a pandemic, companies can help limit the impact of the disease on the economy and society by protecting the health and safety of their employees and the community (CDC, 2016). A functioning infrastructure is imperative during a pandemic, and sectors such as the oil and gas industry have a special responsibility to continue providing goods and services (US Department of Homeland Security Cybersecurity and Infrastructure Security Agency, 2020). ExxonMobil is considered a critical infrastructure organization with global locations and workers. The company's safety and health culture focuses on preventing workplace exposure to disease, swiftly supporting identified cases among workers, and assisting surrounding communities where feasible. Knowing that no one entity can do it all, the company approach is based on global multisectoral (public, private, community, and global health) and intrasectoral partnerships to establish effective local pandemic preparedness and response across its sites (WHO, 2020b).

The company's global multisectoral approach integrates International Health Regulations (IHRs) (WHO, 2005), which are governed by WHO, and the Global Health Security Agenda (GHSA, 2019). Both types of regulations have support from the worldwide public health community and constitute a global health policy framework for local application in countries.

The purpose and scope of the WHO IHRs are to "prevent, protect against, control and provide a public health response to the international spread of disease in ways commensurate with and restricted

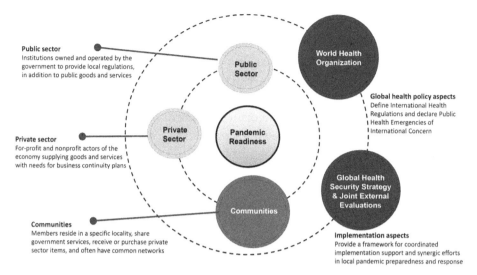

Public sector
Institutions owned and operated by the
government to provide local regulations,
in addition to public goods and services

Private sector
For-profit and nonprofit actors of the
economy supplying goods and services
with needs for business continuity plans

Communities
Members reside in a specific locality, share
government services, receive or purchase private
sector items, and often have common networks

World Health Organization

Global health policy aspects
Define International Health
Regulations and declare Public
Health Emergencies of
International Concern

Global Health Security Strategy & Joint External Evaluations

Implementation aspects
Provide a framework for coordinated
implementation support and synergic efforts
in local pandemic preparedness and response

Figure 6.2. How ExxonMobil perceives the roles of different stakeholders for effective pandemic readiness while considering global enablers (Diara et al., 2019).

to public health risks, and which avoid unnecessary interference with international traffic and trade" (WHO, 2005). The regulations constitute an instrument of international law, with legally binding aspects endorsed by 196 countries. Related rights and obligations include the following:

- The requirement to report public health events.
- Criteria for determining events that represent a PHEIC, such as WHO's declaration of the COVID-19 pandemic in January 2020 (WHO, 2020c).
- Establishing a national IHR focal point for communication with WHO to implement surveillance and response capacities at country entry points.
- Addressing international travel and transportation issues such as required health documents for international traffic.
- Protecting the rights of travelers and other persons regarding their personal data, informed consent, and nondiscrimination in the application of related regulations.

The Global Health Security Agenda has support tools for the IHRs to help countries and key stakeholders identify gaps in their pandemic preparedness and response. The main tool is JEEs (CDC, 2019), which evaluate 19 technical areas related to three objectives:

- Prevention and reduction of the likelihood of outbreaks and other public health risks and events.
- Early detection of unusual health events with a potential large-scale impact.
- A rapid and effective multisector response, including international mobilization (WHO, 2016).

JEEs help countries determine their readiness to manage infectious disease risks, as well as how to coordinate support for local pandemic preparedness while engaging the public and private sectors (WHO, n.d., Joint external evaluation; GHSA, n.d.; Diara et al., 2019). This process helps develop comprehensive local solutions, while enabling targeted partners' investments for effective pandemic preparedness and response with country stakeholders.

ExxonMobil adopted this international health policy framework and global country readiness concept into its site response and mitigation approach and tools, with calibration to the specifics of COVID-19 (fig. 6.2).

Local Site Prevention and Mitigation

Preparing for and responding to a pandemic is a continuous process of planning, exercising, revising, and translating global and local preparedness and response plans into action. The response to a pandemic must be evidence based if possible, and commensurate with the threat, in accordance with the IHRs (European Centre for Disease Prevention and Control, n.d.).

At ExxonMobil, the approach is coordinated by the ESGs, which decide what measures—defined over a decade ago in the company's pandemic flu BCP—to implement at what sites, considering the identified levels of disease risk. This plan has been enhanced by lessons learned during previous public health emergencies such as SARS, MERS, and Ebola.

The ESG is the essential multifunctional company mechanism established for the protection of people (workers, dependents, and the community); environment; assets; and reputation (PEAR). An ESG has structured principles and ingrained processes to manage emergency situations under the lead of company business-line executives, with assistance provided by operations and support organizations such as human resources; law; public and government affairs; and security, safety, health, and the environment.

The objectives of an ESG are to monitor the situation and offer guidance and advice to the business lines with a focus on these areas:

- **Corporate implications:** options for addressing the impact of the emergency and the broader corporate response.
- **Policy and guidelines:** evaluating and adjusting current policy and guidelines as necessary to enable an effective response.
- **Response resources and structure:** reviewing and confirming the adequacy of the management structure and overall resources associated with the emergency.
- **Internal and external communications overview:** a focal point for emergency-related activities and the assumption of responsibility for managing internal and external communications.

In response to the COVID-19 pandemic, ExxonMobil progressively activated ESGs at the country level, triggering the first one in China in January 2020. The company strategically coordinated country ESGs by region—the Americas; Europe, Africa, and the Middle East; and Asia-Pacific—while benefiting from general policy guidance formulated at the corporate level for local consideration and tactical implementation.

Beyond the activation of corporate ESGs, other implemented measures included the execution of the company's pandemic BCP (ExxonMobil, 2006), progressively adapted to evolving knowledge about the COVID-19 pandemic. The BCP is structured in phases, with escalation of preparedness and response measures commensurate with the potential disease impact on the PEAR, and defined triggers are periodically assessed for escalation or de-escalation.

Pandemic Phases and Triggers

ExxonMobil's pandemic flu phase considerations are based on the updated pandemic influenza model outlined in WHO's *Pandemic Influenza Risk Management* document (WHO, 2017) and existing plans adapted to aspects specific to COVID-19, as shown in figure 6.3.

For operational practicality at company sites, there were four phases in ExxonMobil's pandemic flu BCP adapted to COVID-19, instead of the six phases in WHO's *Pandemic Influenza Risk Management* document. The triggers considered for escalation include the following:

- Disease transmission: human to human, proximity to operations, and community spread.
- The number of identified cases of disease transmission in the workplace.
- The local health system's ability to deliver primary health care, manage inpatients, and perform advanced care.
- Local and international health travel restrictions for people and goods.
- The occurrence of local civil unrest or disruption of essential community services.

Although figure 6.3 was developed at the early stages of the pandemic, we modified its contents as we learned more about the disease and the effectiveness of preventive and mitigation measures.

For example, the de-escalation aspects evolved as we learned more about COVID-19 transmission and containment measures applied at the individual, environmental, and policy levels, including the potential results of the stringent application of containment measures by local governments in an attempt to reduce community transmission across countries and subgeographic areas.

The strategic approach for the de-escalation of preventive measures in company sites integrated two major aspects:

- Determine which measures to apply for each pandemic phase.
- Adopt practical and pertinent triggers to adequately define which risk levels and phases to consider, knowing that such

Figure 6.3. ExxonMobil COVID-19 phases.

	MONITORING PHASE	PREPARATION PHASE	
	Human to Human Transmission (HTHT) with New Coronavirus in the region but only rare cases of HTHT or sustained HTHT in remote isolated locations (No HTHT in the country)	HTHT with New Coronavirus in the <u>country</u> but only rare cases of HTHT or sustained HTHT in remote isolated locations and potential to impact EM operations	
WHO PHASES (PANDEMIC)	**PHASES 1, 2, & 3**		
CURRENT OUTBREAK CHARACTERISTICS AND TRIGGERS	Emerging or reemerging human viral infections that have potential for outbreak, severe health consequences, fatality, or operation disruption **AND** Confirmed cases of HTHT in any region **AND** NO/LOW potential to impact EM operations	Emerging or reemerging human viral infections that have potential for outbreak, severe health consequences, fatality, or operation disruption **AND** Confirmed limited cases of HTHT in the region **AND** No civil disruption **AND** No significant government/WHO restrictions **AND** Potential to impact EM operation	

HOT STANDBY PHASE	CRITICAL OPERATIONS PHASE	
Sustained HTHT New Coronavirus in the <u>country</u>; potential to impact EM operations; effective disease containment; potential for local civil unrest or government measures impacting EM operations	Sustained HTHT New Coronavirus in the <u>city/county/ district</u> where there are EM operations; potential failing disease containment has occurred with local threat; significant civil unrest or government restrictions	
PHASE 4	**PHASE 5**	**PHASE 6**
Sustained occurrence of new cases where HTHT has been confirmed in the country and in the city with surrounding area where EM operations are located **OR** 1 or more confirmed cases in workplace or company compound with limited HTHT in the city with surrounding area where EM operations are located **AND** Effective disease containment measures (case management, quarantine, health service delivery) **AND/OR** Potential or limited civil disruption **AND/OR** Potential or limited government/WHO restrictions **AND/OR** Significant influx of population in affected area/region (mass gatherings) with limited HTHT	Sustained occurrence of new cases with HTHT in city/county/district where there are EM operations **AND** Potential failing disease containment measures (case management, quarantine, health service delivery) **OR** Multiple confirmed new cases in the workplace, where sustained HTHT is ongoing within the local area **OR** Widespread local HTHT **AND/OR** Significant civil disruption **AND/OR** Significant government restrictions	

aspects can continue to evolve as more becomes known about the disease and the effectiveness of preventive and control measures.

The preventive measures considered for de-escalation included the following:

- Physical distancing for individuals.
- The use of face coverings.
- Temperature screening where pertinent, knowing its limited effectiveness.
- Facility adjustments, including signage and traffic flow.
- Enhanced cleaning measures.
- Behavioral expectations such as handwashing and staying home if unwell.
- Staffing levels for work sites.
- Restricting site access for visitors and employee travel.

For worksite de-escalation triggers to be used by local ESGs, we proposed recognizing these conditions:

- The vaccination coverage of the local community and of the worksite population, where in progress.
- Community transmission based on the average number of new case rates per one million in the past seven days in the area, and the test positivity rate when available and reliable.
- The ability of the local health system to manage routine and intensive health care services.
- The health authority requirements of the local government, considering security and civil unrest aspects.

Beyond the generic measures defined in the pandemic preparedness plans, ExxonMobil's approach was strengthened by the integration of Infectious Disease Outbreak Management (IDOM) program experience and tools. IDOM was originally designed for remote and offshore sites, with measures and processes built into company operations and safety systems. ExxonMobil provided the program to the oil and gas

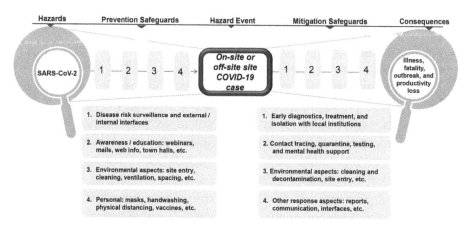

Figure 6.4. ExxonMobil health and safety bow tie for COVID-19 pandemic preparedness and response.

industry as guidelines through the International Association of Oil & Gas Producers/International Petroleum Industry Environmental Conservation Association (International Association of Oil & Gas Producers, 2016). The IDOM program has helped prevent disruptions to operations at platforms and camps since 2010 by helping to quickly detect and control outbreaks of measles, chicken pox, avian flu, and norovirus (Diara et al., 2014).

BCP measures and the integration of IDOM program experience and tools are also framed under what is known as the safety bow-tie concept, which is organized into prevention and mitigation safeguards to minimize the impacts of a pandemic on the health, safety, and security of workers, in addition to company operations and reputation, as indicated in figure 6.4.

Prevention safeguards are designed to limit the occurrence of cases in the workplace and their potential consequences. They are applied at different levels of stringency and intensity based on the phase of the pandemic and include these elements:

- **Hazard identification and disease surveillance** conducted at global, regional, and local levels to understand disease patterns and transmission features, and to anticipate the related risks and adjustment of measures in an informed manner, including for domestic or international business travel. Hazard identification and disease surveillance entails the analysis of international disease-specific scientific information from multiple reliable sources; meetings with external experts; and the establishment of a company-specific reporting system for cases and contacts among workers while consulting community case reports and prediction models.

- **Awareness and education** represents one of the most critical elements of effective workforce engagement at the global, regional, and local levels with the adoption of recommended behaviors. An example is the frequent dissemination of communications using multiple channels, with specific messages sent by defined entities or individuals. Emails, site TV screens, posters, internal websites, town hall meetings, videos, social platforms, and podcasts, when used along with "safety moments" (a brief safety talk about a specific subject at the beginning of a meeting or shift), can raise awareness and communicate with the intended audiences. Content includes information about disease features, trends, and risks, along with the company's approach and recommended or required measures to adopt at work and home based on the prevailing pandemic phase levels using established triggers. From a policy perspective, ExxonMobil already had flexible leave policies in place for its workers. Therefore, employees who were sick with COVID-19 or had contact with a positive case could stay home and where possible work from home, while benefits such as paid time off were made available to sick workers. Audiences include ESG members, key decision-makers including ExxonMobil senior executives, medical and safety personnel, employees, and contractors. The company also issues specific communications to expatriates and their dependents in their assigned location or upon return to their home country.
- **Personal preventive measures** are defined for individuals while at work. Initially, one very important element

promoted by ExxonMobil was advising employees to stay home when they had signs and symptoms compatible with the disease, or if they were identified as having been exposed to a positive case by local health authorities, with MOH review and supervisor engagement before returning to work. Other aspects included social distancing with coworkers, avoiding face-to-face meetings in favor of online meetings, wearing masks or face coverings while in common areas and public spaces, using sanitizers or washing hands with soap for 20 seconds, complying with travel restrictions as applicable and set by ExxonMobil or public health authorities, and avoiding ride sharing to and from work where possible. To support workers and holistically maintain their health for continued productivity, ExxonMobil developed or made more accessible a number of human resources programs and tools, including ergonomic support, telemedicine services, and stress management with mental health services for workers and dependents where applicable. The medical team is continually following up on both vaccines and treatments/chemoprophylaxis developments for use by personnel and dependents, as appropriate. As soon as promising results from COVID-19 vaccine clinical trials emerged, with promised availability by the fourth quarter of 2020, ExxonMobil initiated its workplace vaccination framework. This framework included external and internal policy aspects, supply-and-demand components combined with advocacy, and education to enable workers to make an informed personal decision on COVID-19 vaccines where available. Because vaccine availability would be limited to channels established by government institutions, the company encouraged all its sites across the globe to approach local public health institutions to anticipate vaccine access, prioritization, and the potential for on-site vaccine administration. That approach helped achieve significant global vaccination coverage among our workers. As part of local health authority vaccination campaigns, some of our clinics benefited from an allocation of doses for on-site administration.

- **Site preparedness:** Although the oil and gas sector is usually considered critical infrastructure, the company adjusted personnel levels on-site based on the phase of the pandemic, reducing staff to only critical workers or even shutting down when required by local authorities. In response to COVID-19, ExxonMobil implemented site entry screenings, limited visitor access, reduced or deferred travel, optimized air conditioning and ventilation according to industry standards, enhanced cleaning procedures for frequently touched surfaces, adjusted work and common areas to enable adequate social distancing, and discontinued part of the dine-in service and all self-service at cafeterias. Additional preparedness included identifying medical transportation services, facilities for isolation and quarantine, and locations to test and manage cases while complying with local health regulations and infection prevention and control precautions. For offshore sites and camps, ExxonMobil recommended a 14-day quarantine before deployment. Based on earlier experiences with measles, Ebola, and chicken pox, the MOH group knew that any case could easily spread to others and result in broader health consequences, in addition to a loss of productivity and even disrupted operations, with potential business and reputational damage. In congregate settings with a high risk of secondary transmission and a critical need for business continuity, predeployment measures included a quarantine period coupled with a defined testing regimen when COVID-19 diagnostic methods became more broadly available. The introduction of COVID-19 testing helped with early identification of cases while reducing the risk of outbreaks. Subsequently, using a model estimating the disease and transmission risks with different quarantine durations and testing periodicities, we were able to reduce the quarantine period from 14 to 7 days when combined with serial testing. The subsequent introduction of COVID-19 vaccines and extensive coverage among such workers enabled a further reduction in the number of days in quarantine, down to zero days for locations with very high vaccination rates.

- **Mitigation safeguards** are designed to adequately manage identified cases in the workplace and mitigate the potential impact on employees and contractors, operations, and company business, in coordination with identified health and transportation providers of goods and services while complying with local health regulations. ExxonMobil's mitigation safeguards also embraced community investments and coordinated efforts with other oil and gas companies to support the local health system and civil society organizations, including these elements:

  - **Early diagnosis and treatment** represents a key element of mitigation safeguards and includes asking employees not to come to work when they feel sick or have a fever and to report suspected or confirmed cases to their MOH group contact. ExxonMobil's approach is to have medical and testing services performed in the community while covered by the company or local public health system. For operations in remote areas or where the quality or availability of health services is limited, ExxonMobil supports local health providers with identified supplies for diagnosis and treatment, working with other oil and gas partners as much as possible.

  - **Isolation and contact tracing** are two aspects of case management. Isolation and quarantine capabilities are established internally or externally, depending on the type and location of company sites. ExxonMobil's approach to contact tracing is based on the prevailing disease knowledge obtained from health institutions and initiated locally by ExxonMobil health and safety teams as soon a case is suspected, even before receiving test results. Compliance with local health regulations and coordination with health authorities follows, especially when identifying contacts and instituting and respecting quarantine measures.

  - **Environmental measures** are deployed in the event of a suspected or identified case, with cleaning and decontamination of the employee's work area and any shared spaces that he or she would have used a couple of days before diagnosis. Depending on the type of operation, the company may reduce the on-site employee population or on-site services and perform enhanced disinfection of common areas.

- **Other response measures** include connecting with local health authorities and public health experts to stay informed about the progression of the disease; learning what community measures are in place; and learning what to consider for site preparedness and response, taking into account the local health capabilities and the potential need for community investments that will optimize the ability to prevent and control the impact of the disease. ExxonMobil also encourages coordinated efforts with other oil and gas companies and the private sector where possible and pertinent. Community investments included reconfiguring manufacturing operations to produce and donate medical-grade hand sanitizer to health care providers, first responders, and schools (ExxonMobil, 2020c); applying company knowledge and experience with polymer-based technologies to facilitate the development and third-party production of innovative safety equipment that could be sterilized and worn multiple times (ExxonMobil, 2020a); and donating funds, time, meals, or supplies to charitable organizations that supported communities during the COVID-19 pandemic (ExxonMobil, 2020b).

Challenges versus Implementation Approach

The COVID-19 pandemic has been referred to by WHO as "the defining global health crisis of our time." The evolving pandemic exposed vulnerabilities in global public health but at the same time identified opportunities and solutions that will be useful for future pandemics. The severity and magnitude of the effects of COVID-19 on individuals, families, countries, and economies highlight the reality that we still have a number of challenges in implementing prevention and mitigation safeguards. Although such measures were established, opportunities to evolve more efficient processes were revealed.

Deep-seated policy differences that can exacerbate health and economic incongruities have made it clear that leadership in both the private and public sectors is key to the successful mitigation of outbreaks, especially those with pandemic potential. It is possible to find sources of inspiration from frontline workers, public health officials, and collaborating industries around the world that have all successfully flattened the curve.

With the introduction of COVID vaccines, the experiences to date suggest that successful implementation needs effective leadership and advocacy, with adequate supply to enable equitable distribution; leveraging technology for mobilization, education, and recording of vaccines; and robust monitoring for early identification of adverse events and confirmation of vaccine effectiveness.

With the overall goal to prevent disease and transmission risk among personnel while understanding the global nature of its workforce and varied workplace settings, ExxonMobil encountered challenges related to the effectiveness of its pandemic preparedness and response in four areas: leadership, communication, medical-clinical capacity, and incident management. We will explore these challenges further, while looking at possible solutions and opportunities in accompanying tables.

Leadership

Leadership in a crisis situation maximizes the ability of employees to continue working effectively by providing guidance and spearheading prevention and containment while strategizing resilience and recovery. These efforts are designed not only to keep the employee population healthy but also to minimize disruptions and keep the business going. Key leadership skills include adaptability, empathy, resilience, and relationship management, which are similar to the skills needed in other crisis situations. Key leadership challenges and opportunities are outlined in table 6.1.

Table 6.1. Leadership challenges.

LEADERSHIP CHALLENGES	SOLUTIONS/OPPORTUNITIES
Global leadership challenges outside the company, with limited synergies among countries for optimal containment	Reestablish an influential global health alliance supporting WHO to provide a consensual global technical response, a vaccination strategy, and guidance to countries with aligned efforts and synergic investments, including the adoption of best practices by communities with public and private sectors.
Different company operation types and specific local related leadership perspectives	In a globally integrated oil and gas company, with operations ranging from remote offshore drilling to refining and chemical manufacturing, and with fuel distribution and retail operations, decision-making by leaders may entail different safeguards for different operations. There may also be delays when establishing different mitigation measures across different operations, as all operations are not the same and need a tailored approach. While minimal measures during the COVID-19 pandemic were established by phase, triggers based on critical operations need further risk assessment and management consideration to enable their implementation. One example was deciding to quarantine and test personnel before deployment at operations with offshore or camp locations, while not applying such measures to office-based operations. Drills are also important to allow different operations to identify and mitigate gaps.

Communication

Communication about prevention, containment, treatment, and recovery should occur in phases rather than all at once, and such communications should vary based on the audience. Communication strategies must consider what to communicate to individuals and how; whether specific responses are required; and if so, how to respond effectively. The need for data privacy makes tracking, tracing, and containing the spread of COVID-19 an unprecedented challenge, especially for a global company. A pragmatic and contextual approach that is fit for risk is necessary while respecting fundamental data protection and privacy principles. Communication challenges and opportunities are outlined in table 6.2.

Table 6.2. Communication challenges.

COMMUNICATION CHALLENGES	SOLUTIONS/OPPORTUNITIES
Changing knowledge about the disease with prevailing knowledge gaps	Organize teams able to address knowledge management aspects through continued scientific surveillance and monitoring of external and internal case trends at the headquarters, regional, and country levels. Key disease information includes transmission, symptoms, safeguards, vaccines, treatment, and containment, with the ability to review internal technical guidance documents as knowledge about the disease evolves, and with appropriate communications and management-of-change processes using multiple media and technologies.
Communication dissemination— challenges in reaching all audiences effectively	Effectively use digital platforms and technology to provide targeted and periodic awareness to medical, safety, response, and business-line audiences. With so many unknowns, the COVID-19 pandemic resulted in "infodemics," including rumors and stigma messaging. Monitoring social media data and creating frequently asked questions with myth-busting sections are essential to tracking and addressing misinformation. Communication is also key in optimizing vaccine uptake as a tool to manage complex vaccine hesitancy, focusing on safety and effectiveness while addressing how various audiences process information.
Data privacy constraints for case reporting and contact tracing management	As company sites across countries reported suspected or confirmed cases, it became challenging to maintain a global perspective on the emergence of risk. It is important to engage data-privacy experts and the legal team to address compliance aspects when communicating with affected workers right at the start of the global reporting system. Considering data privacy at the onset ensures the collection of only correct and necessary information, and its appropriate storage in accordance with global data-privacy laws. Recording vaccinations is also key when considering data-privacy requirements, especially as countries resume travel or de-escalation processes.
Pandemic impact on health and work-life balance	The effects of a pandemic include mental and physical health effects, school closures, changes in work situations, limited movement, and economic downturns. To help individuals adjust to their individual situation, it is important to provide and communicate offerings of resiliency and mental health resources, including ergonomic support and assistance with immediate as well as long-term or chronic crisis situations.

Medical-Clinical Capacity (Maintaining Ongoing Medical Services and Periodic Occupational Evaluations)

Medical-clinical systems needed to adjust how they reviewed and cared for patients, especially for preventive aspects, as fewer in-person visits were occurring in favor of virtual consultations. Other changes included the introduction of vaccines and available treatments, the need to reduce staff presence on-site (especially when there was limited personal protective equipment [PPE]), and the challenge of minimizing surges with a limited staff. One challenge was testing gaps for both asymptomatic and symptomatic cases. (table 6.3)

Table 6.3. Medical challenges.

MEDICAL CHALLENGES	SOLUTIONS/OPPORTUNITIES
Knowledge gaps in virus characteristics	Review knowledge and literature on virus characteristics, including the viability of the virus on surfaces. Apply caution when implementing preventive measures with respect to the life cycle of the virus and predictive capabilities.
Lack of effective and readily available treatments earlier in the pandemic and a limited supply of new products	Early on, not having medical preventive measures and specific treatments limited the means to adequately tackle the transmission of COVID-19 and its health impact on affected individuals. Adopted solutions were related to the extensive use of all available and proven methods for prevention, such as social distancing, mask wearing, and handwashing, while swiftly referring suspected and confirmed cases to competent medical providers. Concurrently, it was important to conduct and share surveillance on existing and approved treatments as applicable.

After intensive research efforts by the pharmaceutical industry, some promising medications were introduced in the health sector to aid in the treatment of severe cases. Emergency use authorization allowed convalescent plasma to be among the first medications used initially in patients hospitalized with COVID-19. However, clinical evidence of its effectiveness was limited. This was followed by monoclonal |

Table 6.3. *continued*

MEDICAL CHALLENGES	SOLUTIONS/OPPORTUNITIES
	antibodies and antivirals such as Paxlovid and Remdesivir. Other treatments included symptomatic therapies such as corticosteroids and Tocilizumab, an immunomodulatory agent. Their initial utilization was not extensive because of their limited availability across the globe. Administration methods included infusions with limited outpatient options; patients infected with certain variants did not respond as well; and some medications had extensive drug interactions, with high-cost issues. Solutions to challenges included broader information review and awareness for community prescribers and the general population on medication effectiveness, key properties, and availability. Locations prescribing medication or having direct patient interaction were tasked with establishing a provider relationship with interprofessional health care teams for expanded use of these available treatment options and improved outcomes for patients. In operational locations where urgent care capabilities were limited, we partnered with other oil and gas companies and local health authorities to set up COVID-19 treatment units for workers and dependents while supporting local communities and health systems in the fight against the pandemic.
Introduction of COVID-19 vaccines	Introducing a new vaccine is a multifaceted process that requires detailed planning and coordination. The key drivers that guided COVID-19 vaccine policies, approvals, and availability included strong evidence and leadership oriented in support of vaccines and immunization, at both the international and national levels. Vaccine forecasting should happen early, with orders placed well in advance. It is also essential to plan staffing and administration locations whether you have an internal or third-party provider in the community, while factoring in medical consumables before the campaign. Offering schedules for administration depending on vaccine type, supply, and demand was a critical lesson in managing COVID-19 vaccines.

Table 6.3. *continued*

MEDICAL CHALLENGES	SOLUTIONS/OPPORTUNITIES
	Data collection tools that enabled updated metrics about vaccine coverage represented another important aspect.
	As COVID-19 vaccines were limited in quantities at the time of their introduction, we strongly recommended to our workers that they get vaccinated at sites established in their communities by local health authorities. Concurrently and where appropriate, we interfaced with government institutions for vaccine allocation and on-site administration. Besides efforts to tackle the logistical challenges of the vaccine's initial rollout, we conducted extensive awareness and education campaigns to minimize vaccine hesitancy and misinformation. These were spearheaded by our company health, safety, and business leaders, with several sessions organized with world-renowned infectious disease and vaccine experts.
	As vaccines became more extensively and globally available, we required vaccination for defined types of workers such as those assigned to offshore and camp sites or travelers going to locations where the local health system would have limited advanced health care services. Such a comprehensive approach helped achieve significant vaccination coverage across our global workforce and optimized worker protection against COVID-19 infection and severe episodes.
Testing gaps and knowledge	Testing availability was a challenge across ExxonMobil operations and was progressively addressed as the company identified and engaged more products and providers for related services. One solution entailed reviewing the availability of existing testing methods including polymerase chain reaction or nucleic acid amplification and immunoassay blood tests, along with antibody or serology testing, to determine their reliability and quality. Different tests presented a number of limitations related to their specificity and sensitivity, and how to adequately interpret their results for proper management of cases and their contacts.

Table 6.3. *continued*

MEDICAL CHALLENGES	SOLUTIONS/OPPORTUNITIES
Limited critical care capacity	Limited medical capacity has been a global experience during the COVID-19 pandemic. One of the most effective measures to overcome this challenge was to establish field or secondary hospitals to care for mildly ill patients, and lockdowns to limit infections and allow medical facilities to cope with demand. In one of our locations with limited capabilities for advanced care, ExxonMobil partnered with other oil and gas companies to set up a treatment facility to serve workers and their dependents in coordination with local health authorities.
Travel and telehealth	In the initial phase of a pandemic, it may be prudent to apply more stringent travel and entry restrictions for at-risk sites. After developing the appropriate platforms, migrate the medical staff to various telehealth tools, including electronic information and telecommunication technologies to support and promote long-distance clinical health care, mental education, and public health. The goal is for workers and travelers to interact seamlessly with care providers and make decisions regarding travel.
Prevent outbreaks and operational disruptions while addressing mental health risks at sites with congregate settings such as platforms and camps	During the COVID-19 pandemic, workers continued to be deployed to enable business continuity in areas that could not slow down or shut off. Establishing predeployment procedures with quarantining and testing maintained the health of workers and site operations. The extended duration of assignments with uncertainties related to the pandemic could, however, impact personnel mental health. In order to address such challenges, and as part of company benefits, ExxonMobil made support services for employees and dependents widely available, with extensive communication across locations. As vaccine availability and coverage became more extensive, quarantines before deployment were progressively removed.

Take-Home Message

ExxonMobil would like to share lessons learned from present and past experiences with other private-sector companies so that they can effectively prepare for and respond to pandemics and other large-scale outbreaks. These lessons include the following aspects:

- **Establishing strong public- and private-sector synergies with communities.** It is key to have concerted efforts across and within sectors for effective preparedness and response at the local level, while supporting communities in adopting appropriate behaviors.
- **Monitoring infectious disease threats with a centralized system for early warning across the organization.** Monitoring infectious disease threats at the community and workplace levels through internal and external sources—both to and from country organizations in coordination with a central sharing mechanism—is essential for a swift and effective pandemic response.
- **Engaging at all levels of the corporation.** Obtaining executive-level engagement is excellent but not sufficient; each business line and its administrative chain of command needs to be proactively informed and mobilized at the headquarters, region, country, and site levels for agreement with and implementation of the necessary preventive and mitigation safeguards.
- **Considering local health system capabilities and support for worksite plans.** Taking into account compliance with local health regulations when developing worksite plans is critical. In addition, local investments may be needed for testing and case management, including contact tracing with proper infection control in countries with weaker public health systems.
- **Promoting the use of vaccines, the best preventive measure, wherever safe, effective, and able to prevent or mitigate outbreaks at operational sites.** As SARS-CoV-2 and its variants continue to prevail across the world, vaccines are the most effective and cost-efficient way to eliminate the COVID-19 threat to global public health, particularly with

Table 6.4. Incident management challenges.

INCIDENT MANAGEMENT CHALLENGES	SOLUTIONS/OPPORTUNITIES
Decisions on adequate facility management: workplace setting and staffing levels	It is key to define facility-management practices that can reduce exposure to or transmission of diseases while at work. The solution to this challenge involved risk assessment to review site entry controls, including temperature checks, symptom screenings, de-densification of sites to include social distancing, the use of PPE, and enhanced cleaning and disinfection practices. There should also be a process to manage the admittance of individuals who may be at higher risk of contracting the disease and allow for additional safeguards that may include working from home.
Effective case-management contact tracing and reporting	Establish on-site protocols to identify and manage cases early, including contact tracing. Leverage external partners, governments, private facilities, and technology where practical for additional resources.

the emergence of virulent variants that can evade immunity and be treatment resistant.

- **Using internal and external systems and interfaces for site preparedness and response.** Established internal systems like ESGs with global, regional, and site interfaces facilitated the methodical rollout of pandemic preparedness and response measures at ExxonMobil. For COVID-19, the company strategically linked its internal approach to external systems for disease surveillance, including understanding the characteristics of the virus; detecting, testing, and managing cases; transporting infected cases when necessary; quarantining contacts; and overseeing workers' release with reports to local health authorities when appropriate.
- **Engaging external experts for adequate workplace disease prevention and control.** In addition to in-house public health

experts and medical professionals, for the COVID-19 pandemic ExxonMobil met with external health experts at the global and local levels to confirm disease features, risks, and evolution; to review the appropriateness of applied workplace measures; and to integrate new tools or approaches identified as pertinent to its sites.

- **Anticipating and adapting to COVID-19 vaccine availability.** Vaccinating our workers was a pivotal strategy in battling this historic pandemic. Understanding the multifaceted complexities of global vaccine administration necessitated a strategic, agile process while following a vaccination framework that supported evidence-based and consistent decisions.
- **Communicating often with intended audiences through multiple channels.** Effective risk communication is critical for a composed and continuously productive workforce, engaged business-line executives, supportive first-line supervisors, and competent clinical staff services. Clear, simple, and on-point communications repeatedly issued throughout multiple channels and targeted to specific audiences help reduce knowledge gaps and increase the adoption of recommended practices.
- **Conducting drills, which are the best way to verify preparedness and response capabilities.** Although checklists represent a practical way to verify the necessary elements for effective pandemic preparedness and response, nothing is better than running a real drill on-site to identify potential gaps and allow internal and external stakeholders to work with each other.
- **Applying a global approach with local solutions.** Local regulations differ from one country to another, and workers and communities are also different from location to location. Therefore, it is important to have a global approach with a set of minimum requirements to consider, while being able to tailor them to specific operational needs. Good examples include triggers for preparedness and response phase escalation and de-escalation, the implementation of social distancing, the use of face masks, site entry requirements, travel restrictions, and return-to-work protocols.

Conclusion: Looking Forward

Because the world has metaphorically grown smaller as a result of the volume of international travel, any infectious disease can reach any part of the world within one or two flights, with the potential to spread widely. No one country is immune to a virulent infectious disease, even if it emerged from a country on the other side of the world. No industry or company can adequately address these issues on its own. Therefore, it becomes even more crucial to reestablish an effective global health coalition supporting WHO across sectors, countries, and communities while strengthening local health systems.

Such a coalition will be the only way to avoid a recurrence of the extensive health, economic, and societal impacts of the COVID-19 pandemic. It will also be the best way to further address the pandemic test; treat remaining needs across countries; and, most importantly, equitably distribute effective vaccines with delivery at a large enough scale for successful prevention.

Finally, a coalition is the best way to harmonize guidance for local application, using targeted and consistent communication across sectors and communities, which will ultimately be the key to effective prevention, detection, and early response in private-sector workplaces.

References

Bloomberg. (2022, March 16). More than 11 billion shots given: Covid-19 vaccine tracker. https://www.bloomberg.com/graphics/covid-vaccine-tracker-global-distribution/

CDC (Centers for Disease Control and Prevention). (2016, November 13). Pandemic influenza: Archived documents; businesses and employers. https://www.cdc.gov/flu/pandemic-resources/archived/business-planning.html

CDC (Centers for Disease Control and Prevention). (2019, September 16). Advancing the global health security agenda: CDC achievements and impact 2018; joint external evaluations (JEE) for improved health security. https://www.cdc.gov/globalhealth/security/ghsareport/2018/jee.html

Diara, M., Johnson, C. E., Dockins, R. O., Buford, D. L., Ben Edet, A., Ngunjiri, S., & Brown, A. K. (2013, April 16–18). Mitigating infectious diseases in company workplaces through business partnerships. Paper presented at the Society of Petroleum Engineers European Health, Safety and Environment Conference and Exhibition, London, United Kingdom. https://doi.org/10.2118/164997-MS

Diara, M., Ngunjiri, S., Brown Maruziak, A., Ben Edet, A., Plenderleith, R., Modrick, M., & Buford, D. (2014, March 17–19). Prevention and control of emerging infectious disease outbreaks in global oil and gas workplaces. Paper presented at the Society of Petroleum Engineers International Conference and Exhibition on Health, Safety and Environment, Long Beach, California. https:// doi.org/10.2118/168477-MS

Diara, M., Ngunjiri, S., Aliyu, B., Jones, S., Brown, A., Simmons, C., Miller, G., Plenderleith, R., Gomez, C., & Buford, D. (2016, April 11–13). A global effective Ebola outbreak preparedness and response from an oil and gas company perspective. Paper presented at the Society of Petroleum Engineers International Conference and Exhibition on Health, Safety, Security, Environment and Social Responsibility, Stavanger, Norway. https://doi.org/10.2118/179375-MS

Diara, M., Ngunjiri, S., McAlester, C., & Adesakin, D. (2019, November 19). "Global approach, local partnerships": Private-sector pandemic flu business continuity planning. Scowcroft Infectious Disease Information Platform, Scowcroft Institute of International Affairs, Texas A&M University. http://pandemic.tamu .edu/Blog/Pandemics,-Infectious-Disease,-and-Biosecurity/November-2019/ Global-Approach,-Local-Partnerships-Private-Sector

European Centre for Disease Prevention and Control. (n.d.). Why is pandemic preparedness planning important? https://www.ecdc.europa.eu/en/seasonal -influenza/preparedness/why-pandemic-preparedness

ExxonMobil. (2006). *Pandemic flu preparedness and response manual*, vol. 1. Internal document.

ExxonMobil. (2020a, April 2). ExxonMobil joins Global Center to expedite medical innovation for personal protective equipment. https://corporate.exxonmobil .com/News/Newsroom/News-releases/2020/0402_ExxonMobil-joins-Global -Center-to-expedite-medical-innovation-for-PPE

ExxonMobil. (2020b, April 3). ExxonMobil contributions to Houston-area food banks to provide one million meals. https://corporate.exxonmobil.com/News/ Newsroom/News-releases/2020/0403_ExxonMobil-contributions-to-Houston -area-food-banks-to-provide-one-million-meals

ExxonMobil. (2020c, April 24). ExxonMobil modifies facilities to produce medical -grade sanitizer for COVID-19 response. https://corporate.exxonmobil.com/ News/Newsroom/News-releases/2020/0424_ExxonMobil-modifies-facilities -to-produce-medical-grade-sanitizer-for-COVID19-response

Garrett, T. A. (2007). *Economic effects of the 1918 influenza pandemic: Implications for a modern-day pandemic*. Federal Reserve Bank of St. Louis. https://www .stlouisfed.org/~/media/files/pdfs/community-development/research-reports/ pandemic_flu_report.pdf?la=en.

GHSA (Global Health Security Agenda). (n.d.). Global Health. https://www.cdc.gov/ globalhealth/security/index.htm

GHSA (Global Health Security Agenda). (2019). *Advancing the Global Health Security Agenda: Results and impact of U.S. government investments*. https:// www.state.gov/wp-content/uploads/2019/11/GHSAR-2019_final.pdf

He, W., Yi, G. Y., & Zhu, Y. (2020, November). Estimation of the basic reproduction number, average incubation time, asymptomatic infection rate, and case fatality rate for COVID-19: Meta-analysis and sensitivity analysis. *Journal of Medical Virology, 92*(11), 2543–50. https://doi.org/10.1002/jmv.26041

International Association of Oil & Gas Producers. (2016). *Infectious disease outbreak management: A programme manual for the oil and gas industry* [eBook edition]. https://www.ipieca.org/resources/good-practice/infectious-disease-outbreak-management-a-programme-manual-for-the-oil-and-gas-industry/

Joseph, A. (2020, July 21). Actual COVID-19 case count could be 6 to 24 times higher than official estimates, CDC study shows. STAT. https://www.statnews.com/2020/07/21/cdc-study-actual-covid-19-cases/

Maukayeva, S., & Karimova, S. (2020, April 14). Epidemiologic character of COVID-19 in Kazakhstan: A preliminary report. *Northern Clinics of Istanbul, 7*(3), 210–13. https://doi.org/10.14744/nci.2020.62443

US Department of Homeland Security Cybersecurity and Infrastructure Security Agency. (2020, May 19). *Guidance on the essential critical infrastructure workforce: Ensuring continuity and national resilience in COVID-19 response*, version 3.1 [eBook edition]. https://www.cisa.gov/sites/default/files/publications/Version_3.1_CISA_Guidance_on_Essential_Critical_Infrastructure_Workers_0.pdf

White House, Office of the Press Secretary. (2015, July 28). Fact sheet: The global health security agenda. https://obamawhitehouse.archives.gov/the-press-office/2015/07/28/fact-sheet-global-health-security-agenda

WHO (World Health Organization). (n.d.). IHR procedures concerning public health emergencies of international concern (PHEIC). https://www.who.int/ihr/procedures/pheic/en/

WHO (World Health Organization). (n.d.). Joint external evaluation (JEE) mission reports. https://www.who.int/ihr/procedures/mission-reports/en/

WHO (World Health Organization). 2005. *International health regulations (2005)*. 3rd ed. https://www.who.int/ihr/publications/9789241580496/en/

WHO (World Health Organization). (2016). *Joint external evaluation tool and process overview* [eBook edition]. https://apps.who.int/iris/bitstream/handle/10665/252755/WHO-HSE-GCR-2016.18-eng.pdf?sequence=1

WHO (World Health Organization). (2017). *Pandemic influenza risk management* [eBook edition]. https://apps.who.int/iris/bitstream/handle/10665/259893/WHO-WHE-IHM-GIP-2017.1-eng.pdf

WHO (World Health Organization). (2020a, January 9). WHO statement regarding cluster of pneumonia cases in Wuhan, China. https://www.who.int/china/news/detail/09-01-2020-who-statement-regarding-cluster-of-pneumonia-cases-in-wuhan-china

WHO (World Health Organization). (2020b, January 20). *Novel coronavirus (2019-nCoV) situation report—1.* https://www.who.int/docs/default-source/coronaviruse/situation-reports/20200121-sitrep-1-2019-ncov.pdf

WHO (World Health Organization). (2020c, January 30). Statement on the second meeting of the International Health Regulations (2005) Emergency Committee regarding the outbreak of novel coronavirus (2019-nCoV). https://www.who.int/news-room/detail/30-01-2020-statement-on-the-second-meeting-of-the-international-health-regulations-(2005)-emergency-committee-regarding-the-outbreak-of-novel-coronavirus-(2019-ncov)

WHO (World Health Organization). (2020d, January 31). *Novel coronavirus (2019-nCoV) situation report—11.* https://www.who.int/docs/default-source/coronaviruse/situation-reports/20200131-sitrep-11-ncov.pdf

WHO (World Health Organization). (2020e, March 11). *Coronavirus disease 2019 (COVID-19) situation report—51.* https://www.who.int/docs/default-source/coronaviruse/situation-reports/20200311-sitrep-51-covid-19.pdf

WHO (World Health Organization). (2020f, March 11). WHO director-general's opening remarks at the media briefing on COVID-19—11 March 2020. https://www.who.int/dg/speeches/detail/who-director-general-s-opening-remarks-at-the-media-briefing-on-covid-19---11-march-2020

WHO (World Health Organization). (2020g, May 22). Operational planning guidance to support country preparedness and response. https://www.who.int/publications/i/item/draft-operational-planning-guidance-for-un-country-teams

WHO (World Health Organization). (2020h, June 30). *Coronavirus disease (COVID-19) situation report—162.* https://www.who.int/docs/default-source/coronaviruse/20200630-covid-19-sitrep-162.pdf

WHO (World Health Organization). (2021a, January 27). Weekly epidemiological update—27 January 2021. https://www.who.int/publications/m/item/weekly-epidemiological-update---27-january-2021

WHO (World Health Organization). (2021b, July 13). Weekly epidemiological update on COVID-19—13 July 2021. https://www.who.int/publications/m/item/weekly-epidemiological-update-on-covid-19---13-july-2021

WHO (World Health Organization). (2022a, January 11). Weekly epidemiological update on COVID-19—11 January 2022. https://www.who.int/publications/m/item/weekly-epidemiological-update-on-covid-19---11-january-2022

WHO (World Health Organization). (2022b, February 22). Weekly epidemiological update on COVID-19—22 February 2022. https://www.who.int/publications/m/item/weekly-epidemiological-update-on-covid-19---22-february-2022

WHO (World Health Organization). (2022c, March 1). Weekly epidemiological update on COVID-19—1 March 2022. https://www.who.int/publications/m/item/weekly-epidemiological-update-on-covid-19---1-march-2022

WHO (World Health Organization). (2022d, March 2). Status of COVID-19 vaccines within WHO EUL/PQ evaluation process. https://extranet.who.int/pqweb/sites/default/files/documents/Status_COVID_VAX_02March2022.pdf

Wong, J., Jamaludin, S. A., Alikhan, M. F., & Chaw, L. (2020, September 14). Asymptomatic transmission of SARS-CoV-2 and implications for mass gatherings. *Influenza and Other Respiratory Viruses, 14*(5), 596–98. https://doi.org/10.1111/irv.12767

CHAPTER 7

Resilience and Sustainability of Global Supply Chains in the Post–COVID-19 Era and a Vision for an Integrated North and Central America

ELEFTHERIOS IAKOVOU AND RAYMOND ROBERTSON

RISING TRADE FRICTIONS WITH CHINA, THE COVID-19 CRISIS, AND increasing concerns about supply chain risk motivate a spirited debate about how to balance resilience, sustainability, and efficiency in global supply chains under the new normal. Leading policymakers have suggested "reshoring," or returning production to the United States, as a solution to the supply chain challenges. These calls place a premium on security, possibly at the expense of efficiency, and offer little guidance on sustainability. The goal of this chapter is to offer a vision for how the United States can balance all three concerns and promote regional economic development in a way that addresses other significant US policy concerns, like migration.

The Rise of Global Supply Chains

Supply chains capitalizing on cross-border flows of goods, capital, processes, and information have been at the nexus of globalization. Since the 1990s, most companies have globalized their sourcing and production, while further embracing lean (just-in-time) manufacturing techniques to reduce total delivered costs. Indeed, global trade increased from 39 percent of world GDP in 1990 to 58 percent in 2019 (*Economist*, 2019a) as a result of these changes. Critical to this development has been the inclusion of China in the World Trade Organization (WTO) in 2001, further accelerating the globalization of sourcing and offshore production by many US-based multinational corporations (MNCs). The decision to bring China into the WTO was based on the wishful thinking that economic liberalization would lead to political liberalization. This decision was further based on models that employed rather simplistic and erroneous assumptions, including perfect competition, eternal full employment, fixed exchange rates, no economies of scale, operation of factories at full capacity at all times, no costs attached to opening or closing factories, no technological innovation unique to one country, and so on (Prestowitz, 2021).

Well before the COVID-19 pandemic, technological, geopolitical, and economic forces along with the perceived need for regionalization had already begun reshaping globalization to what is often known as "slowbalization," or deglobalization. The financial crisis of 2008 was an inflection point as MNCs began realizing that the hypertension of their supply chains had left them exposed to a plethora of risks, which led to the shrinkage of global trade from 61 percent of global GDP in 2008 to 58 percent in 2020 (*Economist*, 2020). Such supply chain risks include disruptions resulting from extreme weather events, suppliers, transportation (e.g., the blockage of the Suez Canal by the *Ever Given* container ship in early 2021 and congestion at US ports in the same year), labor issues, cyberattacks, commodity price fluctuations, intellectual property (IP) issues, diverging standards and regulations, the US-China trade war, tariffs, the COVID-19 pandemic, and other geopolitical events.

The pandemic is just another example of this volatile, uncertain, complex, and ambiguous (VUCA) environment that has further brought existing structural supply chain problems to the surface. Exacerbated by the dramatically increased role of e-commerce, demand quickly shifted across industries and regions. During the pandemic, dramatic surges in customer demand for some supply chains (such as groceries, household products, semiconductor chips, personal protective equipment [PPE], and other health care–related products) made logistics and planning much more challenging than normal. Indicatively, in June 2021, when the congestion in US ports finally seemed to be easing, a COVID-19 surge in southern China clogged ports critical to global trade, causing a shipping backlog that would further exacerbate global shortages until at least the end of-year holiday shopping season. Throughout the pandemic (and especially during its onset), sales forecasts were unhelpful, as they did not consider the associated risks and accommodated only sales by customers and products during "normal times."

Additionally, other sources of severe disruptions originated from reductions in supply, production capacity, and transportation capacity as manufacturers and transport operators struggled to adapt to local lockdowns, rising absenteeism of staff, and social distancing restrictions. Furthermore, since supply chains are burdened with complexity and large offerings of essentially the same product, they lacked the flexibility of shifting from the production of one stock keeping unit (SKU) to another within the same product family. A well-advertised example of this was the shortage of toilet paper, with consumers preferring soft multiroll paper as opposed to the thinner paper preferred by businesses. When demand for the latter diminished, chains did not have the agility to quickly increase production of the former. Additionally, well into the second year of the pandemic, anticipation of product shortages and precautionary hoarding at different stages of the supply chain aggravated initial shortages (the "bullwhip effect"), leading to additional supply chain bottlenecks and increased inflation (Rees and Rungcharoenkitkul, 2021).

These stresses further revealed the fragility of the modern global supply chain, mandating a reset in the design of supply chain networks and resulting in a heightened interest in supply chain resilience and sustainability. Companies and federal agencies alike are increasingly realizing that efficiency cannot be the sole economic virtue, as it often comes at the expense of supply chain resilience, agility, and sustainability, and they are rethinking how to execute their six supply chain megaprocesses—namely, plan, buy, make, move, distribute, and sell.

Supply Chain Resilience

Supply chain resilience refers to the adaptive capability of a supply chain to prepare for unexpected events and then to quickly adjust to sudden disruptive changes that can negatively affect its performance.

It does this by recovering quickly to its predisruption state or even growing to a more desirable state in order to increase customer service, market share, and financial performance. To achieve supply chain resilience, the following tenets should be met (Ponomarov & Holcomb, 2009; Vlachos et al., 2012):

1. Agility and responsiveness: supply chains need to be able to respond rapidly to changed conditions.
2. End-to-end (E2E) supply chain integration, transparency, and visibility. In the midst of the COVID-19 pandemic, companies often had to conduct urgent supply chain mappings on paper (mapping the chain from "suppliers' suppliers to customers' customers") to identify vulnerabilities. Such tasks for today's complex global supply chains are extremely laborious and lengthy. Indicatively, following the 2011 tsunami in Japan, a team of 100 executives of a global semiconductor giant needed more than one year to complete this mapping (*Economist*, 2019b).
3. Redundancies, which include emergency stockpiles, safety stocks, and diversified sourcing with offshored, but also nearshored or reshored suppliers. These nearby suppliers will have to provide additional capacity when there are disruptions of supply from offshore suppliers to ensure business continuity (Iakovou, Vlachos, & Xanthopoulos, 2007).
4. Collaboration of private and public supply chain stakeholders.
5. Effective demand planning processes.

The leading MNCs have long recognized that managing supply chain risk is necessary for sustained competitiveness. To this effect, supply chain risk management and mitigation strategies have developed at the intersection of supply chain management and risk management over the last two decades and have attracted growing interest from corporate management and corporate boards (Vlachos et al., 2012). However, rampant deregulation and the financialization of the supply chain, with a single focus on operating margins and asset efficiency—often with engineering of the balance sheet as opposed to the supply chain—have led to the design of brittle, lean, and offshore supply chains (Foroohar,

2016; Lynn, 2020; *American Prospect*, 2022). Unsurprisingly, corporate boards and shareholders have often resisted resilience portfolios that are built on high levels of redundancy (with a negative effect on the bottom line, at least in the short term).

Today, a new paradigm of competitive resilience is necessary for companies to redesign their supply chains for the long haul without bouncing back to their old practices once the pandemic subsides. Assuming a longer-term perspective and embracing all stakeholders (including workers, the wider society, and the nation at large) can help make investing in resilience (but also sustainability) a better value proposition. Indeed, for years there have been calls for corporate governance to move away from shareholder-to-stakeholder capitalism in order for companies to avoid succumbing to short-term pressures to distribute earnings. These pressures sacrifice the investments in R&D, innovation, and capital expenditures necessary for long-term growth. A positive step in this direction was an August 2019 statement by the Business Roundtable (a club of 181 powerful CEOs) that redefined the purpose of a corporation to benefit all stakeholders, including customers, employees, suppliers, communities, and shareholders but also the nation (Mazzucato, 2021).

The level of investment a company makes in addressing risk will depend on (1) the chronically occurring identified supply chain risks; (2) the awareness that some risks are unimaginable "black swans" (Kaplan, Leonard, & Mikes, 2020); and (3) the company's appetite for risk. The challenge for US MNCs is to develop cost-competitive resilient supply chains. The digitalization of supply chains allows organizations to better balance this trade-off of cost efficiency versus resilience. Technologies such as blockchain and artificial intelligence (AI) allow companies to monitor not just tier 1 suppliers but also secondary suppliers and original equipment manufacturers (OEMs) deep within their supply chain, thus offering increased end-to-end supply chain visibility across the global supply chain. This increased visibility further improves communication among supply chain stakeholders and reduces the bullwhip effect (Chang, Iakovou, & Shi, 2020; Bechtsis et al., 2021).

Next-generation resilience will embrace dynamically resilient data-driven supply chain networks that will be able to quickly detect, respond to, and recover from supply chain disruptions by adjusting manufacturing capacity. The resulting supply chains will blend the advantages of distributed supply chain systems having inventory and/ or manufacturing capacity close to demand to enable fast fulfillment, and centralized supply chain systems to enable economies of scale, inventory, "risk pooling," reduced total safety inventory, and reduced total capital expenditures (Iakovou & White, 2020).

Supply Chain Sustainability

While the COVID-19 crisis represents the acute novel risks posed by unusual "black swan" events, further bringing resilience to the forefront of businesses and governments, social risks have become increasingly salient over the last decade and represent another source of a growing chronic supply chain risk. From the 2013 factory collapse in Bangladesh's Rana Plaza to the reports in 2020 that some Chinese factories had forcibly relocated Uighur Muslims working in slave-like conditions, MNCs have increasingly begun to realize that working conditions—broadly defined to include forced labor, child labor, human trafficking, and a wide range of conditions tied to domestic labor law and international labor standards—are a critical component of their risk analysis. Finding ways to ensure that supplier factories are in compliance with both national labor laws and international labor standards is one of the leading sustainability challenges that MNCs face while designing and managing their supply chain networks.

One concern that MNCs must manage is differences in policies across countries. The responses to rising concerns about working conditions across countries have been heterogeneous. The European Union's response has focused primarily on a "due diligence" regulatory approach, which follows nearly two decades of debate over the best way to resolve the tension between lower standards in production countries and higher standards in retail-market countries. Governments, businesses, unions, and nongovernmental organizations (NGOs) often promote very different perspectives about rights and responsibilities of different supply chain stakeholders. To help reconcile competing views, John Ruggie, special representative of the secretary-general of the United Nations, proffered a "protect, respect, and remedy" doctrine to illustrate how governments, corporations, and civil society can all play a role in reducing the "adverse human rights consequences" of supply chains (Ruggie, 2008).

The document that outlined what have come to be known as the Ruggie Principles has several layers. The Ruggie Principles suggest that governments should, and have a responsibility to, use their unique leverage to ensure that human rights standards are applied to workers in global value chains. Corporations have the responsibility to proactively address human rights within their value chain in order to avoid complicity with human rights abuses in factories they do not own or manage but that produce work-in-progress (WIP) or goods sold to lead firms downstream in the supply chain. Relevant countermeasures include monitoring, assessment, and integration of proactive prevention and remediation of violations.

The Ruggie Principles also acknowledge the importance of grievance mechanisms and remediation and advocate for several ways to achieve this goal, including judicial and nonjudicial means, that combine efforts of corporations and the state. Having these procedures in place can help increase the incentives to ensure compliance with national laws and international labor standards.

The COVID-19 pandemic coincided with the beginning of a legal codification of the cumulative push for a regulatory approach toward implementing the Ruggie Principles. This push grew from 2011 to 2020. In 2011, the United Nations Guiding Principles on Business and Human Rights called for explicit steps to ensure that human rights would be protected in global value chains (United Nations, 2011). The Organization for Economic Co-operation and Development (OECD, 2011) offered very specific suggestions, including a focus on due diligence standards and responsible supply chain management. Soon after, in 2014, the European Union released a directive that eventually became binding legislation in 27 member states and required reporting on human rights conditions within supply chains.*

The push for regulations continued to gain strength. In February 2017, the French National Assembly adopted a "Duty of Vigilance Law" for MNCs operating in France that requires them to develop

---

* See Article 1 of Directive 2014/95/EU.

and implement plans to prevent serious violations or mitigate potential risks of violations under the penalty of civil court damages (ECCJ, 2017). Although France's Constitutional Council rejected the civil penalties for failure to develop a diligence plan, it upheld much of the legislation and kept the momentum for increased regulation.

Similarly, in June 2021, Germany officially enacted the "Lieferkettengesetz," which means Supply Chain Law or Distribution Law. This law makes it mandatory for every company with more than 3,000 employees in 2023 and 1,000 in 2024 to have full transparency and control along its entire end-to-end (E2E) supply chain. This is envisioned to further eliminate child work and guarantee quality products from known sources.

The regulatory push is not limited to the European Union. The United Kingdom's 2015 Modern Slavery Act requires that MNCs either implement policies to ensure that slavery and human trafficking are absent from their supply chain or declare the absence of policies to detect slavery and human trafficking in their supply chains. The legislation has neither legally binding requirements to conduct due diligence nor criminal or financial penalties for noncompliance. Several other countries, most notably Australia, have passed similar legislation.

On the other side of the Atlantic, the United States has taken a different approach. In 2010, California passed its Transparency in Supply Chains Act, requiring that applicable companies report their verification, audit, certification, internal accountability, and training activities to mitigate and redress human trafficking and forced labor. Since 2016, US Customs and Border Protection (CBP) has taken a proactive approach toward stopping imports that it deems to have been made with slave labor. When CBP's civil investigative program finds information indicating that foreign goods are made with forced labor, the agency issues a Withhold Release Order that stops the would-be imports. CBP also has the authority to impose monetary penalties for certain forced labor offenses and to refer cases to Homeland Security Investigations for criminal investigation. Since 2016, CBP has issued 29 Withhold Release Orders and blocked more than $100 million in goods from US markets as a result of information indicating forced labor. CBP notes that these enforcement actions are unique in the world (US Customs and Border Protection, 2021). The United States is further working hard to tackle relevant challenges that stem from China. Rising concerns about labor conditions in China have led CBP to limit imports from China that have been linked to forced labor.

In addition to government legislation and administrative enforcement, other stakeholders are pushing for more responsibility on the part of MNCs. One leading example is the International Labour Organization's *Tripartite Declaration of Principles concerning Multinational Enterprises and Social Policy* (ILO, 2017). The declaration offers specific suggestions to help MNCs address potential compliance issues related to training, work and living conditions, industrial relations, and, of course, employment.

Supply Chain Efficiency

One potential approach to address the described challenges regarding both supply chain resilience and labor-related sustainability issues is to promote reshoring or nearshoring or a combination of the two. After the COVID-19 pandemic, policymakers called for production of some critical goods, such as medical supplies and high-tech products (including semiconductor chips and high-capacity batteries), to be reshored back to the United States, but the complete reshoring of such supply chains cannot be the answer. Reshoring may increase security but raises costs. Complete reshoring would make US businesses less competitive and put them at a disadvantage with state-owned enterprises (SOEs) of China and businesses of other (often adversarial) nations that continue to embrace globalization and support key industries with aggressive mercantilism, including industrial policies, subsidies, and currency manipulations (Norris, 2018; Prestowitz, 2021). The result may be reduced appeal of US products in foreign markets, increased costs to US consumers, reduced shareholder value for investors, and erosion of the global innovation leadership of the United States, as complete reshoring would hinder its openness to ideas, people, and sourcing of parts (O'Neil, 2020) and may not make the US economy more resilient to pandemic-type shocks (Bonadio et al., 2020).

Even if the cost concerns are not sufficiently compelling to reconsider calls for complete reshoring, several practical issues still impede the push in that direction. Reshoring to the United States is severely hindered by the lack of the following: (1) a national manufacturing ecosystem of small to medium enterprises tailored to critical industries such as semiconductors; and (2) federal investment in improving the national logistics infrastructure, including the nation's "hard" (ports, roads, rail networks) and "soft" (service industries that underpin logistics) infrastructure with a focus on improvements in supply chain reliability and service quality, cybersecurity, environmental sustainability, and skill shortages. Unfortunately, such investments were not made in the globalization-driven economic boom of the 1980s, when policymakers failed to embrace long-term thinking (Moyo, 2018, 2021).

By contrast, China has made massive investments to improve the competitiveness of its supply chains, investing more than US$1 trillion to develop an advanced logistics network as part of its Belt and Road Initiative (BRI). This network of road and rail routes, ports, airports, and oil and gas pipelines linking Central and West Asia, the Middle East, Europe, and East Africa provides both geostrategic and economic benefits. The BRI has attracted criticism for lacking transparency and accountability and has often been used by China as a tool of "debt trap" diplomacy toward developing countries, where lending leads to the seizure of recipient countries' strategic assets (Gates, 2020; Prestowitz, 2021). On June 12, 2021, the United States and members of the G7 announced the launching of the Build Back Better World (B3W) global initiative, to counter China's BRI. B3W will aim to finance cleaner infrastructure projects (e.g., roads and bridges) for low-income countries (*Economist*, 2021b).

A Vision for an Integrated North and Central America

Instead of complete reshoring focused primarily on mitigating risk, we suggest that the combination of rising trade frictions with China, increasing concerns over sustainability and diligence, and supply chain disruptions creates the opportunity for a "smart reshoring" strategy, with incentives to develop capacity within North America that supports resilience, sustainability, and efficiency within supply chains.

Even before the COVID-19 pandemic, an increasing number of MNCs—taking into account rising wages in China, increased exposure to supply chain risk, and sustainability concerns—were relocating their supply chains away from China to other parts of Asia, further looking to make their supply chains more local (regionalized). Consider the case of Volkswagen. Prior to COVID-19, Volkswagen had already set up regional supply chains in China and Europe so that local companies could quickly fulfill demand for their local plants, supporting just-in-time production. Once the pandemic struck, the company was able to use the added sourcing flexibility to its advantage in order to ensure business continuity by dynamically altering sourcing from China and Europe based on the timing of the shutdowns induced by the pandemic (*Economist* Intelligence Unit, 2021). Similar supply chain strategies may become more common in the post–COVID-19 era, giving rise to quasi-independent supply chains in the Americas, Europe, and China.

The intellectual foundation of our proposed vision lies in what some have called the "flying geese" model of economic development. In the 1930s, Kaname Akamatsu developed a theory of economic development that was similar to the V pattern that geese often follow when flying. In Akamatsu's vision (Akamatsu, 1962), the lead "goose" was Japan. The need for lower-wage labor motivated the shift in Japan's production to its lower-wage neighbors in the form of directed investments and trade. As technology continued to evolve in Japan, Japan shifted older technologies to these neighbors. In turn, these countries, such as South Korea, Singapore, Taiwan, and Hong Kong, would upgrade their technology and shift production using the older technology to third-tier countries, which at the time included China, Vietnam, and the Philippines. This model resulted in Japan-led regional economic development that was based on economic integration.

The driving force of the economic integration was production sharing and technology transfer. This form of directed economic integration provided the guidance and support needed for low-income countries to advance along a development path that moved from agriculture to apparel, to textiles, to light manufacturing, to heavy manufacturing, and eventually to services. The results in East Asia have been very clear, with the first- and second-tier East Asian countries being arguably the most successful examples of rapid economic development in the twentieth century.

In North America, the process of economic integration has been less directed. Production-sharing investments in Mexico increased dramatically in the early 1980s with the reform of the maquiladora program. This program, also known as the "in-bond" industry, created incentives for US companies to set up assembly operations within 20 kilometers of the US border in northern Mexico as early as the 1960s (Castillo and de Vries, 2018). The program led to significant growth in investment and output in northern Mexico, but early legal restrictions and the rather poor transportation infrastructure allowed little spillover into the rest of Mexico (Chiquiar, 2008).

The investment in northern Mexico, as well as the migration that occurred between Mexico and the United States, integrated the Mexican and US labor markets (Robertson, 2000). In fact, some results suggest that Mexico's northern labor market is more integrated with the United States than it is with southern Mexico. The lack of incentives to invest farther south result from policy, an inefficient transportation infrastructure, and a less educated workforce. The North American Free Trade Agreement, which went into effect January 1, 1994, was designed to extend the maquiladora program to the rest of Mexico. As a result, investment, production, and employment grew in regions south of Mexico's northern border but remained concentrated north of Mexico City.

When China joined the WTO on December 11, 2001, Mexico started to face fierce competition in the US market, resulting in falling wages and employment in Mexico (Robertson, Halliday, & Vasireddy, 2020). Since 2001, Mexico has evolved dramatically. Education levels and the technical proficiency of the labor force have increased, and Mexico's production mix has shifted away from apparel and appliances toward automobiles and aerospace. Rising technical capacity and geographic proximity put Mexico in a better position to provide an alternative for supply chain stakeholders leaving China.

Trade frictions with China have several roots. Exchange rates, state-owned enterprises, intellectual property, cyber (and physical) security, and working conditions have motivated companies to seek alternatives to producing in China and motivated the US government to impose punitive trade policies. Since these issues are complex, a concerted effort between government and the private sector is appropriate and possibly necessary. While the need for more robust supply chains is clear, governments with a new focus on resilience and self-reliance should be cautious in their regulatory interventions, as dismantling global supply chains completely could create new supply chain vulnerabilities and undermine free trade and economic growth (*Economist*, 2021a).

While there are calls for the federal government to potentially mirror a few of China's mercantilist policies for critical supply chains (e.g., pharmaceuticals, aerospace, defense), the United States clearly needs to draft a new George Kennan "long telegram" for developing a comprehensive strategy of how to deal with China, while it continues to support free trade. The United States has the opportunity to embark on an ambitious moonshot initiative to fill a pressing gap in global trade and supply chain infrastructure by fostering public-private partnerships and engaging trading partner nations who abide by the rule of law and multilateral agreements, to promote a new generation of diversified, resilient, sustainable, and competitive supply chains. These new supply chains would still have a global footprint with a sophisticated portfolio of offshored, nearshored, and reshored manufacturing and could work in tandem with emerging regionalized supply chains (as described above).

In the vacuum of a directed US policy, China exploited the withdrawal of the United States from the Trans-Pacific Partnership in 2017 and has already increased its investments along the US borders of Mexico and Canada (which both remain in the TPP). Investment is particularly strong in Mexico's maquiladora zones. China's investments in Latin America have grown dramatically (Dollar, 2017), and its investments in Panama and El Salvador were followed by these countries breaking ties with Taiwan and shifting alignment to China.

What steps are necessary to implement a "flying geese" model in North and Central America? The United States has already established a solid foundation. The Central America–Dominican Republic Free Trade Agreement (CAFTA-DR) went into effect in 2006 for El Salvador, Guatemala, Honduras, and Nicaragua (followed by the Dominican Republic in 2007 and Costa Rica in 2009). This agreement, along with the North American Free Trade Agreement and its update, the United States–Mexico–Canada Agreement (USMCA), which went into effect in 2020, provides a foundation for promoting the kind of flying geese–style economic development that helped propel the East Asian region into developed-country status.

But these agreements are far from sufficient. Remaining barriers must be addressed. The barriers to efficiency-enhancing integration with Mexico and Central America include the lack of ancillary activities, the lack of US-led and Mexican-led investments, and political resistance arising from geographically concentrated losses that exist primarily because of trade with China and changes in technology. Ironically, trade with China may explain much of the resistance to expanding trade with Mexico and Central America.

These agreements, and directed policies to support economic integration in North and Central America, support supply chain resilience, efficiency, and sustainability. An integrated North and Central America supports supply chain resilience because proximity to the United States allows quicker transitions to alternatives when risk factors arise. Supply chain integration in North and Central America also potentially increases efficiency. The proximity to US demand allows Mexico and Central America to offer significant time savings and potentially improved supply chain performance (with supply chain postponement and distributed logistics with reduced order lead times). Some companies have realized the advantages of choosing Mexico over China. Polaris, a US vehicle manufacturer, decided to move its factory to Mexico rather than China to allow faster and more flexible deliveries (*Economist* Intelligence Unit, 2021). Chinese wages, by some measures, have already surpassed Mexican wage levels, and Mexican wages are often higher than those in Central America. Furthermore, Mexico and Central American countries spend a higher share of their income on US exports. Rising income in Mexico and Central America increases demand for US imports at a higher rate than in China.

Supply chain integration in North and Central America also promotes sustainability. One key update to the USMCA was to fully incorporate provisions that focus on labor-related sustainability issues and implement new mechanisms to support compliance with national labor law and international labor standards. Dewan and Ronconi (2014) showed that US free trade agreements with Latin America are associated with more labor inspections, which are an important step

Table 7.1. Remittances and US apparel import values.

VARIABLES	FIXED EFFECTS	LAGGED VALUES
US import values	-0.085*	-0.386***
	(0.049)	(0.105)
Lagged imports		0.308***
		(0.102)
Constant	7.117***	7.063***
	(0.861)	(0.866)
Observations	519	503
R-squared	0.006	0.028
Number of countries	20	20

Note: Authors' elaboration using US apparel import data for Latin American countries from OTEXA (https://www.trade.gov/) and remittance data from the World Bank's Understanding Poverty website (https://www.worldbank.org/en/understanding-poverty) and Migration and Remittances dataset (https://www.worldbank.org/en/topic/migration).

* Statistically significant at the 10 percent level.

*** Statistically significant at the 1 percent level.

toward successfully addressing the labor-related sustainability issues that are becoming increasingly important in global policy.

Pursuing supply chain resilience, efficiency, and sustainability through a North and Central American "flying geese" model offers the possibility of addressing other concerns as well, such as the 2021 migration crisis along the US Southwest border (Rooney, 2021).

When the United States imports more apparel from Latin America, remittances from migrants in the United States to Latin America fall. For an illustration of this, consider table 7.1. With respect to US trade and Latin American migration, when proxied with remittances, US apparel imports are negatively related. Table 7.1 depicts the results of a simple fixed-effects panel data regression for 20 Latin American countries from 1990 to 2016. The "fixed effects" are variables that capture country-specific characteristics, such as migration networks and violence, that contribute to migration regardless of trade. The fixed-effects specification also allows us to focus on the year-to-year changes in remittances and US apparel imports, which probably offer a more accurate depiction of the relationship. A short-run increase in the demand for apparel in the United States requires more workers in Latin America, potentially making migration to the United States less attractive.

The results in table 7.1 further demonstrate that US apparel imports are negatively associated with remittances. In other words, rising US apparel imports are associated with falling remittances. Since the pairwise correlation coefficient between migration and remittances is over 0.96, and remittances are often used as a proxy for migration, these results suggest that a "flying geese" model in North America, with the United States leading its neighbors, could not only help balance supply chain resilience, sustainability, and efficiency but also address other policy concerns, such as migration.

References

Akamatsu, K. (1962). A historical pattern of economic growth in developing countries. *Journal of Developing Economies, 1* (1), 3–25. doi:10.1111/j.1746–1049.1962.tb01020.x

American Prospect, 33(1). (2022, February). How we broke the supply chain.

Bechtsis, D., Tsolakis, N., Vlachos, D., & Iakovou E. (2021, August 31). A data sharing framework for data-driven resilient, secure and sustainable supply chains. *International Journal of Production Research*. doi:https://doi.org/10.1080/00207543.2021.1957506

Bonadio, B., Huo, Z., Levchenko, A. A., & Pandalai-Nayar, N. (2020, May). Global supply chains in the pandemic. National Bureau of Economic Research Working Paper No. 27224. doi:10.3386/w27224

Castillo, J. C., & de Vries, G. (2018). The domestic content of Mexico's maquiladora exports: A long-run perspective. *Journal of International Trade & Economic Development, 27*(2), 200–19. doi:10.1080/09638199.2017.1353125

Chang, Y., Iakovou, E., & Shi, W. (2020). Blockchain in global supply chains and cross border trade: A critical synthesis of the state-of-the-art, challenges and opportunities. *International Journal of Production Research, 58*(7), 2082–99.

Chiquiar, D. (2008). Globalization, regional wage differentials and the Stolper–Samuelson Theorem: Evidence from Mexico. *Journal of International Economics, 74*(1), 70–93. https://doi.org/10.1016/j.jinteco.2007.05.009

Dewan, S., & Ronconi, L. (2014). U.S. free trade agreements and enforcement of labor law in Latin America. Inter-American Development Bank Working Paper No. IDB-WP-543. https://publications.iadb.org/publications/english/document/US-Free-Trade-Agreements-and-Enforcement-of-Labor-Law-in-Latin-America.pdf

Dollar, D. (2017). *China's investment in Latin America*. Brookings, Geoeconomics and Global Issues. https://www.brookings.edu/research/chinas-investment-in-latin-america/

ECCJ (European Coalition for Corporate Justice). (2017). FAQs: The French duty of vigilance law. https://corporatejustice.org/publications/faqs-french-duty-of-vigilance-law/

Economist (2019a, January 26). Globalisation has faltered and is now being reshaped.

Economist (2019b, July 13). Slowbalisation: Bumpy new world.

Economist (2020, October 10). Special report: The world economy.

Economist (2021a, April 3). Global supply chains are still a source of strength, not weakness.

Economist (2021b, June 19). China and America are borrowing each other's weapons.

Economist Intelligence Unit (2021, February 25). *The business costs of supply chain disruption*. https://eiuperspectives.economist.com/sites/default/files/the_business_costs_of_supply_chain_disruption_gep_1.pdf

Foroohar, R. (2016). *Makers and takers: The rise of finance and the fall of American business*. New York: Currency.

Gates, R. M. (2020). *Exercise of power: American failures, successes, and a new path forward in the post-cold war world*. New York: Knopf.

Iakovou, E., Vlachos, D., & Xanthopoulos, A. (2007). An analytical methodological framework for the optimal design of resilient supply chains. *International Journal of Logistics Economics and Globalisation, 1*(1), 1–20.

Iakovou, E., & White, C. C., III. (2020). How to build more secure, resilient, next-gen U.S. supply chains. Brookings, TechStream. https://www.brookings.edu/techstream/how-to-build-more-secure-resilient-next-gen-u-s-supply-chains/

ILO (International Labour Organization). (2017, March 17). *Tripartite declaration of principles concerning multinational enterprises and social policy (MNE declaration)*. 5th ed. https://www.ilo.org/empent/Publications/WCMS_094386/lang—en/index.htm

Kaplan, R. S., Leonard, H. B., & Mikes, A. (2020, November–December). The risks you can't foresee. *Harvard Business Review*, 40–46.

Lynn, B. C. (2020). *Liberty from all masters: The new American autocracy vs. the will of the people*. New York: St. Martin's Press.

Mazzucato, M. (2021). *Mission economy: A moonshot guide to changing capitalism*. New York: Harper Business.

Moyo, D. (2018). *Edge of chaos: Why democracy is failing to deliver economic growth—and how to fix it*. New York: Basic Books.

Moyo, D. (2021). *How boards work: And how they can work better in a chaotic world*. New York: Basic Books.

Norris, W. J. (2018). *Chinese economic statecraft: Commercial actors, grand strategy, and state control*. Ithaca, NY: Cornell University Press.

OECD (Organization for Economic Co-operation and Development). (2011). *OECD guidelines for multinational enterprises*. https://www.oecd.org/daf/inv/mne/48004323.pdf

O'Neil, S. K. (2020, April 1). How to pandemic-proof globalization: Redundancy, not re-shoring, is the key to supply-chain security. *Foreign Affairs*. https://www.foreignaffairs.com/articles/2020-04-01/how-pandemic-proof-globalization

Ponomarov, S. Y., & Holcomb, M. C. (2009). Understanding the concept of supply chain resilience. *International Journal of Logistics Management, 20*(1), 124–43.

Prestowitz, C. (2021). *The world turned upside down: America, China, and the struggle for global leadership*. New Haven, CT: Yale University Press.

Rees, D., & Rungcharoenkitkul, P., (2021, November). Bottlenecks: Causes and macro-economic implications. Bank for International Settlements (BIS) Bulletin no. 48.

Robertson, R. (2000). Wage shocks and North American labor-market integration. *American Economic Review, 90*(4), 742–64.

Robertson, R., Halliday, T. J., & Vasireddy, S. (2020). Labour market adjustment to third-party competition: Evidence from Mexico. *World Economy, 43*(7), 1977–2006.

Rooney, M. (2021, May 20). The unexpected solution for immigration from Central America. *Deseret News*. https://www.deseret.com/u-s-world/2021/5/20/22444341/northern-triangle-immigration-border-central-america-trade-free-markets

Ruggie, J. G. (2008). *Protect, respect and remedy: A framework for business and human rights; report of the special representative of the secretary-general on the issue of human rights and transnational corporations and other business enterprises*. United Nations Human Rights Council. https://undocs.org/A/HRC/8/5

Vlachos, D., Iakovou, E., Papapanagiotou, K., & Partsch, D. (2012). Building robust supply chains by reducing vulnerability and improving resilience. *International Journal of Agile Systems and Management, 5*(1), 59–81.

United Nations (2011). *Guiding principles on business and human rights: Implementing the United Nations "Protect, Respect and Remedy" framework*. https://www.ohchr.org/documents/publications/guidingprinciplesbusinesshr_en.pdf

US Customs and Border Protection. (2021, May 4). CBP team selected as finalist for Service to America Medal. https://www.cbp.gov/newsroom/national-media-release/cbp-team-selected-finalist-service-america-medal

PART 4

SOCIAL IMPACTS OF COVID-19

CHAPTER 8

Migrant Communities and COVID-19

*How a Lack of Health Access
Impacts Effective Pandemic Response*

LIDIA AZURDIA SIERRA, SARA ALI, AND
CHRISTINE CRUDO BLACKBURN

Global Migration and the Refugee Crisis

IN THE BEGINNING OF THIS CHAPTER, WE WOULD FIRST LIKE TO
clarify the differences between a refugee, an internally displaced person (IDP), an asylum seeker, an immigrant, and a migrant. These
words are commonly used interchangeably or incorrectly, and the following definitions from the International Organization for Migration
(IOM, 2020) will indicate how we are using them in this context. First,
refugees are persons who flee their country because of armed conflict
or persecution. They must seek safety by crossing national borders and
because of their circumstances are granted limited rights and protections under international law (1951 Refugee Convention). Next, internally displaced persons, or IDPs, have been forced to leave their home
or residence because of armed conflict, violence, or disaster. However,
IDPs have not fled to another country but rather remain within their
country's borders and receive protections from their own government.
An asylum seeker is a person who has applied for sanctuary in another
country, but the application has not yet been approved or denied.
Typically, asylum seekers must go through an interview process that
determines whether they will be granted refugee status. Immigrants
move from their country of residence to another country for at least
one year in order to make that new country their residence. They are

not granted any protections or rights until citizenship in the new country has been established. Finally, migrants move from within a country or across international borders. This move can be temporary or permanent. Reasons typically vary and include economic opportunities, education, climate change, and famine, among others.

Over the last decade, the number of forcibly displaced persons has increased by the tens of millions. By the end of 2022, 108.4 million people had been forcibly displaced worldwide. Of these displaced individuals, 35.3 million were refugees, 62.5 million were internally displaced, and 5.4 million were asylum seekers. Fifty-two percent of forcibly displaced persons originate from just three countries—Syria, Ukraine, and Afghanistan—and 43.3 percent of all forcibly displaced persons are children (UNHCR, 2021a). Additionally, more than 20 million people were displaced in 2020 alone (UNHCR, 2021b). These displacements were the result of persecution, conflict, violence, climate change, economic instability, and famine, which have affected countries on every continent. Although much of the conversation around refugee resettlement centers on wealthy countries, such countries host only about 14 percent of the total refugee population. Seventy-six percent of refugees are hosted in low- and middle-income countries, and 20 percent are provided asylum in the poorest countries in the world (UNHCR, 2021a).

Currently, the largest host country in the world is Turkey, hosting 3.6 million refugees; Iran and Colombia follow, hosting over 3.4 million and 2.5 million, respectively (UNHCR, 2021a). According to a 2020 United Nations (UN) report, "At the end of the decade, just ten countries hosted nearly 3 in 5 of those displaced across borders" (UNHCR, 2020a). It is challenging for low-income countries to provide adequate health care and basic necessities to displaced persons, especially when they have trouble allocating basic necessities for their own citizens. A lack of resources and funding can be detrimental to both the host country and the displaced population. The annual increase in forced migration means that 1 of every 97 people was forced to leave his or her home by the end of 2019 (UNHCR, 2020b). These reports are also prior to COVID-19, which as of January 2022 had resulted in more than 307 million cases and almost 5.5 million deaths worldwide (Johns Hopkins University, 2022). More than two years into the pandemic, as new variants increase the need for vaccine access among the world's poorest countries, COVID-19 continues to pose a dire threat to displaced populations.

Many countries, even prior to COVID-19, had insufficient resources to support the health needs of displaced persons within their borders. For example, Jordan hosts over 658,000 registered Syrian refugees, though estimates that include unregistered refugees put this number closer to 1.3 million (ACAPS, 2020). Thus, approximately one-tenth of Jordan's total population is Syrian refugees, and the country's economy has been substantially impacted by this influx. A 2015 study showed that "$62 million per year is needed to cover the additional demand derived from the influx of Syrian refugees" (Marrouch, 2015). These investments are related mainly to "the provision of municipal services, such as access to running water, connections to the power grid, and road maintenance and construction" (Marrouch, 2015). This figure means that more than 35 percent of Jordan's governmental budget needed to be allocated toward displaced persons residing in the country (Marrouch, 2015). In 2018, 78 percent of Syrian refugees in Jordan were living below the poverty line, leaving many to rely on humanitarian agencies to provide them with basic necessities (ACAPS, 2020). This situation is magnified in middle- and low-income countries like Pakistan, Uganda, and Colombia, which each have over one million resident refugees (UNHCR, 2021b). Providing adequate health care, education, food, water, and housing is a challenge for many host countries.

As the refugee crisis grows, many host countries are finding it more difficult to meet the basic needs of displaced populations. For displaced individuals who integrate into the host society, it can often be even more difficult to access education and health care without significant effort and targeted policies from the host country. For example, more than 5.2 million Venezuelans have migrated to border countries in search of health care, education, and employment (Bahar, Dooley, & Selee, 2020). Colombia, Peru, and Chile together host more than two million displaced persons from Venezuela. Colombia hosts the largest number, with an estimated 1.8 million refugees. Venezuelans have been fleeing insecurity, economic instability, and violence over the last decade. In 2017, 87 percent of Venezuelans lived in poverty, and 80 percent were affected by food insecurity (Freier 2018). The political turmoil in Venezuela has been compounded with hyperinflation, a shortage of medications, an underfunded hospital system, and food shortages (Espinel et al., 2020).

In Colombia, Venezuelans live in the major cities, rather than refugee camps. Colombia hosts Venezuelan refugees with three different destinations. First, there are Venezuelans who intend to settle in Colombia. Second, some displaced persons use Colombia for safe passage to another country. Third, there are those who travel almost daily between Venezuela and Colombia, typically in search of employment, education, health care, and basic necessities in order to take them back to loved ones who cannot make the trek (Bahar, Dooley, & Selee, 2020). Despite its challenges, Colombia has been welcoming to displaced Venezuelans when other countries were turning them away. Colombia offered them a two-year permit, between 2017 and 2020, which would grant them the right to employment and health care access (Frydenlund, Padilla, & Palacio, 2021). Additionally, Colombian agencies that once helped internally displaced Colombians are now helping provide food and shelter to displaced Venezuelans. By integrating displaced Venezuelans into its society, Colombia may reap some benefits. According to survey data, the displaced are, on average, younger and more educated than their host country counterparts (Bahar, Dooley, & Selee, 2020). Colombia serves as a model, albeit imperfect, of a hopeful solution to wide-scale displacement that is both economically and socially beneficial to the host country.

While underinvestment in public health infrastructure, economic instability, political turmoil, and climate change bear responsibility for much of the refugee crisis and migration, the leadership of a host country, or lack thereof, often determines the success and safety of the displaced. Additionally, a country's outlook on health access—that is, whether an individual inherently has a right to health—plays a role in the well-being of displaced individuals and the host country. Considering the COVID-19 pandemic, the policies that were in place beforehand either positively or negatively impacted a country's ability to contain the virus in refugee camps and in the general population. In the following sections we discuss how exclusion of displaced individuals from the health care system and pandemic response policies has been detrimental to countries' ability to contain the COVID-19 pandemic.

Obstacles and Limitations to Health Care Access among Migrants

Access to health care poses one of the biggest obstacles for host countries and migrants. Migrants' legal status is often the central determining factor when it comes to health access within their host countries (WHO, 2018). Those who are legally recognized through employment contracts or protected under international law typically have access to government health care services. However, those who reside in the country without legal documentation "tend not to present to health care institutions because of fear of deportation" (Meer & Villegas, 2020). The laws and practices of some countries deviate from the universal health care responsibilities expected from all countries, while other countries have exceptions that help provide access to their undocumented migrant populations. France and the Netherlands, for example, offer a temporary permit that helps cover health care in the case of a pregnancy. However, having a certain legal status in a country does not necessarily mean that migrants will have access to health care services. In France, "the consequences of social stigmatization, precarious living conditions, and the climate of fear and suspicion generated by increasingly restrictive immigration policies [have] hindered many undocumented migrants from being or feeling entitled to the right to health" (Hacker et al., 2015). In many European studies, migrants have described "concerns regarding appropriate engagement in physical examinations, preserving and respecting religious restrictions on physical contact, and cultural taboos" while receiving treatment (Hacker et al., 2015). This ultimately makes it more difficult to provide adequate quality care and can potentially impact the broader community.

Migrants must overcome social, emotional, physical, and political barriers to access health care. These obstacles range from health policies in the host country to health care financial coverage, health care workforce, availability of medical diagnostics, and health information. First, the host country's legislation on migrant health, again depending on migrants' status, dictates whether they have access to health care. Second, the level of health care coverage and the cost associated with those benefits impact an individual's access to health care. Migrant health policies heavily impact other facets of migrant health as well. For instance, health care workers have a significant effect on a patient's care and experience. If the health care workforce is not representative of the migrant population they serve, then differences in culture and language can cause miscommunication between patients and health care providers. Cultural and linguistic differences are pertinent to understanding health outcomes in migrant communities, yet these services are substandard in many countries all over the world.

Health-related information is often provided to migrants in the host country's primary language and distributed through clinics or mailing services that do not reach the patients who could most benefit from the information. These practices prevent migrants from accessing and understanding pertinent health care information. Additionally, while there are resources on the internet, online information can lead to further misunderstanding and spread of misinformation. A more beneficial way to spread information pertinent to migrants would be through community-based organizations such as places of worship, service organizations, and neighborhood organizations. Additionally, providing information through ethnic and religious media has been effective because they serve as a trusted resource for information among migrant communities (De Vito et al., 2015). In order to overcome these barriers, it is important for host countries to meet migrant communities where they are and work to meet their unique needs, particularly in times of crisis.

In the following sections we will discuss the barriers and limitations migrants have historically faced in accessing health care, the impact of COVID-19 on migrant communities, and policy solutions to address these health inequities.

COVID-19 and Migrant Communities
Global Impact
The COVID-19 pandemic has tested and continues to test health care systems—both strong and weak. Globally speaking, it has disproportionately affected migrants' ability to access care and social assistance to protect themselves from the virus. Containment has been difficult in communities and refugee camps alike. Current data show that lack of action and the barriers to helping displaced persons will cost host countries greatly (Dempster et al., 2020). Refugee and internally displaced

persons (IDP) camps are commonly overcrowded and lack proper sanitary conditions, and children often suffer from malnutrition. The spread of misinformation among community members also works against public health efforts to contain the spread of diseases (Raju & Ayeb-Karlsson, 2020). The COVID-19 pandemic makes it more difficult to ensure the safety and well-being of displaced persons living in camps. Nevertheless, it is possible to take steps to minimize the risk of exposure to COVID-19.

The largest refugee camp in the world is in Cox's Bazar, Bangladesh. This is the second poorest district in the country and home to approximately 890,000 Rohingya refugees who have fled persecution in Myanmar (Vince, 2020; UNHCR, 2021c). While humanitarian efforts are being made to increase water and sanitation and to designate areas to isolate those who have become infected, a modeling prediction by Truelove et al. (2020) urged politicians and the public health community to be proactive in building systems that protect refugees and cater to their needs and do not merely offer a quick or temporary service. In this model, an epidemic was simulated within the camps at low, moderate, and high transmission rates, and the results for each scenario were catastrophic for the already fragile health care system. These predictions were on target with how the pandemic played out in Cox's Bazar. Hospitals did not have enough capacity or health care workers, and not all health care workers had the necessary training or skills to contain the spread of the disease and treat infected patients (Truelove et al., 2020). In a phone survey conducted randomly among the refugee population in Cox's Bazar, 24.6 percent of those surveyed reported having fever, dry cough, and/or fatigue. These are the three most common symptoms of COVID-19 (Barua & Karia, 2020). Some camps have resorted to trying unconventional strategies to treat COVID-19 patients. Cox's Bazar, however, has leveraged its community health workers to aid and respond to confirmed positive cases and educate the community on infection prevention. Despite these efforts, there have been setbacks. In a study conducted by Yale University, only 35 percent of the 120 study participants sought treatment from health care providers at the camp (Lopez-Pena et al., 2020). While suggestions made by the World Health Organization (WHO) and International Rescue Committee—such as mobilizing community health workers, implementing a more hygienic system, and inoculating refugees—will improve disease prevention and containment, large, overcrowded camps still pose a significant threat to refugee health.

Aside from officially designated camps, some host countries are making efforts to include migrant communities in their COVID-19 response plans, while other countries have neglected these communities and failed to include them in their mitigation efforts. For instance, Singapore did not include migrant workers in its COVID-19 containment plan. The government quarantined workers in large groups and excluded them from relief efforts. When the government issued face masks to all Singaporeans in early February 2020, migrant workers were excluded. This neglect quickly hampered containment efforts, as the number of new infections among migrant workers residing in dormitories was 82 times higher than the number of new cases reported among Singapore's permanent residents (Yea, 2020; Beaubien, 2020). Migrant workers are deemed essential to keep our world running but are invisible when it comes to providing them with access to health care and safe working conditions. Disregarding the well-being of migrant workers will lead to higher death rates if they continue to be excluded from the health protections and aid provided to host country citizens.

Though most wealthy countries are moving on from the COVID-19 crisis, conditions in many low-income countries have worsened because of conflict, insufficient health care infrastructure, and lack of vaccine access. In mid-May 2021, a conflict between the Israeli government and Hamas (an extremist Palestinian group) took many lives in the Gaza Strip, creating a dire humanitarian crisis that was worsened by the pandemic. Around 2,000 Palestinians were injured, and 113,000 displaced people sought shelter and protection (OCHA, 2021). Because of this conflict, the primary COVID-19 testing and vaccination center in Gaza, Hala Al Shwa Primary Healthcare Center, was closed and all vaccine administration was halted (Palestinian Ministry of Health, 2021b). Additionally, targeted attacks reduced some Palestinians' access to health care. For example, Israeli warplanes targeted 24 health facilities and their surrounding roads, which caused facility closures and the deaths of health care personnel (Palestinian Ministry of Health, 2021a). Israeli military rockets also struck the Al-Shati refugee camp, which houses around 79,000 refugees. The violence left many people internally displaced, and there is a lack of health care and vaccine access among Palestinians in the Gaza Strip. Additionally, as of summer 2021, only around 5 percent of Palestinians had been fully vaccinated (Doctors Without Borders, 2021), compared to more than 50 percent of Israelis (Rossman et al., 2021). These conditions, coupled with the crowding of many Palestinians into shelters, caused an increase in COVID-19 cases soon after the initial violence. More than 1,000 cases were reported each day in early to mid-May 2021, and these numbers spiked dramatically because of the combination of overcrowding and lack of hospital infrastructure in many areas along the Gaza Strip (Doctors Without Borders, 2021). On May 31, 2021, a few days after the air strikes, 337,191 confirmed cases of COVID-19 and 3,765 deaths had been reported (UN, 2021). Without proper facilities, health care personnel, and aid to displaced people, COVID-19 cases and death tolls will continue to rise.

In India, a growing population, particularly in urban areas, may be a central component contributing to its current COVID-19 crisis. The population of India has increased significantly over the past two decades. A 2019 UN report indicated that India is expected to increase its population by 273 million between 2019 and 2050. It was estimated that India would surpass China as the world's most populous country by 2027 (UN Department of Economic and Social Affairs, Population Division, 2019), but instead this occurred in 2023, four years earlier than predicted. During the week of May 3, 2021, the number of COVID-19 cases increased more than at any previous point in the pandemic. The number of confirmed cases of COVID-19 was 2,738,957, a 5 percent increase from the weeks prior. The spike in cases was a result of the number of people living in overcrowded areas as well as a lack of access to proper treatment. Many visibly sick people were turned away from facilities because they had not yet been tested for the virus. The spike in cases included younger people, in contrast to prior waves when younger populations were not heavily impacted. A new strain of the virus was also spreading. This strain was called B.1.617.2, or the Delta variant. The Delta variant is 60 percent more transmissible than the Alpha variant first detected in the United Kingdom. The Omicron variant, while appearing to be less severe than previous variants, has continued to put a strain on India's health care infrastructure.

On January 5, 2022, India recorded its first death from the Omicron variant, and the health ministry announced a sixfold increase in cases over a one-week period (BBC News, 2022).

Rural populations in India were also heavily impacted. There are not many hospitals or health care services available to rural populations, and there is also a lack of education and public health resources. Many rural young men who traveled into the city for informal labor migrated back to their rural homes because of the second lockdown. Given the large population of India, shifts in the economy, such as lockdowns brought on by COVID-19, impacted many vulnerable populations. This was especially true for individuals who relied on work in the city to provide for their families. During the previous lockdown, men were passing away from illness and dehydration on the journey back to their rural communities. It is likely that during the May 2021 wave, many outbreaks were worsened by workers coming back home and spreading the virus to family members within multigenerational households.

With a lack of pandemic preparedness, India's health care system was quickly overloaded with a plethora of COVID-19 cases and a lack of medical supplies. There was a dire need for ventilators and a shortage of health care professionals. India tried to combat the medical supply shortage by airlifting ventilators and oxygen concentrators from other countries. During this arduous time, many citizens were hoarding supplies like Remdesivir and oxygen in their homes. This contributed to wide-scale panic and ultimately caused a shortage of lifesaving medications (PTI News, 2021). Though this drastic spike in COVID-19 cases impacted the entire country, certain populations were highly vulnerable to infection. As previously mentioned, both men and women from rural areas who traveled to the city for work were at a high risk for infection. Not only were they at higher risk in overcrowded urban dwellings, where there was a lack of proper mask wearing and hygienic practices, but they could also transmit the virus to their rural communities when they returned because of lockdown measures and a lack of work.

Another vulnerable population among migrants in India was the Kashmiri population living in the Kashmir Valley. Prior to the pandemic, and because of political conflicts, this population had been suffering through a communication blackout with no internet or access to the outside world (Shoib & Arafat, 2020). The pandemic began just after the blackout was lifted, but the population was left with only 2G speeds to access the internet (Shoib & Arafat, 2020). According to Riyaz Wani, a contributing author to South Asian Voices at the Stimson Center, this slow internet connectivity delayed doctors' access to important WHO guidelines on preventing the spread of COVID-19 (Wani, 2020). In addition, many citizens who could not read or write and therefore needed access to videos or in-person conversations to understand COVID-19 information were left further in the dark (Wani, 2020). These preventive issues had a profound influence on the spread of cases among the population in the Kashmir Valley. Similarly, hospitals and clinics in the valley also had too few ventilators and insufficient medical equipment, making it difficult to treat COVID-19 patients. Aside from health care, many Kashmiri children do not have access to schooling because of the lack of connectivity, and people in the region cannot work from home (Wani, 2020). In terms of vaccine administration, many Kashmiri residents were not able to register for the state vaccine service because they lacked connectivity. As of June 2021, approximately 2.8 million vaccinations had been administered in the area, most of which went to security and military personnel residing in the valley. Censorship prevented COVID-19 data and statistics from the Kashmir Valley from being confirmed, so the true impact of COVID-19 in this area is difficult to observe.

The crisis across these countries, among others, has illustrated the great need for emergency preparedness, leadership, and consistency among governmental entities regarding health care access and information for migrant populations. It also demonstrates the need for open lines of communication between vulnerable communities and country leaders. Failing to address the unique needs of migrant communities increases their vulnerability to COVID-19 infection and makes it more difficult for countries to contain the spread of the virus within their borders.

United States

As COVID-19 brought much of the United States to a standstill, lawfully present and undocumented migrants in the country continued to work, as many were deemed essential within the agriculture and health care industries. Foreign-born workers make up nearly 20 percent of the total US labor force. They also make up 20 percent of employment in the service industry, which includes health care support, food preparation and serving, building and grounds cleaning and maintenance, and personal care and service. Migrant workers also account for 13 percent of jobs in natural resources, construction, and maintenance, which include farming, fishing, forestry, construction and extraction, installation, maintenance, and repair jobs (US Department of Labor, 2021). As this demonstrates, many migrant workers are employed in jobs that cannot be performed remotely. Additionally, on average migrant workers are paid less than their native-born counterparts and do not receive job benefits. Working physically demanding jobs for little pay and no health insurance made migrant communities particularly vulnerable to COVID-19. With nearly 7.1 million undocumented immigrants lacking health insurance, and a rise in anti-immigrant policies (Page et al., 2020), the COVID-19 pandemic quickly threatened the lives of migrants and made US containment efforts more difficult.

Adults born outside the United States are "nearly three times as likely to be uninsured as native-born Americans: nearly 32 percent versus 13.4 percent" (US Census Bureau, 2001). While most Americans were asked to stay home and use telehealth services, this was rarely, if ever, an option for undocumented immigrants. Even in nonpandemic times, the only access undocumented immigrants often have to medical care is through emergency departments. During the COVID-19 pandemic, these departments were already overburdened with COVID-19 patients, making it nearly impossible for immigrants to receive health care. A lack of access to emergency departments and the inability to afford typical primary or specialist care led many migrants to rely on inaccurate information on the internet (Samra et al., 2019; Page et al., 2020).

In addition to limited health care access, fear among migrant populations seeking care has grown more pronounced in recent years. Undocumented immigrants do not want to fit the stereotype often placed on them and do not want to appear as though they "require assistance." There is a subliminal apprehension about "not wanting to be a burden to society or experiencing shame when seeking services and concerns about being stigmatized when seeking services" (Hacker et al., 2015). Apprehension about accessing benefits such as the Children's Health Insurance Program (CHIP) and Medicaid further erodes the already limited access immigrants in the United States have to health care and public health resources. A study of immigrant communities in the Rio Grande Valley of Texas found that recent anti-immigration policies and anti-immigrant rhetoric are making already vulnerable communities more vulnerable, and this erosion of health access has been compounding for years (Blackburn & Azurdia Sierra, 2021). Additionally, a 2016 study found that "immigrants perceived these policies as a threat not only to them but also to their families and as sources of criminalization" (Martinez et al., 2016).

The combination of positions as essential workers, "high levels of chronic diseases, chronic stress, and less access to preventative health services" (Ross, Diaz, & Starrels, 2020) means that migrants in the United States are at higher risk of severe COVID-19 infection. Immigration and Customs Enforcement (ICE) is known to target places like medical facilities, which are termed "sensitive locations" (US Immigration and Customs Enforcement, 2023), though recent COVID-19 guidance states that it will "not carry out enforcement operations at or near health care facilities" (US Immigration and Customs Enforcement, 2020). Despite these changes in policy, many immigrants may be deterred from accessing health facilities for fear that the policy will not be enforced. Even migrants detained at ports of entry are at risk of contracting COVID-19 and not receiving medical attention. As of January 2022, there had been more than 32,000 confirmed positive cases across all US detention centers since February 2020 (Montoya-Galvez, 2022). The substandard holding facility conditions make infection by the virus likely not only for those being detained but also for ICE agents and other detention facility personnel. Agents and personnel can then spread the virus to their households and communities.

Additionally, many immigrants have lost access to health services because of changes to the Public Charge Rule and the confusion that surrounds it. Immigrant families are removing their US citizen children from vital programs such as the Supplemental Nutrition Assistance Program (SNAP), CHIP, and Medicaid because they fear that use of the program will eliminate their chance of becoming a citizen (Blackburn & Azurdia Sierra, 2021). Fear, criminalization, and a lack of health care access increase the risk of COVID-19 in migrant communities throughout the United States. It makes them less likely to seek care when they fall ill, and because they are more likely to be employed in sectors with limited to no health care benefits, they are less likely to be able to take time off work when they become ill. A lack of sick leave or company policies that support migrant workers means that migrant workers will come to work when sick and have a higher likelihood of transmitting the virus to other employees, customers, or others on their commute to work. While this is an issue for many American citizens, it disproportionately affects low-wage workers and industries that typically employ migrants. According to CDC reports, one in five food service workers has admitted to going to work even while feeling severely sick. A lack of paid sick leave in these industries increases the likelihood that low-wage workers will come to work when ill, making it more difficult to control the spread of disease, especially COVID-19 (Ingraham, 2020).

In the earliest months of the COVID-19 pandemic, substantial attention was drawn to US dependence on migrants for the nation's food supply and the difficult working and living conditions that farmworkers experience. Just 40 counties in the United States are responsible for approximately 75 percent of the country's fruit and vegetable supply (Chandra & Lusk, 2021), and the vast majority of fruit and vegetable harvesting is done by migrants. In fact, roughly half of all farmworkers do not have legal status in the United States (Handal et al., 2020). Thus, the food security of the country depends on a subpopulation with few rights and protections—in either labor or health. Even in nonpandemic times, many farmworkers avoid medical treatment because they fear deportation or lack health insurance (Neef, 2020), and the living and working conditions of many farmworkers greatly increased their risk of COVID-19 infection (Corwin, Sinnwell, and Culp, 2021). During the COVID-19 pandemic, many farmworkers reported that their employers did not provide them with protective gear or information, and some employers even denied the existence of COVID-19, saying that it was a government invention (García-Colón, 2020). Thus, substandard housing, a lack of field sanitation practices, a lack of personal protective equipment, crowded conditions, and fear of seeking medical care put migrant farmworkers in the United States at exceptionally high risk of COVID-19 infection and in turn threatened the overall effectiveness of US containment measures.

The COVID-19 pandemic has tested the US economy, health care system, and social safety net. The federal government and individual state governments alike struggled to find a response plan that would contain the virus and support American families through large-scale unemployment. One subpopulation of American residents who have not received adequate attention or support, however, is migrants, particularly those who are undocumented or perform low-wage labor.

Protecting Immigrant Communities Worldwide

Protecting immigrant communities from the COVID-19 pandemic is vital to their health, but also to a country's ability to contain the pandemic. This need to protect the most vulnerable populations in global society is present now and will also be central to containing pandemics of the future. In order to address the shortcomings of the COVID-19 response as it applies to immigrant communities, significant changes to health care, immigration, asylum, and refugee policy will be needed.

Across the United States, immigrant communities experienced a disproportionate health and economic burden because of the COVID-19 pandemic. Any families in which both taxpayers (married and filing jointly) did not have Social Security numbers were excluded from the first payment of the Coronavirus Aid, Relief, and Economic Security (CARES) Act. For the second payment, which provided $1,200 per adult and $500 per child, the exclusion of mixed-status families was amended, and families were eligible as long as one parent had a Social Security number. However, this payment excluded 2.2 million US citizen children who did not have at least one parent with a Social Security number. For the third round of payments, which provided $1,400 per adult and $1,400 per dependent, payments were given to anyone in the household with a Social Security number (Protecting Immigrant Families, 2021). This allowed payments to go to families that had not previously received checks, such as the families of the 2.2 million children excluded in the second round.

While the federal government excluded many immigrants and immigrant families from eligibility for COVID-19 relief through the

CARES Act, some state and local governments sought to provide protections for these groups. For example, the city of Seattle established a $7.9 million direct cash assistance program called the Seattle COVID-19 Disaster Relief Fund for Immigrants (Office of Immigrant and Refugee Affairs, 2021). The program was designated for immigrants who were ineligible for cash payments through the CARES Act. It paid out awards of $1,000 to $3,000 and maintained strict income eligibility requirements. For example, in order to qualify, a family of four had to have a household income of less than $41,513 between January 1 and September 30, 2020 (Office of Immigrant and Refugee Affairs, 2021). The state of California also created new policies and programs that provided relief to immigrant households. In June 2020, the state amended its tax code to allow individuals who paid taxes but did not have a Social Security number eligibility for a tax benefit aimed at low-wage earners with young children. The state also established a $125 million Disaster Relief Assistance for Immigrants fund, which provided assistance for an estimated 125,000 undocumented immigrants in California (Suro & Findling, 2020). These state and local government efforts were important measures that helped bridge some of the gaps, but not all, in immigrant inclusion in pandemic response plans.

The Coronavirus Immigrant Families Protection Act (NILC, 2020), which was introduced on April 3, 2020, in the US House of Representatives by Representative Judy Chu (D-CA-27), would provide much-needed protections by suspending the new public charge policy, providing COVID-19–related services to uninsured individuals, and providing economic support to immigrant families. Since its introduction in the House, no progress has been made on the bill. Then on May 5, 2020, bill S.3609, the Coronavirus Immigrant Families Protection Act, was introduced in the Senate by Senator Mazie Hirono (D-HI). The purpose of this bill is the same as that of the bill introduced in the House. Its goal is to "ensure that all communities have access to urgently needed COVID-19 testing, treatment, public health information, and relief benefits regardless of immigration status or limited English proficiency" (Hirono, 2020).

One important component of the proposed bill is Section 3, titled "Suspension of Adverse Immigration Actions That Deter Immigrant Communities from Seeking Health Services in a Public Health

Emergency." This section aims to make sure that use of health care services does not count against an individual as a "public charge" and that people cannot be detained or removed when at or traveling to "sensitive locations" such as hospitals and clinics. These restrictions would allow immigrants to seek the medical care they need without fear of deportation or adverse consequences when seeking citizenship in the future.

Actions were also taken by countries and cities around the world to address the unique challenges the pandemic posed to immigrant communities. Overall, 151 countries have created or adapted social programs to combat the social, economic, and health impacts of the COVID-19 pandemic. Despite the expansion of these programs, very few address the needs of immigrant communities, and virtually none provide support for undocumented immigrants. Only six countries developed programs that deliberately included migrants of any kind, and all of these programs focused on work permit extensions for lawfully present immigrants. Although almost all 151 countries provided some sort of cash transfer assistance, undocumented immigrants were left out of all these programs. Some countries did take measures aimed at increasing all individuals' access to testing, treatment, and care for COVID-19 specifically. Thailand stated that all medical costs of those infected with COVID-19 would be covered, and Saudi Arabia stated that all individuals in the country, including undocumented immigrants, would have access to free COVID-19 testing and treatment (Gentilini, Almenfi, & Dale, 2020).

Since the beginning of the COVID-19 pandemic, WHO has worked to provide guidance to member states on protecting the health of migrants. The *Interim Guidance for Refugee and Migrant Health in Relation to COVID-19 in the WHO European Region*, which was released on March 25, 2020, reminds the international community of the rights granted to refugees and migrants in the 1951 Refugee Convention and the 1967 Protocol Relating to the Status of Refugees (WHO, 2020). The guidance argues that health initiatives must be extended to all migrants as the primary method to ensure the human right to health. It also challenges member states to provide information in a multitude of languages and to decrease fear in accessing services (WHO, 2020).

In addition to the guidance put forth by WHO, UNHCR has argued that refugees must be included in response plans, and everyone should have equal access to health services. Further, "we cannot allow fear or intolerance to undermine rights or compromise the effectiveness of responses to the global pandemic" (UNHCR, 2020a). Finally, UNHCR, the International Federation of Red Cross and Red Crescent (IFRC), the International Organization for Migration (IOM), and WHO issued joint interim guidance for preventing the spread of COVID-19 in camp and camp-like settings (IASC, 2020). This document centers around the need to scale up preparedness and response efforts. Despite calls from WHO, UNHCR, and others to include migrant communities in COVID-19 response plans, most countries have not developed policies to meet the needs of these communities.

While addressing the migrant population all over the world, change must be implemented at every level. This translates to increasing health access through policies at the local, state, and national levels. These policies must reduce or eliminate financial barriers, improve health care knowledge, and lessen the stigma or shame many migrants encounter. Governments need to improve their health care systems and invest in public health, so that migrants can access health care without discrimination or unnecessary barriers such as complex paperwork (Scribner, 2017). Changes in public policy are also necessary to avoid the fear and legal barriers that migrants face while seeking health care. All migrants, whether documented or undocumented, whether they were forcibly displaced or immigrated voluntarily, deserve the universal right to health.

References

ACAPS (Assessment Capacities Project). (2020, August 8). Jordan Syrian refugees. Accessed June 16, 2021. https://www.acaps.org/country/jordan/crisis/syrian-refugees

Bahar, D., Dooley, M., & Selee, A. (2020, September 14). Venezuelan migration, crime, and misperceptions: A review of data from Colombia, Peru, and Chile. Migration Policy Institute. Accessed June 2021. https://www.migrationpolicy.org/research/venezuelan-immigration-crime-colombia-peru-chile

Bajekal, N. (2021, April 29). How did India's COVID-19 crisis become a catastrophe? *Time*. https://time.com/5964796/india-covid-19-failure/

Barua, A., & Karia, R. H. (2020, October 6). Challenges faced by Rohingya refugees in the COVID-19 pandemic. *Annals of Global Health*. https://www.annalsofglobalhealth.org/articles/10.5334/aogh.3052/

BBC News. (2022, January 6). Covid-19: India records first death linked to Omicron variant. https://www.bbc.com/news/world-asia-india-59890816

Beaubien, J. (2020, May 3). Singapore was a shining star in COVID-19 control until it wasn't. National Public Radio. https://www.npr.org/sections/goatsandsoda/2020/05/03/849135036/singapore-was-a-shining-star-in-covid-control-until-it-wasnt

Blackburn, C. C., & Azurdia Sierra, L. (2021). Anti-immigrant rhetoric, deteriorating health access, and COVID-19 in the Rio Grande Valley, Texas. *Health Security.* https://doi.org/10.1089/hs.2021.0005

Borjas, G. J. (2013, November 12). The analytics of the wage effect of immigration. *IZA Journal of Development and Migration, 2*(1), 22.

California Department of Social Services. (2020). Coronavirus (COVID-19) disaster relief assistance for immigrants. Accessed July 18, 2020. https://www.cdss.ca.gov/inforesources/immigration/covid-19-drai

Callahan, M. (2021, May 12). The COVID19 crisis in India could cause a global economic chain reaction. Northeastern Global News. https://news.northeastern.edu/2021/05/12/the-covid-19-crisis-in-india-could-cause-a-global-economic-chain-reaction/

Chandra, R., & Lusk, J. L. (2021). Farmer and farm worker illnesses and deaths from COVID-19 and impacts on agricultural output. *PLoS ONE.* https://doi.org/10.1371/journal.pone.0250621

Corwin, C., Sinnwell, E., & Culp, K. (2021). A mobile primary care clinic mitigates an early COVID-19 outbreak among migrant farmworkers in Iowa. *Journal of Agromedicine.* https://www.tandfonline.com/doi/full/10.1080/1059924X.2021.1913272

Dempster, H., Ginn, T., Graham, J., Guerrero Ble, M., Jayasinghe, D., & Shorey, B. (2020, July 8). Locked down and left behind: The impact of COVID-19 on refugees' economic inclusion. Center for Global Development. Accessed August 25, 2020. https://www.cgdev.org/publication/locked-down-and-left-behind-impact-covid-19-refugees-economic-inclusion

DeSilver, D. (2017). Immigrants don't make up a majority of workers in any U.S. industry. Pew Research Center. Accessed July 21, 2020. https://www.pewresearch.org/short-reads/2017/03/16/immigrants-dont-make-up-a-majority-of-workers-in-any-u-s-industry/

De Vito, E., de Waure, C., Specchia, M. L., & Ricciardi, W. (2015). *Public health aspects of migrant health: A review of the evidence on health status for undocumented migrants in the European region.* Health Evidence Network Synthesis Report 42. Copenhagen: WHO Regional Office for Europe.

Dickerson, C., & Jordan, M. (2020, April 15). South Dakota meat plant is now country's biggest coronavirus hot spot. *New York Times.* https://www.nytimes.com/2020/04/15/us/coronavirus-south-dakota-meat-plant-refugees.html

Doctors Without Borders—USA. (2021, May 3). Palestinian territories: Alarming increase in COVID-19 cases further strains Gaza's overstretched health care system. https://www.doctorswithoutborders.org/what-we-do/news-stories/news/palestinian-territories-alarming-increase-covid-19-cases-further

Enchautegui, M. E. (2015, October 14). Immigrant and native workers compete for different low-skilled jobs. Urban Wire. Accessed July 21, 2020. http://www .urban.org/urban-wire/immigrant-and-native-workers-compete-different -low-skilled-jobs

Espinel, Z., Chaskel, R., Berg, R. C., Florez, H. J., Gaviria, S. L., Bernal, O., . . . Shultz, J. M. (2020). Venezuelan migrants in Colombia: COVID-19 and mental health. *Lancet Psychiatry, 7*(8), 653–55. doi:10.1016/s2215–0366(20)30242-x

Freier, L. F. (2018, June 28). Understanding the Venezuelan displacement crisis. E-International Relations. Accessed June 2021. https://www.e-ir.info/pdf/74606

Frydenlund, E., Padilla, J. J., & Palacio, K. (2021, April 14). Colombia gives nearly 1 million Venezuelan migrants legal status and right to work. *The Conversation.* Accessed June 2021. https://theconversation.com/colombia-gives-nearly-1 -million-venezuelan-migrants-legal-status-and-right-to-work-155448

García-Colón, I. (2020). The COVID-19 spring and the expendability of guestworkers. *Dialectical Anthropology, 44,* 257–64. https://link.springer .com/content/pdf/10.1007/s10624-020-09601-6.pdf

Gentilini, U., Almenfi, M., & Dale, P. (2020, April 23). Social protection and job responses to COVID-19: A real-time review of country measures. https:// www.ugogentilini.net/wp-content/uploads/2020/04/Country-SP-COVID -responses_April23-1.pdf

Hacker, K., Anies, M., Folb, B., & Zallman, L. (2015, October 30). Barriers to health care for undocumented immigrants: A literature review. National Library of Medicine. Accessed August 26, 2020. https://www.ncbi.nlm.nih.gov/pmc/ articles/PMC4634824/

Haedicke, M. (2020). How coronavirus threatens the seasonal farmworkers at the heart of the American food supply. *The Conversation.* https://theconversation. com/how-coronavirus-threatens-the-seasonal-farmworkers-at-the-heart-of -the-american-food-supply-135252

Handal, A. J., Iglesias-Rios, L., Fleming, P. J., Valentin-Cortes, M. A., & O'Neill, M. S. (2020). "Essential" but expendable: Farmworkers during the COVID-19 pandemic—the Michigan Farmworker Project. *American Journal of Public Health.* https://ajph.aphapublications.org/doi/full/10.2105/AJPH.2020.305947

Hirono, M. K. (2020, May 5). S.3609—Coronavirus Immigrant Families Protection Act. Congress.gov. https://www.congress.gov/bill/116th-congress/senate-bill/ 3609/text

IASC (Inter-Agency Standing Committee). (2020). Scaling-up COVID-19 outbreak readiness and response in camps and camp based settings. IASC, IFRC, IOM, UNHCR, and WHO. https://www.who.int/publications/m/item/scaling-up -covid-19-outbreak-readiness-and-response-in-camps-and-camp-based -settings-(jointly-developed-by-iasc-ifrc-iom-unhcr-who)

Ingraham, C. (2020, March 3). Our lack of paid sick leave will make the coronavirus worse. *Washington Post.* https://www.washingtonpost.com/business/2020/03/ 03/our-lack-paid-sick-leave-will-make-coronavirus-worse/

IOM (International Organization for Migration). (2020). Key migration terms. https://www.iom.int/key-migration-terms

Irwin, R., Gastelum, J., & Burgess, H. (2020, April 21). Coronavirus Immigrant
Families Protection Act targets crucial gaps in COVID-19 relief legislation.
National Immigration Law Center. Accessed July 20, 2020. https://www.nilc
.org/2020/04/03/coronavirus-immigrant-families-protection-act-introduced/
Johns Hopkins University. (2022, January 10). COVID-19 dashboard. Accessed
January 10, 2022. https://coronavirus.jhu.edu/map.html
Kaiser Family Foundation. (2022). Health coverage and care of immigrants. https://
www.kff.org/racial-equity-and-health-policy/fact-sheet/health-coverage-and
-care-of-immigrants/
Katella, K. (2023, January 6). 9 Things Everyone Should Know about the Coronavirus
Outbreak. Yale Medicine. Accessed July 27, 2023. https://www.yalemedicine.org/
news/2019-novel-coronavirus
Kuppalli, K., Gala, P., Cherabuddi, K., Kalantri, S. P., Mohanan, M., Mukherjee, B.,
. . . Pai, M. (2021). India's COVID-19 crisis: A call for international action.
Lancet, 397(10290), 2132–35. https://doi.org/10.1016/s0140-6736(21)01121-1
Lopez-Pena, P., Austin Davis, C., Mushfiq Mobarak, A., & Raihan, S. (2020, May 11).
Prevalence of COVID-19 symptoms, risk factors, and health behaviors in host
and refugee communities in Cox's Bazar: A representative panel study. *Bulletin
of the World Health Organization.* doi:http://dx.doi.org/10.2471/BLT.20.265173
Marrouch, A. (2015, November 10). The economic impacts of Syrian refugees:
Challenges and opportunities in host countries. Accessed August 26, 2020.
https://www.georgetownjournalofinternationalaffairs.org/online-edition/
the-economic-impacts-of-syrian-refugees-challenges-and-opportunities-in
-host-countries (site discontinued)
Martinez, O., Wu, E., Sandfort, T. G. M., Dodge, B., Carballo-Dieguez, A., Pinto,
R. M., Rhodes, S. D., Moya, E. M., & Chavez-Baray, S. M. (2016, December 28).
Evaluating the impact of immigration policies on health status among undocumented immigrants: A systematic review. *Journal of Immigrant and Minority
Health, 17*(3), 947–70.
McQuaid, G., & Fishbein, D. (2020, May 7). COVID-19's distinctive footprint on
immigrants in the United States. *The Hill.* https://thehill.com/opinion/
immigration/496414-covid-19s-distinctive-footprint-on-immigrants-in-
the-united-states
Meer, N., & Villegas, L. (2020, May 27). The impact of COVID-19 on global
migration. GLIMER (Governance and the Local Integration of Migrants and
Europe's Refugees). Accessed August 25, 2020. https://www.glimer.eu/wp
-content/uploads/2020/06/Global-Migration-Policies-and-COVID-19.pdf
Mehrotra, A., and Konina, M. (2020). Situational analysis of internally displaced
persons (IDPs) in the context of international law, Indian law and COVID-19.
International Journal of Law Management and Humanities, 3(6), 334–40. http://
doi.one/10.1732/IJLMH.25113
Misgar, U. L. (2021, June 8). Kashmir: Surviving COVID-19 under the military boot.
Al Jazeera. https://www.aljazeera.com/opinions/2021/6/8/kashmir-surviving
-covid-19-under-the-military-boot

Montoya-Galvez, C. (2022, January 14). Coronavirus infections inside U.S. immigration detention centers surges by 520% in 2022. CBS News. https://www.cbsnews.com/news/immigration-detention-covid-cases-surge/

Neef, A. (2020). Legal and social protection for migrant farm workers: Lessons from COVID-19. *Agriculture and Human Values, 37,* 641–42.

NILC (National Immigration Law Center). (2020, April 3). Coronavirus Immigrant Families Protection Act targets crucial gaps in COVID-19 relief legislation. https://www.nilc.org/2020/04/03/coronavirus-immigrant-families-protection-act-introduced/

NYC Mayor's Office of Immigrant Affairs. (2020). Resources for immigrants during COVID-19. City of New York. https://www1.nyc.gov/site/immigrants/help/city-services/resources-for-immigrant-communities-during-covid-19-pandemic.page

OCHA (Office for the Coordination of Humanitarian Affairs). (2021, May 27). *Occupied Palestinian Territory (oPt): Response to the escalation in the oPt, situation report no. 1, 21–27 May 2021.* https://www.ochaopt.org/content/response-escalation-opt-situation-report-no-1-21-27-may-2021

Office of Immigrant and Refugee Affairs. (2021). Seattle COVID-19 Disaster Relief Fund for Immigrants. https://www.seattle.gov/iandraffairs/programs-and-services/covid-19-disaster-relief-fund-for-immigrants

Page, K. R., Venkataramani, M., Beyrer, C., & Polk, S. (2020). Undocumented U.S. immigrants and Covid-19. *New England Journal of Medicine, 382*(21).

Palestinian Ministry of Health. (2021a, June 9). Dr. Youssef Abu Al-Rish briefs ICRC director-general on the damage to the health system as a result of the recent Israeli attacks. https://www.moh.gov.ps/portal/dr-youssef-abu-al-rish-briefs-icrc-director-general-on-the-damage-to-the-health-system-as-a-result-of-the-recent-israeli-attacks/

Palestinian Ministry of Health. (2021b, May 11). Israeli airstrikes levelled Hala Al Shwa Primary Healthcare Center—Gaza. https://www.moh.gov.ps/portal/israeli-airstrike-levelled-hala-al-shwa-primary-healthcare-centre-gaza/

Passel, J. S., & Cohn, D. (2019). Occupations of unauthorized immigrant workers. Pew Research Center, Hispanic Trends Project. Accessed July 20, 2020. https://www.pewresearch.org/hispanic/2015/03/26/chapter-1-occupations-of-unauthorized-immigrant-workers/

Protecting Immigrant Families. (2021, March 26). Immigrant eligibility for public programs during COVID-19. https://protectingimmigrantfamilies.org/immigrant-eligibility-for-public-programs-during-covid-19/

PTI News. (2021, April 26). Hoarding of oxygen, medicines creates panic shortage: Experts. *Indian Express.* https://indianexpress.com/article/india/hoarding-of-oxygen-medicines-creates-panic-shortage-experts-7289367/

Radford, J. (2020). Key findings about U.S. immigrants. Pew Research Center. https://www.pewresearch.org/fact-tank/2019/06/17/key-findings-about-u-s-immigrants/

Raju, E., & Ayeb-Karlsson, S. (2020). COVID-19: How do you self-isolate in a refugee camp? *International Journal of Public Health, 65*(5), 515–17. doi:10.1007/s00038-020-01381-8

Ross, J., Diaz, C., & Starrels, J. (2020). The disproportionate burden of COVID-19 for immigrants in the Bronx, New York. *JAMA Internal Medicine, 180*(8): 1043–44. doi:10.1001/jamainternmed.2020.2131

Rossman, H., Shilo, S., Meir, T., Gorfine, M., Shalit, U., & Segal, E. (2021). COVID-19 dynamics after a national immunization program in Israel. *Nature Medicine, 27,* 1055–61.

Samra, S., Taira, B., Pinheiro, E., Trotzky-Sirr, R., & Schneberk, T. (2019). Undocumented patients in the emergency department: Challenges and opportunities. *Western Journal of Emergency Medicine, 20*(5), 791–98.

Sanche, S., Lin, Y., Xu, C., Romero-Severson, E., Hengartner, N., & Ke, R. (2020). High contagiousness and rapid spread of Severe Acute Respiratory Syndrome Coronavirus 2. *Emerging Infectious Diseases, 26*(7), 1470–77. doi:10.3201/eid2607.200282

Schoch-Spana, M., Bouri, N., Norwood, A., & Rambhia, K. (2009). Preliminary findings: Study of the impact of the 2009 H1N1 influenza pandemic on Latino migrant farm workers in the U.S. Johns Hopkins Center for Health Security. https://www.centerforhealthsecurity.org/our-work/publications/preliminary -findings-study-of-the-impact-of-the-2009-h1n1-influenza-pandemic-on -latino-migrant-farm-workers-in-the-us

Scribner, T. (2017). You are not welcome here anymore: Restoring support for refugee resettlement in the age of Trump. *Journal on Migration and Human Security, 5*(2), 263–84. doi:10.1177/233150241700500203

Shoib, S., & Arafat, S. M. (2020). COVID-19 and the communication blackouts in Kashmir, India. *Lancet Psychiatry, 7*(9), 738. https://doi.org/10.1016/s2215 -0366(20)30338-2

Suro, R., & Findling, H. (2020, July 8). State and local aid for immigrants during the COVID-19 pandemic: Innovating inclusion. Center for Migration Studies. https://doi.org/10.14240/cmsesy070820

Truelove, S., Abrahim, O., Altare, C., Lauer, S. A., Grantz, K. H., Azman, A. S., & Spiegel, P. (2020). The potential impact of COVID-19 in refugee camps in Bangladesh and beyond: A modeling study. *PLoS Medicine, 17*(6), 1–15. doi:10.1371/journal.pmed.1003144

UN (United Nations). (2021, June 2). Staggering health needs emerge in Gaza, following Israel-Hamas conflict. United Nations News. https://news.un.org/ en/story/2021/06/1093262

UN Department of Economic and Social Affairs, Population Division. (2019). *World population prospects 2019: Highlights.* ST/ESA/SER.A/423. https://population. un.org/wpp/publications/files/wpp2019_highlights.pdf

UNHCR (United Nations High Commissioner for Refugees). (2018). Global trends: Forced displacement in 2018. https://reliefweb.int/report/world/unhcr-global -trends-forced-displacement-2018-0#:~:text=Over%20the%20past%20decade %2C%20the,mainly%20by%20the%20Syrian%20conflict.

UNHCR (United Nations High Commissioner for Refugees). (2020a). *UNHCR global trends 2019.* Accessed August 26, 2020. https://www.unhcr.org/statistics/ unhcrstats/5ee200e37/unhcr-global-trends-2019.html

UNHCR (United Nations High Commissioner for Refugees). (2020b, June 18).
1 percent of humanity displaced: UNHCR global trends report. Accessed
August 26, 2020. https://www.unhcr.org/en-us/news/press/2020/6/5ee9db2e4/
1-cent-humanity-displaced-unhcr-global-trends-report.html

UNHCR (United Nations High Commissioner for Refugees). (2021a). Refugee data
finder. Accessed January 10, 2022. https://www.unhcr.org/refugee-statistics/

UNHCR (United Nations High Commissioner for Refugees). (2021b). Refugee data
finder—population figures. Accessed January 10, 2022. https://www.unhcr.org/
refugee-statistics/download/?url=g1pF2Y

UNHCR (United Nations High Commissioner for Refugees). (2021c). Rohingya refugee crisis explained. Accessed January 10, 2022. https://www.unrefugees.org/
news/rohingya-refugee-crisis-explained/

US Census Bureau, Department of Commerce, Economics and Statistics Administration. (2001). *Survey of income and program participation users' guide.* https://
www2.census.gov/programs-surveys/sipp/guidance/SIPP_USERS_Guide_
Third_Edition_2001.pdf

US Department of Labor (2021, May 18). Foreign-born workers: Labor force characteristics—2020. Accessed June 2021. https://www.bls.gov/news.release/archives/
forbrn_05182021.pdf

US Immigration and Customs Enforcement. (2020). ICE guidance on COVID-19.
https://www.ice.gov/coronavirus

US Immigration and Customs Enforcement. (2023). Protected areas enforcement
actions Accessed July 27, 2023. https://www.ice.gov/about-ice/ero/protected
-areas

Vince, G. (2020, March). The world's largest refugee camp prepares for Covid-19.
BMJ Clinical Research. doi:10.1136/bmj.m1205

Wani, R. (2020, May 3). COVID-19 and the interplay of disease and conflict in
Kashmir. Stimson, South Asian Voices. https://southasianvoices.org/covid-19
-and-the-interplay-of-disease-and-conflict-in-kashmir/

WHO (World Health Organization). (2018). Health of refugees and migrants.
Accessed August 25, 2020. https://www.who.int/publications/i/item/health
-of-refugees-and-migrants---who-european-region-(2018)

WHO (World Health Organization). (2020, March 25). Interim guidance for refugee
and migrant health in relation to COVID-19 in the WHO European Region.
Regional Office for Europe. https://apps.who.int/iris/handle/10665/359103

WHO (World Health Organization). (2021). India: WHO coronavirus disease
(COVID-19) dashboard with vaccination data. https://covid19.who.int/region/
searo/country/in

Yea, S. (2020). This is why Singapore's coronavirus cases are growing: A look inside
the dismal living conditions of migrant workers. *The Conversation.* https://
theconversation.com/this-is-why-singapores-coronavirus-cases-are-growing
-a-look-inside-the-dismal-living-conditions-of-migrant-workers-136959

CHAPTER 9

The Contemporaneous COVID-19 Infodemic

RACHEL-PAIGE CASEY

We're not just fighting an epidemic; we're fighting an info-demic. Fake news spreads faster and more easily than this coronavirus and is just as dangerous.
—DR. TEDROS ADHANOM GHEBREYESUS,
director-general of the World Health Organization

SARS-CoV-2 is transmitted through 5G networks. The novel coronavirus is a biological weapon deployed by a nation-state. Genetically modified organisms caused the COVID-19 pandemic. Injecting, swallowing, or bathing in bleach protects against SARS-CoV-2 infection. The pandemic is a hoax fabricated for profit. Masks do not help prevent transmission. The COVID-19 vaccines insert microchips into patients. The pandemic is an elaborate scheme to depopulate the Earth.

ABOVE ARE JUST A HANDFUL OF EXAMPLES OF THE FALSE information disseminated about SARS-CoV-2 and the pandemic it triggered. These ideas, among many others, have spread rapidly throughout the world thanks to pervasive global social media usage. Nearly half the worldwide population uses social media, the primary ecosystem for the spread of conspiracy theories, fake news, disinformation, and misinformation regarding all things related to COVID-19.

This chapter focuses on the infodemic that arose alongside the ongoing COVID-19 pandemic, which has claimed the lives of more than 6 million and infected over 632 million people worldwide, as of this writing (Johns Hopkins University, n.d.). The COVID-19 infodemic consists of the widespread perpetration of erroneous, distorted, or misrepresented information related to SARS-CoV-2 or COVID-19 (the disease it causes). Specifically, the chapter includes a description of infodemiology and its elements, characterization and examination of the COVID-19 infodemic, discussion of the impacts from the COVID-19 infodemic, and an overview of potential approaches and tools to combat the COVID-19 infodemic and mitigate the risk of infodemics in future public health emergencies.

The Ins and Outs of an Infodemic

An infodemic (portmanteau of "information" and "epidemic") is a glut of information that occurs during an epidemic and is characterized by the swift and widespread dissemination of misinformation and disinformation through a plethora of media and informational channels, primarily via electronic or online platforms (Center for Health Security, 2020). The World Health Organization (WHO) further describes an infodemic as the emergence of "too much information including false or misleading information in digital and physical environments during a disease outbreak" (WHO, 2021). The false narratives and advice associated with the disease spur confusion and risk-taking behaviors and increase mistrust in health authorities, thereby undermining public health responses. The uncertainty that many people suffer regarding how to protect their health contributes to intensifying and prolonging infectious disease outbreaks (WHO, 2021).

Misinformation and Disinformation

Misinformation and disinformation both involve the sharing of erroneous information. However, misinformation is not the result of malicious intent, whereas malicious intent is a component in the spread of disinformation (Wayne State University, 2020). Misinformation and disinformation are omnipresent these days, especially on social media platforms like Facebook, Twitter, and TikTok, which provide inaccurate or distorted information about various topics such as vaccine safety and efficacy, genetically modified organisms (GMOs), and COVID-19. Prior to the COVID-19 pandemic, these types of campaigns targeted vaccines, particularly childhood inoculations, and genetically modified (GM) foods to weaken confidence in their safety and utility. These inaccuracies can take many forms: manipulated content, misleading content, fabricated content, imposter content, satire or parody, false connection, and false context (University of Iowa Libraries, 2021).

FAKE NEWS AND DEEPFAKES

Within the ecosystem of misinformation and disinformation lie fake news and deepfakes. Fake news encompasses a broad spectrum of media used to provide erroneous information: product reviews and endorsements, articles, videos, websites, blogs, satirical pieces, and social media posts or comments. Deepfakes are a form of synthetic media in which videos and presentations are developed using artificial intelligence to present fictional depictions of a person or event. The dissemination of false narratives or statements is a detriment to public health in general, but it has an especially disastrous effect in public health emergencies.

The Power of Social Media

In 2020, an estimated 3.6 billion people worldwide used some form of social media, a number projected to swell to 4.4 billion by 2025 (Statista, 2020a). The ubiquity of social media offers a fertile platform for misled or malicious actors to share misinformation and disinformation related to any topic. These platforms serve as powerful amplifiers of rumors and unsubstantiated material and can also be a vehicle for the weaponization of disinformation.

From a technological perspective, tools such as bots are available to broaden the transmission of content. Internet bots are software often employed to perform repetitive tasks. Bots come in a variety of forms: spider, scraper, spam, and, of course, social media. The Overclock Intelligence Agency (OCIA) defines social media bots as "programs that vary in size depending on their function, capability, and design; and can be used on social media platforms to do various useful and malicious tasks while simulating human behavior" (National Protection and Programs Directorate, 2018). Social media bots are programmed to generate messages and posts on platforms that support the ideas of users and behave as a follower. These bots can be programmed to create fake accounts that artificially inflate the number of followers another account has. Common attack methods of social media bots include hashtag hijacking to focus hashtags to attack a specific audience; using a repost storm to repost something under the guise of a parent or martyr; and trendjacking of top-trending topics to target an intended audience (National Protection and Programs Directorate, 2018). A team of researchers at Carnegie Mellon University has been monitoring and analyzing social media bot activity, specifically the activity surrounding the pandemic. This team collected over 200 million tweets discussing the novel coronavirus or COVID-19 pandemic and found that among the top 50 influential "retweeters," 82 percent were bots. Among the top 1,000 "retweeters," 62 percent were bots. These findings reveal that social media is being used to tailor the content that users see, and these tools can be leveraged to spread disinformation about COVID-19 or any other topic.

Sources of Spuriousness

The sources of spurious information are varied and include coordinated campaigns by states or organizations, close-knit communities on the fringes of society, malevolent ne'er-do-wells with self-serving objectives, and misinformed individuals without bad intentions.

STATE ACTORS

Arguably, the most prolific and well-known state to conduct disinformation campaigns is Russia. Other state perpetrators of disinformation campaigns include China, Iran, and North Korea.

NONSTATE ACTORS

Purveyors of disinformation (as well as misinformation) also come in the form of individuals, groups, or communities. An individual or a group may be localized and niche, but even a single person can bend the ear of millions.

THE DISINFORMATION DOZEN

An analysis of antivaccine content pulled from Facebook and Twitter in early 2021 attributed 65 percent of such content on the COVID-19 inoculations to a mere 12 antivaxxers, dubbed the Disinformation Dozen. Related research showed that social media platforms failed to act on 95 percent of the reported COVID-19 and vaccine misinformation. Ongoing tracking of vaccine disinformation on social media reveals that the 20 most prominent antivaxxers account for over two-thirds of the total cross-platform following of 59.2 million users. Additional tracking of 425 antivaccine accounts calculated the total number of followers across platforms at nearly 60 million in December 2020, an increase of over 877,000 from June (Center for Countering Digital Hate, 2021).

Vulnerability to Disinformation

An individual's vulnerability to disinformation is influenced by a variety of factors, both intrinsic and extrinsic.

ADROIT ALGORITHMS

An algorithm, put simply, is a set of instructions constructed to perform a specific task. Social media algorithms are designed to inundate users with targeted advertisements or material. Algorithms have become increasingly ingrained in social media platforms as tools to keep people interacting with the platform.

A 2021 report titled *Malgorithm*, from the Center for Countering Digital Hate (2020), discovered that Instagram's algorithm actively recommends antivaccine and COVID-19 misinformation to users. Additionally, the Instagram algorithm was found to be nudging certain types of users toward extremist content (Center for Countering Digital Hate, 2020). For example, users who interacted with antivaccine content were directed toward anti-Semitic and election conspiracy posts. Similarly, users who interacted with far-right content were directed toward COVID-19 and vaccine misinformation and disinformation.

PSYCHOLOGICAL FACTORS

Emotional factors or cognitive biases can sway beliefs and behaviors. The desire for social acceptance and inclusion is an essential human motivation that often directs interpersonal behavior. Social media sites facilitate connection between geographically dispersed people with congruent interests, values, or beliefs and provide a sense of belonging. These connections can create positive psychosocial welfare, increase social capital, and spur offline interpersonal interactions. Though these effects are often beneficial to an individual or a society, there are pitfalls as well. Given that many people rely on their social networks—family and friends—for what they deem to be trustworthy information and sources, their susceptibility to disinformation rises when it is delivered by someone in their network (Nemr & Gangware, 2019).

The sheer volume of information a person encounters in a day can be overwhelming and confusing, especially when contradictions arise. This inundation can lead an individual to seek cognitive closure for whatever seems unclear. Seeking this closure creates an opening for extremism and polarization to fill in the gaps (Nemr & Gangware, 2019). Confirmation bias is the tendency to seek out or favor information that substantiates a preexisting belief. This can create a vacuum in which people never encounter any challenges to their ideas and assumptions.

The COVID-19 infodemic comprised a creative array of unfounded origin stories, bogus remedies, perilous prevention practices, and outlandish explanations for viral transmission. This section offers an overview of the untrue claims that circulated regarding COVID-19 prevention, treatment, transmission, vaccines, and origin.

Prevention and Treatment

Because this was a novel virus, there was a dearth of both preventive and treatment options. Additionally, the lack of cultural memory and experience with highly pathogenic infectious diseases rendered the population unfamiliar with, if not skeptical of, nonpharmaceutical medical countermeasures and public health interventions to contain the spread of infectious disease. Nonpharmaceutical medical countermeasures include the wearing of personal protective equipment (PPE) like face masks and gloves; public health interventions include social distancing and community shielding.

Masks became a point of contention as inaccurate claims of their inefficacy abounded. The science shows that face masks are an effective countermeasure to significantly reduce the spread of a pathogen transmitted through respiratory droplets, such as SARS-CoV-2. Although prior to COVID-19, the research on face mask efficacy focused on health care workers and various types of masks commonly found in clinical settings, the evidence is mounting in support of the wearing of cloth masks by the general public in subduing the transmission of droplet-borne infectious disease. If masks are worn properly over the mouth and nose, droplets are less likely to spread from the wearer to infect others and to spread to the wearer from an infected individual. Regrettably, the disinformation surrounding masks ranges from simply inaccurate to outrageous, including statements that masks are wholly ineffective, masks increase the risk of contracting the virus, and masks activate the coronavirus hidden in influenza vaccines.

Additionally, the uniqueness of SARS-CoV-2 meant that when it first emerged, there was a critical lack of medical interventions to prevent or treat the infection. Unfortunately, this gap and people's desperation to stay healthy allowed unqualified medical advice to reach the ears of many. For example, several anecdotes involved consuming or bathing in bleach to prevent or treat SARS-CoV-2 infection.

Hydroxychloroquine and chloroquine are immunosuppression and antiparasite medications that are commonly used to prevent and treat malaria but may also be used to treat lupus and rheumatoid arthritis. These drugs were given emergency use authorization by the Food and Drug Administration (FDA) after a request from the Biomedical Advanced Research and Development Authority (BARDA) (FDA, 2020). Lamentably, a number of patients suffered cardiac events and other severe adverse effects as a result of taking these treatments. Though these antimalarial medicines seemed like viable possibilities to control COVID-19, clinical evaluations ultimately concluded that the risks related to the administration of hydroxychloroquine and chloroquine for COVID-19 outweighed the benefits (FDA, 2020).

Transmission

The transmission of SARS-CoV-2 has been falsely attributed to 5G mobile technologies and network infrastructure. 5G is the next-generation cellular communication network that improves on existing 2G, 3G, and 4G infrastructures. The 5G network, along with its predecessors, utilizes radio frequencies to transmit communication data across mobile devices. Radio frequencies are a subset of the electro-magnetic frequency (EMF) spectrum, which is not capable of trans-mitting virions or parasites. Despite this scientific fact, fear remains that the 5G network is being exploited to transmit SARS-CoV-2, stim-ulating the pandemic. Meese, Frith, and Wilken (2020) described two types of COVID-19 conspiracy theories related to 5G. The first is that radiation from 5G weakens the immune system and renders a person more susceptible to the virus. The second is that 5G directly causes COVID-19. The former theory is a derivative of a long-held belief within the anti-5G community that continual exposure to EMF can cause cancer. The latter theory has several variations, but the more prominent offshoots include claims that the COVID-19 pandemic is an attempt to cover up the "deleterious effects of 5G radiation"; that the pandemic emerged from Wuhan, China, the supposed "guinea pig city for 5G"; or that Bill Gates engineered the outbreak to "depopulate an overcrowded planet" (Meese, Frith, & Wilken, 2020).

COVID-19 Vaccines

Vaccine hesitancy predates the pandemic, but a worrisome propor-tion of the US population has reported unwillingness to get vacci-nated against COVID-19. Monmouth University conducted a poll of 800 adults in the United States from April 8 to 12, 2021, and found that about one-fifth of Americans did not intend to get a COVID-19 vaccine (Monmouth University, 2021). This significant prevalence of vaccine hesitancy is attributed partially to concerns about safety and adverse effects; however, fears that the vaccines are a vehicle to insert microchips into patients may also contribute to the issue. Indeed, stud-ies have shown that individuals who depend on social media platforms for information are less willing to be vaccinated (Jennings et al., 2021).

SARS-CoV-2 Origin

A topic of particular scrutiny is the origin of the specific coronavirus that causes COVID-19. Coronaviruses are endemic in bats, pigs, and birds, and bats are known to transmit pandemic-potential coronaviruses to humans. The Coronaviridae family of viruses is large, and its members typically cause mild to moderate upper respiratory tract illnesses, such as the common cold. At present, how the novel coronavirus emerged remains a scientific mystery, but there are several unsupported suppositions regarding its beginning, such as its creation as a biological weapon and its release as a catalyst for pharmaceutical profits.

Perhaps the most terrifying conspiracy theory behind the origin of SARS-CoV-2 is the claim that it is a biological weapon. This fabrication has taken several forms: the virus is a bioweapon deployed by (1) China, (2) the United States in China, or (3) a "deep state" of powerful people with malicious intent.

Less grand is the theory that SARS-CoV-2 was a profit-mongering attempt by the pharmaceutical industry in either the United States or the European Union. This conspiracy states that the virus was concocted by "Big Pharma" to generate new markets for medications and vaccines. Accusations have been made that pharmaceutical patents were submitted prior to the onset of the pandemic or in its earliest days.

The dangers of disinformation, whether in the form of poor medical advice or a conspiracy theory, need significantly more study and evaluation; however, some domino effects are already emerging.

Infodemic Impacts—Public Health and Health Security

Additional research is needed to develop a more comprehensive picture of the effects of an infodemic, both for epidemics in general and for COVID-19 specifically. Erroneous information or advice regarding a disease, its treatment, or its prevention could stimulate vaccine hesitancy, spur panic prescribing, and cause higher rates of morbidity and mortality for other diseases.

Elevated Morbidity and Mortality from the Pandemic Agent

Reluctance or refusal to seek professional medical help for either oneself or others could have negative health consequences, including death. Further, the specious medical advice proffered on the internet and elsewhere may lead people to try hazardous remedies, instigating other health issues and injury. For example, in the United States, there were reports of people misusing cleaning products in attempts to kill the virus. The Centers for Disease Control and Prevention (CDC) conducted an online survey of 502 adults in May 2020, finding that nearly 40 percent of respondents had misused cleaning products, including putting bleach on food, applying household cleaners to skin, misting themselves with disinfectant sprays, inhaling vapors from the cleaners, and drinking or gargling diluted bleach solutions (Gharpure et al., 2020). In summary, this survey showed that one of every three adults in the United States was using chemicals and disinfectants in an unsafe manner in hopes of protection from SARS-CoV-2. Drinking bleach can damage the esophagus, create respiratory problems that can damage airways, or lead to death. Using bleach on the skin can cause chemical burns, and bleach on the eyes can cause permanent nerve damage.

Anecdotal evidence is showing that in the summer of 2021, cases of and fatalities from the novel coronavirus were occurring largely, if not primarily, in people who did not receive a COVID-19 vaccine. Further data collection and analysis are needed to obtain a better picture of the relationship between vaccine hesitancy and COVID-19 incidence and outcomes.

Vaccine Hesitancy

Vaccine hesitancy is a delay in the acceptance of vaccines or a refusal to take them despite availability of vaccine services (WHO, 2014). Vaccine hesitancy not only leaves the person refusing or delaying a vaccination at greater health risk, but also increases the risk of illness for those around them. As more and more people opt out of vaccinations, herd immunity—a form of indirect protection of a population from an infectious disease—will become an unattainable dream. As previously noted, heightened vaccine hesitancy is a trend seen in the COVID-19 pandemic, which has compromised efforts to contain transmission. Given the arguable endemicity of antivaccine sentiments, particularly in the United States, an uptick in delaying or refusing vaccines—either approved and scheduled or emergency authorized—should be expected in future outbreaks.

Panic Prescribing

In a public health emergency like the COVID-19 pandemic, there is great urgency to reveal or formulate prevention and treatment options. The improper prescription of medications could put patients at risk of unpleasant side effects or adverse events. All drugs carry risk, and the use of unnecessary medications heightens those risks. Additionally, a patient's preexisting health issues or comorbidities could conflict with an ill-fitting medication used to combat an infection. In another direction, a sudden surge in the use of a medication for an off-label purpose can result in significant changes in the accessibility and availability of that drug for those who require it for approved applications. For instance, the surge in prescriptions of antimalarial medications created a boom in demand for which supply could not keep up, leaving many without access to much-needed interventions.

Malaria is a life-threatening disease caused by the bites of infected female *Anopheles* mosquitoes; however, it is preventable and curable with vector control and drug treatment. In 2019, there were nearly 230 million cases of malaria worldwide and over 400,000 deaths (WHO, 2021). A survey found that among 3,872 individuals taking antimalarial medications, 6.2 percent were forced to discontinue their medication regimen because of a shortage of the medication at pharmacies (Sirotich et al., 2020). Most of these patients resided in Southeast Asia and Africa, signaling that the repurposing of medications like hydroxychloroquine and chloroquine impeded access of malaria patients to these drugs during the COVID-19 pandemic. These patients reported worse mental and physical health outcomes compared to those who were able to take their antimalarial medications. Though it is understandable, especially in a crisis, to desire a speedy solution to an ailment, the science behind the safety and utility of a medical intervention against a specific disease and the supply of said intervention are unlikely to be instantaneous. Initially, the antimalarials were reasonably proposed as a treatment option for SARS-CoV-2 infections, but studies eventually revealed that they were not a satisfactory option. Indeed, massive studies in which patients are randomly assigned to receive either a drug or a placebo are the gold standard for evaluating the efficacy (and safety) of a drug against a disease, but these trials require a great number of resources, including time, which is in short supply during an emergency.

Elevated Morbidity and Mortality for Other Diseases

Another concern is the opportunity for other diseases, chronic or acute, to worsen or arise with paused medical campaigns and compromised medical care. For instance, cancer care has been inhibited by the COVID-19 pandemic, leaving many patients without adequate treatment or diagnosis. Richards et al. (2020) outlined several reasons for the degradation of cancer care during COVID-19. Preliminary data show that cancer patients seem to be more vulnerable to severe outcomes from infection with SARS-CoV-2, including a greater need for ventilator support and higher mortality rates. Reduced clinical and hospital operations may be postponing proper screening for cancer, thereby delaying diagnosis. For those with a diagnosis, treatment pathways have been modified to reduce the risk of exposure to SARS-CoV-2. The prioritization of COVID-19 has relegated other diseases and care to low importance, leaving many patients with suboptimal or belated care. Finally, clinical trials and other research activities were suspended, limiting therapeutic options and advancement.

Additionally, especially in poor areas with tenuous health care systems, the disruption caused by the pandemic has had severe impacts for tuberculosis, measles, and polio. Tuberculosis (TB), a bacterial infection that attacks the lungs, remained the biggest killer in low- and middle-income countries in 2020. Treating TB generally entails a half-year medication regimen, which can extend to two years if a drug-resistant strain is contracted. As the pandemic began, physicians and other health care providers focused their attention on COVID-19 patients, and TB facilities were repurposed into COVID-19 sites. Additionally, lockdowns created obstacles for TB patients in reaching care and pharmacies (Roberts, 2021). Joint research between the Stop TB Partnership and Imperial College London modeled the impact of COVID-19 on the TB burden, and their worst-case scenario of a three-month lockdown of prepandemic TB services with a 10-month recovery period gave rise to 6.3 million additional cases and 1.4 million excess TB deaths worldwide between 2020 and 2025 (Stop TB Partnership, 2020). In hindsight, we know that the worst-case scenario woefully underestimated the protracted timeline of the COVID-19 pandemic.

Measles is caused by a highly contagious virus typified by a fever, dry cough, runny nose, sore throat, Koplik's spots, and the telltale measles rash. There was a steep rise in measles cases and deaths, especially in young children, in 2019; 413,308 confirmed cases and 207,500 measles-related deaths, compared with 140,000 deaths in 2018, 110,000 deaths in 2017, and 89,780 deaths in 2016 (Rana et al., 2021). This surge is attributed to a lack of measles immunizations, which suffered a further setback when WHO suspended all mass vaccination campaigns at the start of the pandemic and many nations canceled or postponed their own campaigns (Roberts, 2021). Experts assert that we should expect increases in the number of unvaccinated children left susceptible to measles, as well as increases in the case fatality ratios for the disease.

Poliovirus causes a disabling and life-threatening disease that can lead to paralysis. The global efforts to eradicate polio have been significantly undermined as a result of COVID-19. The disease remains endemic in Pakistan and Afghanistan, where cases of wild poliovirus emerged in 2019 and 2020 (Roberts, 2021). In late March 2020, the Global Polio Eradication Initiative suspended all supplementary polio immunization activities and recommended modifications to polio surveillance (Zomahoun et al., 2021). These pauses are leaving the disease largely unchecked and have delayed the goal of eradication.

Infodemic Impacts—Bioeconomy and Biotechnology

The bioeconomy is a growing subset of the overall economy that encompasses an array of fields: biological, physical, agricultural, social, engineering, computer, and information sciences as well as mathematics, medicine, and psychology. Because it is a fledgling concept and unit of study, a universally accepted definition of the bioeconomy remains undetermined; however, it can be roughly described as the employment of research, development, and innovation in the biological sciences in ways that generate economic activity in the production of goods, services, or energy from biological products or processes (Lewandowski, 2018). The Committee on Safeguarding the Bioeconomy at the National Academies of Sciences, Engineering, and Medicine (NASEM) defines the bioeconomy as "economic activity that is driven by research and innovation in the life sciences and biotechnology, and that is enabled by technological advances in engineering and in computing and information sciences," including all products, processes, and services that relate to research, development, and innovation in the life sciences and biotechnology fields (National Academies of Sciences, Engineering, and Medicine, 2020). At present, there is no standardized and universally accepted definition of the bioeconomy, specifically regarding the sectors and products it includes, nor is there a metric for measuring the bioeconomy. According to the committee, there are four primary drivers of the bioeconomy: (1) life sciences, such as biological, biomedical, environmental biological, and agricultural sciences; (2) biotechnologies, such as advanced sequencing, metabolic engineering, epigenetic modulation of gene expression, and gene editing; (3) engineering in areas such as robotics, microfluidics, tissue engineering, and cell culture; and (4) computing and information sciences to include mathematical modeling of experiments to predict outcomes (National Academies of Sciences, Engineering, and Medicine, 2020).

Given the debates—both accurate and otherwise—around medical countermeasures for COVID-19, it is likely that interest in and scrutiny of the biotechnology field as a whole will continue to rise, with consequences reverberating on the bioeconomy. Accurate and clear communication regarding biotechnologies is critical but is made much more complicated with the misinformation and disinformation broadcasted in an infodemic, especially on social media, but also on traditional media platforms. If a large portion of the public becomes uncomfortable with or wary about these powerful tools and techniques, then confidence in their safety and efficacy, and trust in the institutions within the biotechnology sector, will deteriorate. Such erosion could result in significantly negative effects on public health. The antivaccine movement, a quintessential example, and the growing unease about genetic engineering show the potential effects of misinformation and disinformation on the bioeconomy and biotechnology sector.

Antivaccine Movement

The modern campaign aimed at besmirching vaccinations found its roots in the late 1990s when Andrew Wakefield published an unethical study that falsely linked the measles, mumps, and rubella (MMR) vaccine with autism. Wakefield and his colleagues were found to be falsifying major components of the paper, even committing fraud to back up their fabricated results. Despite a retraction of the paper and sound refutations of the results, MMR vaccination rates dropped. Even today, this incident resonates across the media, with antivaxxers using it as evidence to support their stance.

Genetic Engineering

Research on the perceptions of genetically modified organisms (GMOs) and foods finds that reservations about biotechnology tend to govern purchasing behavior. Specifically, consumers are willing to pay a premium for a product free of GMOs (Lusk, 2004). The US Department of Agriculture (USDA) certifies produce as organic if it was grown in soil that had no prohibited substances applied for three years prior to harvest. For organic produce, prohibited substances include most synthetic fertilizers and pesticides (US Department of Agriculture, 2012).

Among the general population, there is limited understanding of the technical aspects of genetic modification along with widespread misconceptions of and unfamiliarity with these foods (Wunderlich & Gatto, 2015). The lack of trust in GM foods is exacerbated by disinformation. An analysis of nearly 95,000 unique online articles about GMOs found that a small collection of alternative health and proconspiracy sites received more total engagements on social media than sites generally regarded as media outlets (*Mother Jones*, NPR, and the *Washington Post*) on the topic of GMOs (Ryan et al., 2020).

Dorius and Lawrence-Dill (2018) found distinct patterns in Russian news that served as evidence of a coordinated information campaign aimed at pivoting US public opinion against genetic engineering, specifically GMOs. In recent years, Russia has been working to brand its own agricultural sector as the "ecologically clean" alternative to genetically engineered foods, indicating an economic motive behind the information campaign against Western biotechnologies. At present, the United States is the top exporting country of agricultural products, with agricultural exports totaling about $140 billion in 2018, according to the USDA (US Department of Agriculture, 2019). In 2019, the US agricultural trade balance was a surplus of US$5.7 billion while Russia held a deficit of almost US$4.2 million (US Department of Agriculture, 2020; Statista, 2020b). The leading theory behind this anti-GMO campaign is that Russia is working to position itself as the "ecologically clean" alternative to the American agriculture industry, in which the majority of farmers produce crops that have been genetically modified to repel insects, survive droughts, and require minimal herbicides for weed control (Cremer, 2018).

Infodemic Impacts—National Security

An infodemic can potentially create national security concerns, such as social instability as a result of distrust in local, regional, and national authorities and entities. Public trust and confidence in science and public health is waning, adding more risk to a disease crisis. The primary concern revolves around vaccine hesitancy. If a large enough proportion of the population chooses to not vaccinate, the country could be left vulnerable to resurgent outbreaks of COVID-19. This would compromise public health but also the economic health of households and the nation. Additionally, the long reach of social media provides political actors with ample opportunity to spread incendiary rhetoric and imagery, which could catalyze mob violence, riots, and vigilante behavior (Ward & Beyer, 2019).

Possible Paths to Improvement

The omnipresence of disinformation in the COVID-19 era requires a variety of tools and techniques to combat its effects.

Infodemiology and Infoveillance

Infodemiology, a concept developed by Gunther Eysenbach (2009), is the "science of distribution and determinants of information in an electronic medium, specifically the Internet, or in a population, with the ultimate aim to inform public health and public policy." Infodemiology examines events and patterns related to infectious diseases and public health in general, such as internet queries in search engines related to disease; status updates of individuals on social media platforms (e.g., Twitter, Instagram, TikTok, and Facebook) for syndromic surveillance; and internet monitoring for the publication of information relevant to public health (e.g., antivaccine movement sites and news outlets).

Studying how people navigate online to find health-related information, what they search for regarding health and disease, and how they communicate and share this information via digital media platforms reveals valuable insights into health behavior (Eysenbach, 2009). Infodemiology includes tools that measure the circulation of information and knowledge translation, which is the "dynamic and iterative process that includes the synthesis, dissemination, exchange and ethically sound application of knowledge to improve health, provide more effective health services and products, and strengthen the health care system" (Straus, Telroe, & Graham, 2009). The basic metrics used in infodemiological study include information prevalence, concept occurrence ratios, and information incidence. Information prevalence and concept occurrence ratios, basic indicators of content published on the internet, "measure the absolute or relative number of occurrences of a certain keyword or concept in a pool of information." Information incidence rates describe the number of new information units created per unit of time (Eysenbach, 2009).

Infoveillance (portmanteau of "information" and "surveillance") is a form of online syndromic surveillance to monitor and detect disease outbreaks. Infoveillance can be active or passive. Active techniques entail user participation in surveillance, such as responding to a survey. Passive infoveillance includes collecting data on search engine queries or website activity.

Disinformation Detection and Deplatforming

Content authentication helps certify the integrity of content and can also verify the identity of the content's originator. Machine learning algorithms can be employed to detect fake news using crowdsourced datasets or other frameworks. Deplatforming is the removal of an account on social media (i.e., Twitter, Facebook, Instagram, YouTube, Reddit) for flouting platform rules regarding extreme content or hate speech. This is an option that platforms themselves can take to remove sources of falsities.

Effective and Efficient Public Health Communication

The effective and efficient communication of accurate information during infectious disease events is a crucial component of a public health response. In such a situation, messaging should help guide and encourage behaviors that protect the population against infection, further transmission, and adverse medical events. Relating health and safety information to the entire population is a delicate task in normal conditions, and even more difficult in a public health emergency. Sadly, communication from health and government authorities in the COVID-19 pandemic lacked consistency and clarity, prompting many to turn to alternative—albeit unreliable and often invalid—sources for insight and advice, provoking the concurrent infodemic. Beyond communication from authoritative sources, communication from the media—traditional and social—can play a detrimental role in a crisis. Ideally, as a primary source of information for many, social media should serve as a far-reaching venue for the dissemination of reliable health information. To improve public health communication, new and improved strategies are needed for public health communication in general, messaging via media platforms, and messaging to counter health misinformation or disinformation.

To improve messaging during a public health crisis, Sauer et al. (2021) recommend rapid and accurate communication with the population, and a focus on "building credibility and trust and showcasing empathy" by using a unified voice. Their recommendation is based on an analysis of the US government's adherence to the Crisis and Emergency Risk Communication (CERC) manual created by the CDC. The six communication principles of CERC are (1) be first, (2) be right, (3) be credible, (4) express empathy, (5) promote action, and (6) show respect (Sauer et al., 2021).

Murthy et al. (2021) developed a novel framework to aid public health experts in tailoring messages that promote health and prevent disease before, during, and after a public health emergency. Their Review, Recognize, and Respond (3 Rs) framework is a systematic process in which health communicators review the target audience, recognize the health communication needs, and respond with tailored messages. Each of the three steps entails specific actions to guide communicators toward effective messaging. The Review step includes identifying the target population in a community, the specific target audience, the social media communication platforms used by the target audience, the literacy levels of the target audience, and the followers and relevant influencers. The Recognize step involves identifying the needs of the target audience following an emergency, conducting rapid surveillance of social media for misinformation or disinformation, and identifying the social media influencers shaping communication. The Respond step entails disseminating customized messages to the relevant target audience, expressing empathy in a bid to build trust and credibility, and analyzing social media metrics and discourse to evaluate the impact of messaging.

Health and Science Literacy

Health literacy is the ability to access, understand, appraise, and apply health information (Okan et al., 2020). Okan et al. (2020) recommend favoring consistency over completeness in information gathering and outputs; seeking primary sources and original data; prioritizing the accuracy of information over being the first to report it; including gray literature (reports from the National Academy of Medicine or congressional legislation, conference abstracts, posters, and other unpublished data); and pursuing collaboration across disciplines.

Scientific Situational Awareness

Scientific situational awareness is generally defined as the "monitoring of citation databases and newer repositories such as preprint servers for publication of new findings and sharing relevant references within organizations or emergency response structures" (Iskander & Bianchi, 2021). Types of scientific repositories and platforms include data dashboards, source codes, and clinical trial databases. Scientific situational awareness is a necessity in the formulation of science-informed policies, especially in response to a public health emergency. In a public health crisis, such awareness would encompass public health surveillance and laboratory testing data, information on relevant health infrastructure, population data, and environmental exposure data (Iskander & Bianchi, 2021).

Conclusion

The COVID-19 infodemic is ongoing, but it can provide lessons learned that can help mitigate the next one. Disinformation and misinformation are rampant and persuasive but can be countered and attenuated through tools and techniques such as infodemiological interventions, disinformation detection and deplatforming, efficient and effective public health communication, health and science literacy, and scientific situational awareness. This list, of course, is far from exhaustive, and additional research is needed to better refine the methods we can employ to improve the integrity of information before it is shared, the public's ability to differentiate between valid and invalid sources of information, and the level of health literacy across the population.

The COVID-19 infodemic should serve as both a dire warning to the health and life sciences community about the dangers that disinformation and misinformation can pose to the health of the population, and a source of motivation to exploit the opportunities afforded by social media to disseminate sound information and advice to the masses.

References

Center for Countering Digital Hate. (2020). *Malgorithm: How Instagram's algorithm publishes misinformation and hate to millions during a pandemic.* https://252f2edd-1c8b-49f5-9bb2-cb57bb47e4ba.filesusr.com/ugd/f4d9b9_89ed644926aa4477a442b55afbeaco0e.pdf

Center for Countering Digital Hate. (2021). *The Disinformation Dozen: Why platforms must act on twelve leading online anti-vaxxers.* https://252f2edd-1c8b-49f5-9bb2-cb57bb47e4ba.filesusr.com/ugd/f4d9b9_b7cedc0553604720b7137f8663366ee5.pdf

Center for Health Security, Johns Hopkins Bloomberg School of Public Health. (2020). *Call for special feature papers: Infodemiology and infodemics.* https://www.liebertpub.com/doi/10.1089/hs.2020.29001.cfp

Cremer, J. (2018, February 28). Russia uses "information warfare" to portray GMOs negatively. Alliance for Science. https://allianceforscience.cornell.edu/blog/2018/02/russia-uses-information-warfare-portray-gmos-negatively/

Dorius, S. F., & Lawrence-Dill, C. J. (2018). Sowing the seeds of skepticism: Russian state news and anti-GMO sentiment. *GM Crops & Food, 9*(2), 53–58. https://doi.org/10.1080/21645698.2018.1454192

Eysenbach, G. (2009). Infodemiology and infoveillance: Framework for an emerging set of public health informatics methods to analyze search, communication and publication behavior on the internet. *Journal of Medical Internet Research, 11*(1), e11. https://doi.org/10.2196/jmir.1157

FDA (US Food and Drug Administration). (2020, June 15). Coronavirus (COVID-19) update: FDA revokes emergency use authorization for chloroquine and hydroxychloroquine. https://www.fda.gov/news-events/press-announcements/coronavirus-covid-19-update-fda-revokes-emergency-use-authorization-chloroquine-and

Gallagher, F. (2020, April 22). Tracking hydroxychloroquine misinformation: How an unproven COVID-19 treatment ended up being endorsed by Trump. *ABC News.* https://abcnews.go.com/Health/tracking-hydroxychloroquine-misinformation-unproven-covid-19-treatment-ended/story?id=70074235

Gharpure, R., Hunter, C. M., Schnall, A. H., Barrett, C. E., Kirby, A. E., Kunz, J., Berling, K., Mercante, J. W., Murphy, J. L., & Garcia-Williams, A. G. (2020). Knowledge and practices regarding safe household cleaning and disinfection for COVID-19 prevention—United States, May 2020. *Morbidity and Mortality Weekly Report, 69*(23), 705–9. https://doi.org/10.15585/mmwr.mm6923e2

Iskander, J. K., & Bianchi, K. M. (2021). Changes in the scientific information environment during the COVID-19 pandemic: The importance of scientific situational awareness in responding to the infodemic. *Health Security, 19*(1), 82–87. https://doi.org/10.1089/hs.2020.0194

Jennings, W., Stoker, G., Willis, H., Valgardsson, V., Gaskell, J., Devine, D., McKay, L., & Mills, M. C. (2021). Lack of trust and social media echo chambers predict COVID-19 vaccine hesitancy. *Health Policy* preprint. https://doi.org/10.1101/2021.01.26.21250246

Johns Hopkins University. (n.d.). COVID-19 dashboard by the Center for Systems Science and Engineering (CSSE) at Johns Hopkins University (JHU) [map]. https://coronavirus.jhu.edu/map.html

Lewandowski, I. (2018). *Bioeconomy: Shaping the transition to a biobased economy.* Berlin: Springer Nature.

Lusk, J. L. (2004). Effect of information about benefits of biotechnology on consumer acceptance of genetically modified food: Evidence from experimental auctions in the United States, England, and France. *European Review of Agriculture Economics, 31*(2), 179–204. https://doi.org/10.1093/erae/31.2.179

Meese, J., Frith, J., & Wilken, R. (2020). COVID-19, 5G conspiracies and infrastructural futures. *Media International Australia, 177*(1), 30–46. https://doi.org/10.1177/1329878X20952165

Monmouth University. (2021). *National: One in five still shun vaccine.* Monmouth University Poll. https://www.monmouth.edu/polling-institute/documents/monmouthpoll_us_041421.pdf/

Murthy, B. P., LeBlanc, T. T., Vagi, S. J., & Avchen, R. N. (2021). Going viral: The 3 Rs of social media messaging during public health emergencies. *Health Security, 19*(1), 75–81. https://doi.org/10.1089/hs.2020.0157

National Academies of Sciences, Engineering, and Medicine. (2020). *Safeguarding the bioeconomy.* Washington, DC: National Academies Press. https://doi.org/10.17226/25525

National Protection and Programs Directorate. (2018). Social media bots overview. Department of Homeland Security. https://niccs.cisa.gov/sites/default/files/documents/pdf/ncsam_socialmediabotsoverview_508.pdf?trackDocs=ncsam_socialmediabotsoverview_508.pdf

Nemr, C., & Gangware, W. (2019). *Weapons of mass distraction: Foreign state-sponsored disinformation in the digital age.* Park Advisors. https://www.state.gov/wp-content/uploads/2019/05/Weapons-of-Mass-Distraction-Foreign-State-Sponsored-Disinformation-in-the-Digital-Age.pdf

Okan, O., Bollweg, T. M., Berens, E.-M., Hurrelmann, K., Bauer, U., & Schaeffer, D. (2020). Coronavirus-related health literacy: A cross-sectional study in adults during the COVID-19 infodemic in Germany. *International Journal of Environmental Research and Public Health, 17*(15), 5503. https://doi.org/10.3390/ijerph17155503

Rana, M. S., Alam, M. M., Ikram, A., Salman, M., Mere, M. O., Usman, M., Umair, M., Zaidi, S. S. Z., & Arshad, Y. (2021). Emergence of measles during the COVID-19 pandemic threatens Pakistan's children and the wider region. *Nature Medicine, 27*(7), 1127–28. https://doi.org/10.1038/s41591-021-01430-6

Richards, M., Anderson, M., Carter, P., Ebert, B. L., & Mossialos, E. (2020). The impact of the COVID-19 pandemic on cancer care. *Nature Cancer*, *1*(6), 565–67. https://doi.org/10.1038/s43018-020-0074-y

Roberts, L. (2021). How COVID hurt the fight against other dangerous diseases. *Nature*, *592*(7855), 502–4. https://doi.org/10.1038/d41586-021-01022-x

Rogers, R. (2020). Deplatforming: Following extreme internet celebrities to Telegram and alternative social media. *European Journal of Communication*, *35*(3), 213–29. https://doi.org/10.1177/0267323120922066

Ryan, C. D., Schaul, A. J., Butner, R., & Swarthout, J. T. (2020). Monetizing disinformation in the attention economy: The case of genetically modified organisms (GMOs). *European Management Journal*, *38*(1), 7–18. https://doi.org/10.1016/j.emj.2019.11.002

Sauer, M. A., Truelove, S., Gerste, A. K., & Limaye, R. J. (2021). A failure to communicate? How public messaging has strained the COVID-19 response in the United States. *Health Security*, *19*(1), 65–74. https://doi.org/10.1089/hs.2020.0190

Sirotich, E., Kennedy, K., Surangiwala, S., Semalulu, T., Larche, M., Liew, J., . . . Hausmann, J. (2020, November 6). Antimalarial drug shortages during the COVID-19 pandemic: Results from the Global Rheumatology Alliance Patient Experience Survey. American College of Rheumatology Convergence 2020. https://acrabstracts.org/abstract/antimalarial-drug-shortages-during-the-covid-19-pandemic-results-from-the-global-rheumatology-alliance-patient-experience-survey/

Statista. (2020a). Number of social media users worldwide from 2017 to 2027. https://www.statista.com/statistics/278414/number-of-worldwide-social-network-users/#:~:text=In%202020%2C%20over%203.6%20billion,almost%204.41%20billion%20in%202025

Statista. (2020b, January 23). Annual agricultural trade balance of Russia from 2014 to 2018. https://www.statista.com/statistics/1071708/agricultural-trade-balance-in-russia/

Stop TB Partnership. (2020). The potential impact of the COVID-19 response on tuberculosis in high-burden countries: A modelling analysis. http://www.stoptb.org/assets/documents/covid/TB%20and%20COVID19_Modelling%20Study_5%20May%202020.pdf

Straus, S. E., Tetroe, J., & Graham, I. (2009). Defining knowledge translation. *Canadian Medical Association Journal*, *181*(3–4), 165–68. https://doi.org/10.1503/cmaj.081229

University of Iowa Libraries. (2021, January 19). Evaluating online information: Types of misinformation. https://guides.lib.uiowa.edu/c.php?g=849536&p=6077637

US Department of Agriculture. (2012). Organic 101: What the USDA organic label means. https://www.usda.gov/media/blog/2012/03/22/organic-101-what-usda-organic-label-means

US Department of Agriculture. (2019, August 20). Agricultural trade. https://www.ers.usda.gov/data-products/ag-and-food-statistics-charting-the-essentials/agricultural-trade/#:~:text=U.S.%20agricultural%20exports%20were%20valued,percent%20increase%20relative%20to%202017.&text=These%20shifts%20in%20U.S.%20agricultural,the%20smallest%20surplus%20since%202006

US Department of Agriculture. (2020, December 7). US agricultural trade data update. https://www.ers.usda.gov/data-products/foreign-agricultural-trade -of the united-states-fatus/us-agricultural-trade-data-update/#Total%20 value%20of%20U.S.%20agricultural%20trade%20and%20trade%20balance ,%20monthly

Ward, M., & Beyer, J. (2019). *Vulnerable landscapes: Case studies of violence and disinformation*. Wilson Center. https://www.wilsoncenter.org/sites/default/ files/media/documents/publication/vulnerable_landscapes_case_studies.pdf

Wayne State University. (2020). Fake news and its intents: Propaganda, disinformation and misinformation. https://guides.lib.wayne.edu/c.php?g=401320&p=2729574

WHO (World Health Organization). (2014). *Report of the Sage Working Group on Vaccine Hesitancy.* https://www.asset-scienceinsociety.eu/sites/default/files/ sage_working_group_revised_report_vaccine_hesitancy.pdf

WHO (World Health Organization). (2021, April 1). Malaria. https://www.who.int/ news-room/fact-sheets/detail/malaria

WHO (World Health Organization). (n.d.). Infodemic. https://www.who.int/health -topics/infodemic#tab=tab_1

Wunderlich, S., & Gatto, K. A. (2015). Consumer perception of genetically modified organisms and sources of information. *Advances in Nutrition, 6*(6), 842–51. https://doi.org/10.3945/an.115.008870

Zomahoun, D. J., Burman, A. L., Snider, C. J., Chauvin, C., Gardner, T., Lickness, J. S., Ahmed, J. A., Diop, O., Gerber, S., & Anand, A. (2021). Impact of COVID-19 pandemic on global poliovirus surveillance. *Morbidity and Mortality Weekly Report, 69*(5152), 1648–52. https://doi.org/10.15585/mmwr .mm695152a4

CHAPTER 10

The Most Deadly Death

COVID-19 and the Spectacle of Media Crises

NATALIE BAKER

The Ghosts of Hobbes and Rousseau

PHILOSOPHER THOMAS HOBBES FAMOUSLY WROTE THAT THE natural state of human behavior in the absence of government is "solitary, poor, nasty, brutish, and short" (Hobbes, 1994). He uses this to justify one of his primary contentions, that formal governance is needed as a way to keep in check the natural urges of humans, who are at their core motivated by selfishness and chaos. In stark contrast to Hobbes's pessimistic views on the natural state of humans is the contention of Jean-Jacques Rousseau that people, by default, are good; it is society that ruins them (Rousseau, 2011). The problem for Rousseau was the advancement of civilization through the development of agriculture, which was how social inequities, and thus human evils, originated. For Rousseau, even though people are good, they are also inherently driven to self-preservation as their end goal. Both Hobbes and Rousseau have made major, if not some of the greatest, impacts on how we have structured governance in the Western world (Graeber & Wengrow, 2021). Either people behave terribly when ungoverned, à la Hobbes, or they are "good" yet always self-interested, in the perspective of Rousseau. Their views have also been some of the fundamental philosophies underpinning how we study and understand human behavior. We can see their dichotomies reverberating in societal responses to crises large and small, most profoundly in popular culture.

William Golding's *Lord of the Flies* is one example. The book and film recount a story in which shipwrecked and stranded boys must create their own version of society (Golding, 1954). Their efforts quickly devolve into tribalism and abject human violence. Golding's story intended to demonstrate that the core of human nature is evil and civilized society is necessary to tame our inner devils. The novel represents what the author believed humans behaved like in the absence of formal governance—a very stark vision of total depravity. Golding falls well in line with Hobbesian thinking, which is rooted in Western Judeo-Christian dichotomies of human good and evil (Khan, Shah, & Bilal, 2021). Yet Dutch historian Rutger Bregman flew to the South Pacific to talk to a few boys from Tonga who went out on a stolen fishing boat one night in 1965. The six boys ended up shipwrecked on a deserted island. Rather than devolving into the debased chaos depicted in Golding's book, the group survived by immediately establishing order and setting rules for cooperation until their serendipitous rescue 15 months later (Bregman, 2019). Their experience directly challenges the depiction of behavior in the book. Bregman underscores that *Lord of the Flies* is fiction; Golding made it all up.

Civic perspectives on approaches to major crises, both domestic and international, embrace a Golding-like, Hobbesian approach to human behavior. Should the landscape of governance and social order be disturbed, then what is assumed to be our natural instincts of panic, pillage, and violence will naturally take over. Hobbes's ideas are written all over *veneer theory*, which informs this approach. As Bregman (2019) explains, veneer theory is "the notion that civilization is nothing more than a thin veneer that will crack at the merest provocation." However, we find case after case of orderly, altruistic behavior when disaster strikes, despite what we are led to believe (see, for example, Dynes, 1994; Mawson, 2005; Rodríguez, Trainor, & and Quarantelli, 2006; Wachtendorf & Kendra, 2006; Kendra & Wachtendorf, 2007; Baker and Denham, 2020). Yet this is still little known to mass media, politicians, and the public, who mostly assume social chaos is normal and Hobbes is right. And even if they do not undergo total degradation into brutishness, people will always act from self-interest. With COVID-19 in early 2020, we saw similar dynamics play out in real time.

COVID-19 in the US Media

"We are all in this together," said Gal Gadot. Six days into a self-imposed lockdown, Gadot, a Hollywood star, blessed her Instagram followers with a celebrity-laden rendition of the John Lennon song "Imagine." Although it seemed like a thoughtful gesture, Gadot was soon derided for her cringeworthy spectacle of celebrity self-indulgence and disconnection from the regular person's experience. As Doyle Greene wrote in 2020:

> After ruminating on how the self-imposed isolation most of us currently endure during the pandemic has made her "philosophical," there is an *a cappella* version of "Imagine" which starts with Gadot singing the first line of the song followed by jump cuts of twenty-one celebrity actors, comedians, and musicians each contributing a line of the song until the sequence cuts back to Gadot delivering the final line. To be sure, the video had good intentions but no matter how melismatic (Sia) or monotone (Zoë Kravitz) the singing is, whether a performance takes itself too seriously (Eddie Benjamin) or not seriously enough (Sarah Silverman), there is a continual air of self-importance and even condescension.

Gadot's oblivious display of communal narcissism and out-of-touch disregard marked the beginning of the parade of ill-informed pontifications about the course of the impending multiyear pandemic that made its rounds on social media. What it seemed to say was not that we are all in this together, but rather that *we all need to keep ourselves together, lest we all fall apart and die.* What really happened was that we ended up apart. Or so we are told. Echoing Gadot's vision of a peaceful, utopian pandemic experience, and similarly packaged, branded, and marketed on TV commercials and in corporate newscasts in the United States, were the "we are all in this together" tropes, much like Gadot's sentiments. The ghost of Hobbes bellowed from his grave, where contrasting discourses of human hatred and political vitriol emerged during the course of the pandemic as amplified in communicative media. "We are all in this together," the commercials and newscasters said, but not really. We were not together, but six feet apart. If not six feet apart, then six feet deep.

With COVID-19, one's closest friends and family were a potential vector of death. Media discourses set the stage for the perfect conditions for humanity to crumble through an apocalyptic plague. In the pandemic we had a mix of the Hobbesian-Rousseauian every man for himself in the so-called toilet paper panics of mid-2020 (Andrew, 2020; Moore, 2020; Taylor, 2020). In reality, it is not unreasonable to purchase supplies in an impending disaster; it is in fact recommended. Repeated diametric rhetorics used in the media response to the pandemic evoked images of war and destruction, panic and fear, contrasted with the need for some form of togetherness. There was no in-between, no nuance.

We are on the frontlines in the war against the virus. Frontline, essential workers are the *heroes of the pandemic.* Much of this echoed post–Cold War and 9/11 good-versus-evil polemics, which have been capitalized on over decades to create the neoliberal security state (Masco, 2014). Indeed, *we are all in this together in a conflict against an invisible enemy in a new normal yet unprecedented situation of potential horrific death and destruction, greater than we have ever known* is no new set of rhetorics. Replace "pandemic" with "communism" or "terrorism," and it is the same set of constructs. In reality, a virus is not an enemy and it does not know of the war against it. It just goes on its way, replicating. The virus does not care whether we live or die; it wants to replicate only out of pure self-interest.

COVID-19 did kill many people. However, mundane deaths still occurred and were overshadowed by a pandemic elevated to the most important story of all. In 2020, heart disease killed almost 700,000 and cancer followed in a close second, taking the lives of 598,932 people. The pandemic took over 300,000 lives in 2020, which was the third leading cause of death that year in the United States (Ahmad & Anderson, 2021). Missing from the top 10 causes of death in the same year were drug overdoses. In 2021, the Centers for Disease Control and Prevention (CDC) stated, "There were an estimated 100,306 drug overdose deaths in the United States during the 12-month period ending in April 2021, an increase of 28.5% from the 78,056 deaths during the same period the year before" (CDC, 2021). These deaths, even without COVID-19, happen all the time, statistically speaking. During the pandemic, however, the deaths from heart disease and cancer combined topped over a million people, as they do every year. Yet in 2020, they barely seemed to matter in media discourse, where COVID-19 was elevated to the status of an existential threat within media and political discourse, reinforcing the core philosophies underpinning American society. This gets at answering the question, How is it that one version of death becomes much more important than others?

Crises as Hobbesian Spectacle

While the pandemic was without question a very real experience, the ways it was portrayed in mass media and its influence on both government and even civic perspectives were pure spectacle. As Guy Debord (1995) explained, "The spectacle appears at once as society itself, as a part of society and as a means of unification. As a part of society, it is that sector where all attention, all consciousness converges.... The spectacle is not a collection of images; rather, it is a social relationship between people that is mediated by images." Spectacle is closely connected to the ideas of Jean Baudrillard, in particular those of hyperreality and simulacra. Baudrillard and his contemporaries (e.g., Gilles Deleuze, Jean-François Lyotard, Michel Foucault, Jacques Derrida, and Ferdinand de Saussure) generally accepted that human reality is constructed through symbols and signs. This is part of what we believe to be reality. Mediated culture, including television, news, and now social media, is a major component of what shapes reality, which is also simulated; it is not actual reality (Baudrillard, 1994). What this means is that how we understand shared experiences and what we perceive as *reality* are highly influenced by mediated culture.

The *hyperreal*, combined with a fixation on the *extraordinary*, or in this case crisis and catastrophe, is created in popular culture. It is highly influential in what people come to know of the world. As Bregman (2019) writes, "Most books are also about the exceptional. The biggest history bestsellers are invariably about catastrophes and adversity, tyranny and oppression. About war, war, and to spice things up a little, war." This is no surprise, given the role of spectacle in how people make sense of world events, which is especially amplified in modern communication technologies. However, it is troubling when considering an argument brought forth by Achilles Mbembe (2016) in his book *Necropolitics*. He suggests, "No impenetrable separation exists between the screen and life. Life now transpires on the screen, and the screen is now the plastic and simulated form of living."

Hyperreality, simulacra, and spectacle influence both national and international security concerns. This also applies to pandemics (Masco, 2014; Ehsen & Alam, 2021). Critical security studies scholars have argued for decades about the alarming ease with which reality and fantasy become conflated (Hansen, 1997). Lene Hansen (1997) points out, "Security has now entered the realm of hyperreality, it does not refer to anything real but is part of a self-referring system, which is per-ceived as more real than reality." Security, in the face of the unknown, is positioned as a fundamental human need. Ekberg (2007) argues, "Risk can be real or imaginary, but people believe the threats are real whether or not they actually exist. It is clear from a large body of relevant schol-arship such perceived risks actually exist in the private consciousness of individuals and public consciousness of society." This is irrespective of whether or how they actually affect people.

Societal security, then, is in many cases a performance, and one that emphasizes control. This is reinforced and reiterated within medi-ated popular culture, especially within rhetorics shared in mass and social media that reinforce good-versus-evil polemics, permeated with Hobbesian (and to some extent Rousseauian) undertones. Good and evil discourses bombard mass media in matters of security (Baker & Jones, 2019). The concept of societal crises as represented in the exis-tential security threat, vis-à-vis disaster, calamity, apocalypse, and now pandemics, creates spaces for problematic discourses (e.g., COVID as apocalypse) that influence how reality is experienced on the ground in the form of human action.

Modern threat spectacle is made possible because of inherent polemics that constitute modern America, with origins in the philoso-phies that underpin the structure of society. In this case, safety and its associates (e.g., security and its presumed rationality) are superior to their opposite states, as they are dependent on the exclusion and marginalization of their subordinate counters (Farmer, 1997). The United States and other modern, high-income societies imagine themselves as constantly under threat of existential elimination. Post–World War II North American history in particular is intimately tied to the idea of fighting some version of an enemy (Ambrose & Brinkley, 1997). This enemy has shifted forms from communism in the post–World War II and Cold War contexts, to nuclear obliteration, Islamic terrorism, and now infectious disease.

Many of us believed we were threatened by the greatest enemy of all. An invisible, not well understood, pervasive, unbeatable, all-powerful, nonhuman enemy. The pandemic saturated 24/7 news discourse for almost two years—that is, until the next global threat took over. We were all living a full-time apocalypse simulacrum of the security society Kabuki theater. Despite the damage it caused, the pandemic was not existentially threatening to the extent that it would have wiped out humanity, which is what is meant by "existential threat." However, a simple Google search combining terms such as "COVID" and "existential threat" (or similar terms) yields countless hits that declare the virus to be a world ender, or something even more sinister.

A COVID-19 Zombie Apocalypse

Many discussions in the media treated COVID-19 as an unprecedented apocalypse and the deaths resulting from infection as unprecedented. In this sense, COVID-19 was a little different from most typical crises in the prepandemic context, such as natural disasters or terrorism, in that it was on a global scale. However, the factors that determine which risk one is to worry about more than another depend on the security discourses elevated as crucial by those in power and their mouthpieces— that is, media who have control over information and how it is shared. COVID-19 was presented as an existential threat to humanity in many ways, and this set the stage for "requiring emergency measures and justifying actions outside the normal bounds of political procedure" (Buzan, Wæver, & de Wilde, 1998).

One particularly tenacious set of discourses that pervaded the early days of the pandemic demonstrates this point. In the United States, the brain-hungry undead have formed a culture of their own, and there is even a subgenre of academic literature dedicated to the topic (McIntosh & Leverette, 2008; Hubner, Leaning, & Manning, 2015; Payne 2017). In this alternate world created by Hollywood and fiction, "zombies engender mass panic, social dislocation and collapse, conflict, terror, catastrophe of apocalyptic proportions" (Hannah & Wilkinson, 2016). Zombie mythologies creak into the shady precipices of human desire that long to know what might happen should there be a collapse of modern society in the wake of an external threat (Drezner, 2014). Enter, yet again, a Hobbesian-Rousseauian hellscape of every man for himself—but now with zombies. COVID-19 fits well into the bizarre and unfortunately undying collective fetish for zombies left by the 2014 Ebola virus nonevent in the United States.

Ebola perhaps had a more obvious connection with these fictional monsters given its grotesque hemorrhagic qualities. The number of references to the zombie apocalypse and both Ebola and COVID-19 is uncountable. As much as zombies are not real, something about crisis pandemics brings a bit of humanity's propensities for darkness to the forefront. The 2014 case of Ebola in the United States provides some insight. Certain government actors and members of the public wanted to shut down society and take away liberties to prevent disease spread, but that did not happen because there was no real pandemic. Polemics were a major undercurrent of the reaction to Ebola, which was emblematic of what occurs when infections are "foreign": nationalism versus globalism, capitalism versus socialism, racism versus anti-racism, all dichotomies considered, ad infinitum (Baker, Samonas, & Artello, 2015). It was similar for COVID-19, although it looked much different given the extent of the pandemic.

Once it was certain that COVID-19 was going to materialize as a pandemic, but not a zombie apocalypse, it seemed reasonable to justify limitations on human freedoms (i.e., societal lockdowns) in the name of the greater good. This arises from the perspective that people must be controlled through government intervention in the Hobbesian sense. Despite evidence, many, including Gal Gadot, self-isolated on their own without harsh laws, strict lockdowns were possibly not terribly effective (Herby, Jonung, & Hanke, 2022), and government intervention via public health was the only effective solution to the pandemic. Black-and-white thinking such as that which so deeply pervades the Hobbesian/Rousseauian perspectives on human behavior prevents visionary solutions and approaches to societal problems. It is also unfortunate that both Hobbes and Rousseau in their general philosophies about the natural state of humans were very wrong.

Lessons Learned

> It is the same with man as with the tree. The more he seeketh to rise into the height and light, the more vigorously do his roots struggle earthward, downward, into the dark and deep—into the evil.
>
> (NIETZSCHE, 2016)

David Graeber and David Wengrow (2021) contend that both Hobbes's and Rousseau's arguments about the natural state of humans were just thought experiments. The authors, an anthropologist and an archaeologist, substantiate their claims with over 500 pages of evidence-supported alternatives to contemporary human history. We are actually quite altruistic, as the prior research on crisis response over decades demonstrates. We also operate from a broad spectrum of behaviors and are generally more inclined to kindness overall, as Bregman (2019) shows. Evil is very difficult for most humans to enact, even though we do it in small ways every day; it is part of the spectrum of traits that constitutes being human. We love to talk about good and evil in our discourses, and there is something about the prospect of the end of the world that we find appealing. The never-ending loom of apocalypse serves as both the paradoxical end of everything and a beginning; it is the potential for "something better" to replace what was not great before.

In the case of the COVID-19 pandemic, there has been a constant nauseating double call and warning to be prepared for whatever the "new normal" will be once it is over, though it will inevitably be replaced by another existential crisis. But worse. Something about modern culture, at least in the United States, really seems to want a crisis to happen. There is a dual intense longing for a crisis to materialize as a way to crack the facade of safety and order that are constituted in the practices of everyday life (de Certeau, 1988). As some scholars argue, safety and order and that very act of day-to-day living can be deeply boring.

Boredom creates spaces for destructive acts to take place, especially in the fictions or even nonfictions we tell to satisfy our need for uncertainty. Or as Kierkegaard (1987) put it: "Since boredom advances and boredom is the root of all evil, no wonder, then, that the world goes backwards, that evil spreads. This can be traced back to the very beginning of the world. The gods were bored; therefore, they created human beings." The advancement of total security and safety as an essential component of society suggests that there is also an equal need for danger and its analogues to justify the need for such security. In this sense, security cannot exist without danger and the continued perpetuation of the notion that somehow society is always at risk of inevitable doom. In this existence, the citizenry must always need governmental intervention in some form to protect itself from itself; humans are inherently evil and or self-interested, according to Hobbes and Rousseau, respectively. But we now know this is not true. Much of our societal disposition toward the good and evil nature of humans (aside from religion) is rooted in a sixteenth-century thought experiment conducted by European philosophers.

There are a few calls to action here. First, psychiatrist Frank Ochberg, one of the progenitors of the concepts of post-traumatic stress disorder and Stockholm syndrome, argues about treatment of traumatic situations in the media. He writes: "When we, the audience, tire of the formulaic, repetitive treatment of trauma in the news, the formula will change. But we may not tire. We may be destined by biology to feed endlessly on other people's horror, distorting our perceptions and understanding of reality. And if that, indeed, is true, a new journalism and new journalist is needed to help us overcome ourselves." Mediated popular culture is a major issue with respect to how it amplifies problematic information, and how this in turn influences action.

This problem goes beyond purposeful misinformation and into the realm of the media shaping how people conceive of perceived reality. It includes public health issues such as pandemics. How do we turn off the simulacrum? By removing our attention from the spectacle, as Ochberg suggests. We give it life through our attention, and when we do not, it goes away. Even further, with respect to popular discourses of public health and crises, Sandset (2021) calls for us to "become more attuned to the mundane, the slow, and the chronic more so than the usual focus of necropolitics on the moment of crisis, the extraordinary, and those spaces that are marked as exceptional." While none of these requests is likely realistic, all of them are a call for those who shape the narratives to be accountable for the fictions and misunderstandings they peddle.

Misconceptions of the natural state perpetuated by Hobbes and Rousseau over centuries are fictions. These stories make sense when we tell crisis narratives in mediated popular culture because if people are inherently unruly and self-interested, then to some extent they require institutional control. If they are not controlled, society falls apart. We see these things happen in news and social media and believe they are real. We believe those who say there were toilet paper panics during COVID-19, when this was a gross exaggeration. We even entertain the prospect that infectious disease might turn us into zombies, or that COVID-19 might kill us all. None of these prospects is even remotely supported by science. However, the threat of ever-impending crises justifies a security state, where safety takes center stage. But when the spectacle is questioned, we realize that it is not our everyday selves that are brutish and selfish; it is the stories that we tell about ourselves that are. In continuing on this path, we miss the opportunities to capitalize on and advance human goodwill, which is much more common than not, especially in crises.

References

Ahmad, F. B., & Anderson, R. N. (2021). The leading causes of death in the US for 2020. *Journal of the American Medical Association, 325*(18), 1829–30. doi:10.1001/jama.2021.5469

Ambrose, S. E., & Brinkley, D. G. (1997). *Rise to globalism: American foreign policy since 1938.* London: Penguin Books UK.

Andrew, S. (2020). The psychology behind why toilet paper, of all things, is the latest coronavirus panic buy. CNN. https://www.cnn.com/2020/03/09/health/toilet-paper-shortages-novel-coronavirus-trnd/index.html

Baker, N. D., & Denham, M. (2020). For a short time, we were the best versions of ourselves: Hurricane Harvey and the ideal of community. *International Journal of Emergency Services, 9*(1).

Baker, N. D., and Jones, N. (2019). A snake who eats the devil's tail: The recursivity of good and evil in the security state. *Media, War and Conflict*. https://doi.org/10.1177%2F1750635219846001

Baker, N., Samonas, S., & Artello, K. (2015). (Not) welcome to the US: Hyper-Ebola and the crisis of misinformation. Short Paper—Ethical, Legal and Social Issues. In L. Palen, M. Büscher, T. Comes, & A. L. Hughes, (Eds.), *Proceedings of the International Association for Information Systems for Crisis Response and Management (ISCRAM) 2015 Conference*, Kristiansand, Norway, May 24–27, 2015.

Baudrillard, J. (1994). *Simulacra and simulation—the body in theory: Histories of cultural materialism*. Translated by S. F. Glaser. Ann Arbor: University of Michigan Press.

Beck, U. (1992). *Risk society: Towards a new modernity*. Newbury Park, CA: Sage Publications.

Beck, U. (1999). *World risk society*. Cambridge, UK: Polity Press.

Bregman, R. (2019). *Humankind: A hopeful history*. New York: Back Bay Books.

Buzan, B., Wæver, O., & de Wilde, J. (1998). *Security: A new framework for analysis*. Boulder, CO: Lynne Rienner.

CDC (Centers for Disease Control and Prevention). (2020). Leading causes of death. https://www.cdc.gov/nchs/fastats/leading-causes-of-death.htm

CDC (Centers for Disease Control and Prevention). (2021). Drug overdose deaths in the U.S. top 100,000 annually. Centers for Disease Control and Prevention. https://www.cdc.gov/nchs/pressroom/nchs_press_releases/2021/20211117.htm

Debord, D. (1995). *The society of the spectacle*. Translated by Donald Nicholson-Smith. Brooklyn, NY: Zone Books.

de Certeau, M. (1988). *The practice of everyday life*. Translated by Steven Rendall. Los Angeles: University of California Press.

Dellamora, R. (1995). *Postmodern apocalypse: Theory and cultural practice at the end*. Philadelphia: University of Pennsylvania Press.

Der Derian, J. (1995). The value of security: Hobbes, Marx, Nietzsche, and Baudrillard. In Ronnie D. Lipschutz (Ed.), *On security* (pp. 24–45). New York: Columbia University Press.

Drezner, D. (2014). *Theories of international relational politics and zombies*. Princeton, NJ: Princeton University Press.

Dynes, R. (1994). Community emergency planning: False assumptions and inappropriate analogies. *International Journal of Mass Emergencies and Disasters*. https://udspace.udel.edu/handle/19716/1626

Ehsen, Z. R., & Alam, K. (2021). Covid-19: An age of fear, simulacra, or reality? *Contemporary Social Science*. doi:10.1080/21582041.2021.1942964

Ekberg, M. (2007). The parameters of the Risk Society: A review and exploration. *Current Sociology, 55*, 343–66.

Farmer, D. (1997). Derrida, deconstruction, and public administration. *American Behavioral Scientist, 41*(1), 12–27. https://doi.org/10.1177/0002764297041001003

Foucault, M. (2008). *The birth of biopolitics: Lectures at the College de France, 1978–1979*. Translated by Graham Burchell. London: Palgrave.

Giddens, A. (1991). *Modernity and self-identity: Self and society in the late modern age.* Palo Alto, CA: Stanford University Press.

Golding, W. (1954). *Lord of the flies.* New York: Perigee Books.

Graeber, D., & Wengrow, D. (2021). *The dawn of everything: A new history of humanity.* New York: Farrar, Straus, and Giroux.

Greene, D. (2020). "Imagine" there's a Covid-19 pandemic. *Film Criticism, 44*(4). https://quod.lib.umich.edu/f/fc/13761232.0044.404?view=text;rgn=main

Hannah, E., & Wilkinson, R. (2016). Zombies and IR: A critical reading. *Politics, 36*(1), 5–18.

Hansen, L. (1997). A case for seduction? Evaluating the poststructuralist conceptualization of security. *Cooperation and Conflict, 32*(4), 369–97.

Herby, J., Jonung, L., & Hanke, S. (2022). A literature review and meta-analysis of the effects of lockdowns on Covid-19 mortality. *Studies in Applied Economics* 200. Johns Hopkins Institute for Applied Economics, Global Health, and the Study of Business Enterprise.

Hobbes, T. (1994). *Leviathan.* Indianapolis, IN: Hackett.

Hubner, L., Leaning, M., & Manning, P. (2015). *The zombie renaissance in popular culture.* New York: Palgrave Macmillan.

Kendra, J., & Wachtendorf, T. (2007). Improvisation, creativity, and the art of emergency management. In C. E. Cummings & E. Stikova, *NATO Security through the Sciences Series: Human and societal dynamics* (vol. 19, pp. 324–35). Amsterdam: IOS Press.

Khan, N. S., Shah, S. Q., & Bilal, M. (2021). Evil in human nature and its reflections in society: With reference to "Lord of the Flies" by Golding. *Sir Syed Journal of Education & Social Research, 4*(1), 72–76.

Kierkegaard, S. (1987). *Either/or, part I.* Edited and translated by Howard V. Hong and Edna H. Hong. Princeton, NJ: Princeton University Press.

Masco, J. (2014). *The theater of operations: National security affect from the Cold War to the War on Terror.* Durham, NC: Duke University Press.

Mawson, A. R. (2005). Understanding mass panic and other collective responses to threat and disaster. *Psychiatry, 68*(2), 95–113.

Mbembe, A. (2016). *Necropolitics.* Durham, NC: Duke University Press.

McIntosh, S., & Leverette, M. (2008). *Zombie culture: Autopsies of the living dead.* Lanham, MD: Scarecrow Press.

Moore, A. (2020). How the coronavirus created a toilet paper shortage. College of Natural Resources News, North Carolina State University. https://cnr.ncsu.edu/news/2020/05/coronavirus-toilet-paper-shortage/

Nietzsche, F. W. (2016). *Thus spoke Zarathustra: A book for all and none.* Translated by Thomas Common. Digireads.com.

Ochberg, F. (1999). Three acts of trauma news, PTSD resources for survivors and caregivers. https://studylib.net/doc/18906284/three-acts-of-trauma

Payne, R. (2017). Laughing off a zombie apocalypse: The value of comedic and satirical narratives. *International Studies Perspectives, 18*(2), 211–24. https://doi.org/10.1093/isp/ekv026.

Rodríguez, H., Trainor, J., & Quarantelli, E. L. (2006). Rising to the challenges of a catastrophe: The emergent and prosocial behavior following Hurricane Katrina. *Annals of the American Academy of Political and Social Science, 604*(1), 82–101.

Rousseau, J. J. (2011). *A discourse upon the origin and the foundation of the inequality among mankind*. San Francisco, CA: Bottom of the Hill Publishing.

Sandset, T. (2021). The necropolitics of COVID-19: Race, class and slow death in an ongoing pandemic. *Global Public Health, 16*(8–9), 1411–23.

Taylor, C. (2020). Here's why people are panic buying and stockpiling toilet paper to cope with coronavirus fears. CNBC. https://www.cnbc.com/2020/03/11/heres -why-people-are-panic-buying-and-stockpiling-toilet-paper.html

Wachtendorf, T., & Kendra, J. (2006). Improvising disaster in the city of jazz: Organizational response to Hurricane Katrina. Social Science Research Council. https://items.ssrc.org/understanding-katrina/improvising-disaster -in-the-city-of-jazz-organizational-response-to-hurricane-katrina/

CHAPTER 11

The Impact of COVID-19 on K–12 Education in the United States

MATTHEW ETCHELLS, LILLIAN BRANNEN, JORDAN DONOP, ERICA MOORHEAD, ERIN A. SINGER, AND TAMRA WALDERON

Introduction

THE DEVASTATING GLOBAL SPREAD OF COVID-19 AND ITS IMPACT on the K–12 education system ravaged face-to-face schooling for educators, students, and parents alike and, in many countries, forced national school closures, leaving educators scrambling to maintain a semblance of structure. As a result, the impact on educator, student, and parent mental health and student growth and achievement will be prolonged and far reaching. Contrary to common assumption, global school closures were not in lockstep with the spread of COVID-19, and the United States only partially closed schools—there was no national school closure in the country during COVID-19. According to the United Nations Educational, Scientific and Cultural Organization (UNESCO), the first recorded national school closure was in Mongolia on February 17, 2020, with 843,766 affected K–12 learners. China's schools were highly affected but remained partially open, with 233,169,621 affected learners. At its most bellicose on April 27, 2020, COVID-19 had led to 163 countrywide closures, affecting 1.2 billion learners (UNESCO, 2021c). For context, this equated to 69.3 percent of the total global enrolled learners experiencing displacement from their traditional learning environment.

This chapter focuses on how COVID-19 impacted US education. Specifically, it focuses on the effects on educators, teacher recruitment and retention, students, parents, mental health, schooling, and K-12 funding and policy, as well as the global impact of COVID-19.

COVID-19 Impact on US Education

In the United States, many schools moved to virtual learning and some schools remained partially open; this meant that 58,663,970 K-12 learners experienced displacement from their traditional learning environment (UNESCO, 2021c). For example, in Texas all K-12 public schools, charter schools, and universities were closed during March and the first part of April 2020 because of COVID-19. As we reached the April 10 deadline to go back to school, the governor of Texas announced that schools would remain closed until the end of the school year in May or June. At that point, school operations shifted from school buildings to synchronous and asynchronous home learning. Texas educators were given a two-week window to create all online content needed for their students, regardless of grade, age range, or special needs, and then were asked by their districts to teach those students entirely virtually.

This dynamic shift in protocol left many teachers across the United States at a loss; without proper training and equipment, instruction in virtual classrooms would be limited, and 66 to 72 percent of mathematics, science, and arts educators reported that teaching their subject during school closures was somewhat to very difficult (Kurtz, 2020). Indeed, teachers showed increased anxiety, stress, and depression during this period because they felt they could not teach their students effectively (Etchells et al., 2021). Katie, a teacher who participated in a study by Etchells et al. (2021), stated that the low participation of her high school students was most likely the result of school not being their first priority, "*because [it's] summer and they're at that age where they can work to help their families. And if you know someone in their family isn't working, they're going to step up, you know.*" She also noted that many of her students could not afford a computer or internet service at their homes and relied on the school and district to provide access to technological services. The school district she worked for eventually provided laptops to students, but she said it took more time than the district had expected to distribute the computers, which most likely contributed to the low student attendance. Danielle, a teacher from a neighboring district, commented that it was almost impossible to engage and maintain the attention of first graders in a virtual classroom (Etchells et al., 2021). Throughout this process, teachers were asked to call parents and students at home and to create physical "packets" for those students who did not have access to computers or the internet.

This narrative was echoed across the country, with 41 percent of all US schools moving to a distance-learning format using paper materials (Berger et al., 2022), The strain of stakeholders was emphasized by Suzanne B. Goldberg, acting assistant secretary for the Office of Civil Rights in the US Department of Education, when she wrote:

> Educators, staff, and school leaders at all educational levels and in all parts of the country have made extraordinary commitments and dedicated their talents, energy, and resources to address the needs of students and families in their communities. Parents, family members, and caregivers have done the same, supporting their students while responding to profound challenges in their own lives. (US Department of Education, 2021c)

The longitudinal effects of the pandemic on the structure of and stakeholders in K–12 education have led to significant impacts and changes in education. The understanding that global K–12 education will flex back to its pre–COVID-19 shape is erroneous. The school systems and people therein have been forever changed by the trauma created by the COVID-19 pandemic (Etchells et al., 2021).

Impact on Educators

School districts across the country tried to keep teachers in schools despite rising cases of COVID-19 and the initial lack of vaccines available for children. Over 139,000 teachers had tested positive for

COVID-19 since the beginning of the pandemic as of mid-March 2022, and the week with the highest number of staff and student cases was the week of January 16, 2022, with 24,995 staff cases and 93,830 student cases as a result of the Omicron variant (Texas Department of State Health Services, 2022). Teachers expressed frustration, exhaustion, and hopelessness as the school year progressed (Etchells et al., 2021; Jotkoff, 2022), and in many cases, teachers and principals decided to leave education altogether (McMurdock, 2022). In an effort to stem the exodus, some states and school districts provided financial bonuses and other support initiatives to teachers. The state of Utah, for example, gave a $1,500 bonus to teachers during the spring of 2021. In North Carolina, Governor Roy Cooper included a May 2021 teacher bonus of $2,000 in his budget proposal, and in Texas, Houston ISD's superintendent initiated a $10,000 recruitment and retention initiative (KHOU-11, 2022). In some states, "proposed teacher pay raises that were shelved in 2020 have been reintroduced in budget bills" (Schwartz, 2021). However, despite the COVID-19 pandemic, graduating preservice teacher college students in Texas are still required to take an additional exam to complete their teacher certification. Some teachers do not think a pay raise will make any difference, saying that it just will not be enough to offset the workload (Schwartz, 2021). Governor Greg Abbott of Texas ordered the Texas Education Agency (TEA) to put together a task force to investigate why teachers were leaving the classroom and what policy changes could help stem the shortage, and recommended flexibility in the alternative teacher certification program in Texas. A study of 919 Texas teachers stated that the COVID-19 pandemic was not the largest reason that teachers had considered leaving the classroom; rather, it was recurrent issues such as being underpaid, overworked, and undervalued (Charles Butt Foundation, 2021).

Teachers saw an increase in the hours they worked during the 2020–21 school year as compared to other fields, which saw a decrease in daily hours worked. This was because many teachers suddenly needed to learn multiple online platforms, increase family communication standards, and potentially juggle multiple forms of synchronous and asynchronous learning. (Gicheva, 2021). A study by the National Council on Teacher Quality analyzed 148 large school districts across the United States and found that more than 40 percent of the districts offered some type of monetary bonus to help with teacher retention, ranging from $350 to $2,500 (Saenz-Armstrong, 2021). More recently, school districts in some states such as Missouri moved to a four-day week in an effort to ameliorate the strain on educators, and "school districts report that when they go to a four-day week, they're attracting veteran teachers from five-day weeks" (Gunn, 2022). Despite these recruitment and retention interventions, the preexisting conditions of teacher attrition in the United States were dialed up during the pandemic. The exodus of educators from the field is set to continue as schools of education see lower enrollment, with 13 percent of institutions claiming significantly lower numbers of students, especially in rural communities (Maxouris & Zdanowicz, 2022).

During the height of the COVID-19 pandemic, reports of teacher deaths from COVID-19 seemed to be on the rise; however, "there is no definitive number that records exactly how many teachers, administrators and school employees have died of COVID-19, though new reports of deaths seem to surface with increasing frequency" (Kaur, 2021). Teachers were understandably apprehensive about returning to schools and campuses for the 2021–22 school year with very little information available about how schools would reopen safely. For example, in Louisiana, despite the rise in cases around the state, the decision to wear masks in schools for the 2021–22 school year was placed on the shoulders of the school districts and not mandated at the state level (Associated Press, 2021). In 2021, the rise of the Alpha and Delta variants of COVID-19 in the United States was recorded, especially among undervaccinated populations, and the transmission rates for the two variants were 50–70 percent higher than that of the original COVID-19 (Sparks, 2021). The most marked indicators that the school system's fuel gauge light was flashing empty were mass teacher shortages (Breslin, 2022), administrators returning to teach in classrooms (WCVB, 2022), and the deployment of the National Guard in New Mexico as classroom support to educators (Green, 2022). While the image of military uniformed personnel was widely reported by the media, the shortage faced by Governor Michelle Lujan Grisham was by no means isolated. Other states were "recruiting any qualified adult to take over classrooms temporarily," with National Guard members in Massachusetts driving school buses, and police in one Oklahoma school serving as substitutes (Green, 2022)

Impact on Students

By the end of the first quarter of 2022, there had been a total of 12,711,006 diagnosed and reported cases of COVID-19 in children, equaling 16,888 cases per 100,000 children. Nineteen percent of all COVID-19 cases reported to states were among children (American Academy of Pediatrics, 2022). Fortunately, children are overall not as adversely affected by COVID-19 as adults (CDC, 2021a). Only 0.1–1.5 percent of all child cases resulted in hospitalization, and children made up 1.3–4.7 percent of hospitalizations (American Academy of Pediatrics, 2022).

Even though COVID-19 does not adversely affect children's physical health at the rates it affects adults (CDC, 2021a), there is no doubt that children have had their lives upended by the pandemic and will bear its consequences for many years to come. Collectively, their mental health deteriorated, and many students are showing increased rates of depression and anxiety and are at risk for unhealthy weight gain from the months spent at home (Meyers, 2021; Nissen, Højgaard, & Thomsen, 2020; Rundle et al., 2020). Suicide attempts by adolescents increased at the onset of COVID-19 and subsequently increased further when students largely returned to school, driven mainly by suicide attempts among adolescent girls (Yard et al., 2021). In winter 2021, this change was most pronounced; emergency department visits for suspected suicide attempts among girls aged 12–17 increased by 50.6 percent compared to the same time in 2019 (Yard et al., 2021). Although the onset of COVID-19 and the rapid transition to virtual learning from home clearly took its toll on the mental health of American teenagers, the extended period of virtual learning and, for some, readjustment to returning to in-person learning presented significant consequences. Furthermore, many students encountered incredible losses and continue to struggle with their mental health amid the ongoing COVID-19 pandemic, according to a press release from the CDC. For example, by October 2021, approximately 143,000 American children had lost a parent or caregiver to COVID-19. More than five million children worldwide suffered similar losses of caregivers (Hillis, N'konzi, & Msemburi, 2022). Additionally, educators continued to report "social and emotional challenges" for their students who were learning virtually (US Department of Education, 2021c).

At the beginning of June 2021, the Office for Civil Rights in the US Department of Education published one of the first reports on the disparate impacts of COVID-19 on American students (US Department of Education, 2021c). The report outlined several observations on the impact of COVID-19 on K–12 and higher education, including the following:

- The pandemic negatively affected academic growth, especially in core subjects, widening preexisting disparities among students.
- Students of color faced greater barriers in accessing and staying engaged with virtual classrooms and technology.
- English language learners met greater challenges in trying to virtually master grade-level content as well as learn English.
- Students with disabilities and special needs experienced significant disruption to the services and aid provided by their school. This increased long-standing disability-based disparities in academic achievement.
- LGBTQ+ students experienced a dual negative effect during COVID-19. First, they experienced higher levels of stress and anxiety from being isolated from their school-based support network of peers, teachers, services, and student organizations. Second, they were at increased risk of an actively negative home environment.
- Nearly all students experienced challenges to their mental health, and these were greater for some students based on their race, gender, and sexual orientation.
- Students experienced increased rates of harassment, violence, and discrimination both in person and online. This was experienced more by girls, LGBTQ+ students, and Asian and Pacific Islander students, affecting their access to educational opportunities.

How these disparities will manifest over time in a traditional class-room setting is yet to unfurl. It is to be expected that challenges experienced during at-home learning will be tracked to the students' school and classroom, and students should not be expected to automatically return to their pre–COVID-19 identity. The need for students to learn to transition from feeling isolated to experiencing the increased anxiety of returning to being close to others, with increased ambient noise, should be considered by educators, administrators, and parents.

Impact on Child Development

Understanding the effect of COVID-19 on child development is important because in early childhood, the involvement and emotional state of primary caregivers has a profound impact on a child's ability to trust and his or her sense of self-confidence or self-sufficiency (Bowers & Yehuda, 2016; Erikson, 1959). Not only have parents and caregivers been more stressed than normal because of COVID-19 (McKegney, 2021), but children have also not had the usual access to other care-givers, such as grandparents, daycare providers, and preschool teachers (Tomlinson, Richter, & Slemming, 2021). Grandmothers in particular play a crucial role in infant survival by helping a new mother by providing a secondary support system of care to a toddler while the mother takes care of her infant (Gopnik, 2016). Because COVID-19 social distancing affected how often young children could see the other caregivers in their lives as well as other high-risk community members, children were at greater risk of experiencing post–COVID-19 delayed and diminished capacity to trust in others and exhibited lower self-efficacy.

Once children reach school age, their development is affected primarily by their interactions with peers and mentors (Erikson, 1959; McKegney, 2021). COVID-19 interrupted this developmental process for children who did not have consistent proximal access to their peers for a variety of reasons. It should be noted that during the first wave of COVID-19 in the spring of 2020, 77 percent of public and 73 percent of private schools reported moving classes to online distance-learning formats (Berger et al., 2022). This meant that students who attended face to face while their friends attended virtually experienced disruption from mandatory quarantines and school closures. Many elementary schools had rotations in recess to keep students within their own classes and limit the potential spread of the virus (Meyers, 2021). Even those fully in person had to maintain their distance and did not have full access to their peers as they would in a typical school year. Because of COVID-19, these cohorts of children did not have the opportunity to discover how to have positive relationships with their peers for over a year, nor could they explore their identity with other children or nurture peer-to-peer relationship skills. This will be especially important to bear in mind as students return to full in-person school and interact with peers after spending a larger, more developmentally integral proportion of their lives with significantly fewer opportunities for peer-to-peer interaction and play than is typical.

Impact on Parents

From the disruption of daily routines; the fusion of school, childcare, and recreational activities; and the shift of roles and relationships, families were thrust into turmoil by COVID-19. In many ways, COVID-19 acted like a catalytic magnifying glass, amplifying preexisting family structures, whether positive or negative. For parents, COVID-19 presented unique challenges as they found themselves at the forefront of their children's education.

Research indicates that family dynamics were intensified by the pandemic. Achterburg et al. (2021) reported a significant increase in negative feelings, such as anxiety, depression, hostility, and sensitivity, in parents during the COVID-19 lockdown. Combined with food scarcity, financial insecurity, and social isolation, these negative feelings translated into an increase in child abuse and neglect as well as the severity of abuse reported (Swedo et al., 2020). Consequently, the family dynamics that were apparent prior to the outbreak of COVID-19 were often reinforced during the lockdown.

Impact on Parents as Pedagogists

Despite their lack of knowledge of pedagogy—the methods and practices of teaching—parents found themselves acting as teachers or facilitating their child's or children's learning. This atypical relationship of children to their learning created a new dynamic because students typically learn from a qualified teacher acting in loco parentis. However, the pandemic inverted this dynamic en masse and positioned parents as pedagogists, placing them in the role of the teacher *in loco magister* (Johnston et al., 2021). According to Nietzel (2021), approximately one-third of Americans aged 25 and older possess a college degree. Therefore, a large portion of American schoolchildren relied on parents with a high school education for support in their learning during COVID-19. Even parents who were properly versed in the content did not possess the pedagogical knowledge to scaffold their child's learning with fidelity. Furthermore, new academic content was introduced in 74 percent of schools during the school closures (Henderson et al., 2020), and parents were "struggling to juggle their jobs and help their children, especially younger ones" (Lambert, 2020). The labor markets were also negatively impacted, with many caregivers needing to work part time rather than full time to compensate for their roles as facilitators of their child's education, as well as providing supervision (Garcia & Cowan, 2022). Parents of younger children, from preschool through grade 2, were often more involved in facilitating their children's learning opportunities (Tal, Tish, & Tal, 2021). In some states, such as California, alternative routes of education other than at-home learning provided directly by a school were home-school programs offered by independent school districts and charter school providers. These programs offered a hybrid between state-provided education and traditional home-school models, supplying teaching guidance from an advisory teacher for support and a curriculum framework for parents to teach themselves. School closures created an influx of children being home-schooled in both traditional and nontraditional home-school designs (Lambert, 2020, 2021).

According to Berger et al. (2022), about half of public school principals in urban areas reported working with internet providers to help students access the internet at home. This was more than the 36 percent of public school principals in rural areas. In addition, public school principals in urban areas sent home hot spots or other internet devices at rates that were a third higher than those of their rural counterparts.

As a result of these challenges, student growth and achievement were hindered during this period, with major implications for future learning and achievement. Furthermore, the inequities in education were exacerbated by COVID-19, imposing more threat to students of historically underrepresented and marginalized populations. Dorn et al. (2021) estimated that students were an average of four months behind in reading and five months in mathematics. Based on student achievement on the state's standardized tests for grades 3–8, the Texas Education Agency (2021) found an increase in the number of students not meeting grade level across all subject areas and grade levels, with only two exceptions. Additionally, face-to-face learners achieved higher levels of proficiency than their virtual counterparts, especially in reading. Many states, such as California, Ohio, and Georgia, filed exemptions and opted out of testing altogether during the 2020–21 school year.

Impact on Educator and Parent Mental Health

Teachers, along with others who serve traumatized populations, are vulnerable to "compassion fatigue" and "shared trauma"—the vicarious experience of trauma through caring for and hearing the stories of people who have gone through potentially traumatic events (Berger, Abu-Raiya, & Benatov, 2016; Cohen, Gagin, & Peled-Avram, 2006; Etchells et al., 2021; Saakvitne, 2002). This can lead to secondary traumatic stress (STS), in which people who have vicarious trauma show symptoms of post-traumatic stress disorder (PTSD) themselves (Berger, Abu-Raiya, & Benatov, 2016; Boscarino, Figley, & Adams, 2004; McCann & Pearlman, 1990). With the onset of COVID-19 came myriad traumatic events for teachers in their own lives, as well as vicarious experiences of traumatic events in the lives of their students. From the first days of the COVID-19 pandemic, teachers exhibited the physical, emotional, and cognitive responses typically seen in people diagnosed with PTSD (Etchells et al., 2021). Many teachers also existed at the nexus of parent and educator; not only did they worry for their own children's mental health response in coping with new heights of uncertainty, but they also had dozens of children under their charge whose well-being they could not guarantee (Etchells et al., 2021). As seen in table 11.1, comparative data on adults in the United States provide evidence that adults overall felt an increase in symptoms of anxiety and depression after the onset of COVID-19.

Table 11.1. Incidence of symptoms of anxiety and depression in adults between 2019 and 2021.

SYMPTOM	AVERAGE IN 2019 (Terlizzi & Schiller, 2021)	LOWEST PERCENTAGE DURING COVID-19 AND THE CORRESPONDING PERIOD (CDC, 2022)	HIGHEST PERCENTAGE DURING COVID-19 AND THE CORRESPONDING PERIOD (CDC, 2022)
Adults who reported feeling symptoms of general anxiety disorder (GAD)	8.1%	24.5% June 23–July 5, 2021	37.2% November 11– November 23, 2020
Adults who reported feeling symptoms of depressive disorder	6.5%	20.9% Both May 26– June 7, 2021, and June 23–July 5, 2021	30.2% December 9–21, 2020
Adults who reported feeling symptoms of GAD and/ or depressive disorder	10.8%	29.0% June 23–July 5, 2021	42.6% November 11– November 23, 2020

At a minimum, three times as many adults reported frequent feelings of anxiety and/or depression during COVID-19 as compared to the average in 2019. At the lowest point in morale during November 2020 and the months following, four to five times as many adults reported showing symptoms. The lowest incidence was at the beginning of the pandemic in spring 2020 and in summer 2021, despite the rise in cases of the Delta variant. Even during the height of the Omicron variant, adults did not show symptoms of anxiety or depression at the levels they did during November 2020 (CDC, 2022).

Caregivers of school-aged children experienced higher levels of "psychological distress and work/social impairment" as compared to their counterparts without children or without school-aged children (Calear et al., 2022). At the beginning of the pandemic and remote learning, the perceived support from the child's school also played a role in the caregiver's mental health. When the school offered flexibility, communication, and connection to the student's peers and school community, parents perceived the school and their new role more positively (Calear et al., 2022).

Impact on Schooling

At the outset of COVID-19, areas with a higher population density, such as large cities, had higher rates of infection because of the proximity in which people lived and worked, but it slowly spread outward to rural areas with lower population density (Penuliar et al., 2020). COVID-19 initially spread to pockets of people in rural areas who worked in close proximity, such as a meatpacking plant in Amarillo, Texas, and then spread to the community, because rural areas tend to have larger populations of older adults with medical conditions and less access to medical care (CDC, 2017; Penuliar et al., 2020). In addition, rural areas do not have equitable access to the internet compared to their urban counterparts, with a third of rural schools having little to no access to the internet (Siegler, 2020b). In Texas, where the total population is 29 million people, an estimated 1.2 to 4.3 million people do not have access to the internet (Busby, Tanberk, & Cooper, 2021; Casselman, 2021; Siegler, 2020a). The lack of access to the internet in rural areas created significant barriers to the logistics and infrastructure of implementing distance education (Siegler, 2020b), and how this affected post–COVID-19 student growth and achievement is yet to be manifested.

Innovative and durable programs and structures have emerged during COVID-19 that may redefine the framework of American education for years to come. In response to the increased demands and decreased resources districts and administrations were presented with during the 2019–21 school years, dispersed education allowed nontraditional approaches to be explored. The role of technology in a student's average school day went from being encouraged to being absolutely critical in order for students to be reached safely. Face-to-face instructional delivery shifted to virtual online platforms such as Zoom, Schoology, Google Meet, and many other virtual conferencing platforms (Etchells et al., 2021). Technological alternatives to the submission of assignments, assessments, and exams were also necessary to reduce physical contact between students and educators, resulting in preexisting learning platforms having to adapt exponentially quickly to meet district needs, as well as other platforms emerging to bridge the dearth of services being offered by myriad competing providers.

Another area reconsidered and redesigned was academic and extracurricular enrichment in schools, such as the daily special rotations schools offered—PE, art, music, theater, and so forth—as well as field trips, summer camps, tutoring sessions, and place-based educational opportunities. Schools were now offering virtual help sessions, Zooming with field experts for research projects, traveling across the world on virtual field trips, integrating different artistic disciplines, and even running full summer camps designed to help fill educational gaps students might be facing, as well as enrich their experiences, all virtually synchronously. Even educators who were teaching in a hybrid model, or fully face to face for certain periods, were embracing the added benefits that new platforms and utilizations of technology could bring to their classroom.

Summer school received an update and redefinition, with new federal funding resulting in "more than $1.2 billion of the $129 billion for public schools [being] flagged for summer and extended-learning programs" (Richards, 2021) through the American Rescue Plan Act of 2021 (Yarmuth, 2021). Many districts across the country are now offering online as well as in-person options for summer school to try to accommodate student academic needs and provide credit recovery options, social opportunities, and placed-based education opportunities by partnering with local experts (Heim, 2021). Although summer school has long needed reevaluation because it has been seen mainly as a punitive and stopgap measure for struggling students (Heim, 2021; Richards, 2021), districts and policymakers discovered that teachers were not signing up to teach summer school in 2021 because they were exhausted and needed rest after the previous two school years (Heim, 2021; Will, 2020). Districts provided incentives for educators to engage in summer school by increasing financial compensation, funded largely by the American Rescue Plan Act of 2021 (Yarmuth, 2021), only to be met by exhausted teachers who were unable to pour more out of their own empty cups (Heim, 2021; Thompson, 2021; Will, 2020). COVID-19 pinpointed areas in education that needed to be redesigned to be more effective and meaningful for learners after COVID-19.

Areas of positive lasting impact, summarized and identified globally, are outlined in an Organization for Economic Co-operation and Development (OECD) report, including increased autonomy of students to manage their own learning, strengthened involvement and cooperation of parents, improved multisectoral coordination in society, increased pedagogical autonomy of teachers, innovative technologies and solutions, and greater social interest in education, as well as strengthened public-private partnerships (Reimers & Scheicher, 2020). Moreover, reflection about all the ways schools had to adapt to ever-changing conditions shows that there could also be possible future implications of more flexible accommodations for nontraditional students whose needs may be better met through programs and methods explored and implemented throughout the pandemic. Students with medical conditions that need to be accommodated as well as other nontraditional needs may be better served with a blend of some of these more flexible options.

Impact on K–12 School Funding and Policy

Throughout federal, state, and local administrations' responses to COVID-19, teachers had to quickly familiarize themselves with a plethora of platforms—some obvious and some less so. Many teachers found themselves unprepared for the responsibilities of teaching in a virtual environment but adapted nonetheless (Etchells et al., 2021). In navigating their districts' online conferencing or learning platform; creating online classes, lessons, and editable assignments that were still developmentally appropriate; converting previously tactile assignments and lessons into a digital format; and learning how to use all the other filler platforms and converters in between, teachers spent countless hours becoming experts in running classes only to have to change or switch platforms later in the school year. Teachers also had to grapple with interacting with and checking on their students online to help ensure their social and emotional development. A greater focus on mental health training, as well as technology training, was being added to the already full plates of educators. As a result of COVID-19, digital literacy and virtual learning dominated teacher professional development.

Although certification and licensure programs relaxed or even waived some of their requirements at the beginning of the pandemic (AACTE, n.d.; Dooley, 2020; Saenz-Armstrong, 2020; Slay, Riley, & Miller, 2020), in response to all the increased demands, educator preparation programs and certification programs had to contemplate how to best prepare their graduates to enter this new career with new job descriptions. Districts attempted to fill the gaps in teacher preparation by assigning district-made technology training, Google teacher certifications, and other training replacements throughout the already hectic school year. In response, educator preparation programs began adding technological knowledge or certifications to their graduates' requirements after teachers were thrown into new teaching modalities during COVID-19 (AACTE, 2020). In Texas, Senate Bill No. 226, enacted into law on September 1, 2021, states that preservice teachers must receive instruction in digital learning, virtual learning, and virtual instruction as part of their certification. The bill also stated that this instruction must (a) align with the teaching standards of the International Society for Technology in Education (ISTE), (b) provide evidence-based strategies to assess and evaluate students' digital literacy, (c) follow best practices in grading students receiving virtual learning, (d) develop curriculum for synchronous and asynchronous virtual instruction, and (e) develop resources to address identified deficiencies in students' digital literacy (Senate Bill No. 226, 2021).

To support policy changes and meet the needs of the American educational system, significant national funding was unlocked. The Coronavirus Aid, Relief, and Economic Security Act, or CARES Act, passed on March 27, 2020 (Office of Postsecondary Education, 2020). The $2 trillion stimulus package included $30.75 billion for an Education Stabilization Fund (Office of Elementary and Secondary Education, 2021). On December 27, 2020, the Coronavirus Response and Relief Supplemental Appropriations Act, 2021 (CRRSA Act) was signed into law and allotted an additional $81.9 billion to the Education Stabilization Fund (Office of Elementary and Secondary Education, 2021). These funds were assigned to state educational agencies to address the impact of COVID-19, including the reopening of schools and addressing academic, social, emotional, and mental health needs during and after the COVID-19 pandemic (US Department of

Education, 2021b). Funds were encouraged to be used to "safely reopen schools, maximize in-person instructional time for all students, and provide opportunities to address the impacts of lost instructional time resulting from the COVID-19 pandemic" (US Department of Education, 2021b). In a transition in the US government, President Joe Biden signed the $1.9 trillion American Rescue Plan, which allocated $130 billion in grants to K–12 schools (White House, 2021). These funds were specifically earmarked to help address "learning loss, social and emotional needs of students disproportionately impacted by COVID-19, including students of color, English learners, and students with disabilities" (White House, 2021). Funds were allocated to states based on need, and many states that were identified as COVID-19 hot spots such as New York, California, Florida, and Texas received more funds than other states. For example, California received the most, $28.6 billion, and had spent $3.4 billion of that as of August 1, 2021. Texas received a total of $25.8 billion and had spent $2.8 billion as of that same date (US Department of Education, 2021a). These funds have been distributed among state educational boards, school districts, and other educational institutions to allow them to decide where to invest.

COVID-19 also produced the first national break in state-mandated testing with Secretary of Education Betsy DeVos's waiver regarding state testing in the spring of 2020 (Olson, 2020). In February 2021, President Biden announced that states would be responsible for state testing during the 2020–21 school year, with flexibility to decide on how to give assessments, including changes such as shortening tests and giving tests in the summer and the following school year (Ujifusa, 2021). The Department of Education urged mandatory state testing for that school year, claiming that it was "vitally important that parents, educators, and the public have access to data on student learning and success" (Rosenblum, 2021). In addition to this resumption, the Department of Education was mandating that states "publicly report other indicators, like chronic absenteeism, as well as, where possible, information on students' access to computers and the Internet for remote learning" (Kamenetz, 2021) in order to "address the educational inequities that have been exacerbated by the pandemic, including by using student learning data to enable states, school districts, and schools to target resources and supports to the students with the greatest needs" (Rosenblum, 2021).

Global Impact of COVID-19

Globally, no two countries have followed the same COVID-19 mitigation policies in education, although there have been parallels. According to the United Nations Children's Fund (UNICEF), one in seven children had missed more than three-quarters of in-person learning since the onset of the COVID-19 pandemic (UNICEF, 2021), before countries moved to return students to in-person learning. From March 2020 to February 2021, schools in 14 countries remained mostly closed, including Bolivia, Panama, and Bangladesh (UNICEF, 2021). While the majority of schools opened in some capacity, the regulations constantly fluctuated in accordance with recommendations from local, state, provincial, and federal governments, as well as health organizations. The response of the general educational system to the pandemic meant that many countries including the United States, Canada, England, and China required face coverings for staff and students, social distancing in the classroom, additional cleaning measures, and daily screenings for those entering schools. However, in the United States, responses varied by state and had an effect on both K–12 and higher education mandates to wear masks, practice social distancing, and engage in other COVID-19 measures, even though the data were clear that "high adherence to mask wearing could be a key factor in reducing the spread of COVID-19" (Fischer et al., 2021).

As the battle against COVID-19 continued, several vaccines were authorized for the general public, and later for children aged 12 and older. There was a global call to prioritize educator health and safety, with the International Task Force on Teachers for Education launching a program for that purpose. Nineteen countries immediately prioritized their educators, and Russia and China both included educators as a priority group with one of their vaccine rollouts (Morrison, 2021). The other countries included a scattering of middle- and low-income countries supported by the COVAX program. For example, Chile's large emphasis on vaccinating teachers led to more than half of its 513,000 teachers being vaccinated by April 2021 (Vargas-Tamez & Wallet, 2021). Several states and provinces included educators in their subnational priority group 1 vaccine rollouts. The United States and 18 other countries placed teachers in priority group 2, right below frontline health care workers and at-risk individuals (UNESCO, 2021b). Other countries, including Canada and many countries in Europe such as Italy, included their educators in priority group 3 or lower (UNESCO, 2021b). However, as of March 2021, 54 countries had not prioritized teachers in their rollout plans or were still developing their plans. These countries included several sub-Saharan countries, Japan, Belgium, Sweden, and a few other East Asian and European countries; in total, 25 percent of teachers worldwide did not have access to a vaccine (UNESCO, 2021b). A recent study suggested that widespread immunization would not occur until 2023 or later in countries experiencing economic challenges linked to vaccine diplomacy, financial costs, and production (*Economist Intelligence Unit*, 2021).

Internationally, governments have a wide-ranging strategy of financial and government aid for K–12 education. While many countries have received COVID-19 relief aid, one-third of affluent and economically secure countries have slashed their education budget, along with two-thirds of countries experiencing economic challenges and less economically secure countries (UNESCO, 2021a). Although the United States has been a leader in global vaccine distribution, these decisions have widened the financial disparities that already existed between affluent countries and countries experiencing economic challenges in their educational systems. In Finland, the government had earmarked €68 million (US$80.6 million) as of August 2021 for educational inequalities resulting from the pandemic (Yle News, 2021). Provincial governments in Canada differed in their choices, with Ontario opting to invest CA$656.5 million in infrastructure improvements for its schools (Ontario Newsroom, 2021). Alberta also promised CA$45 million to support young students affected by the pandemic (Bourne, 2021). Mexico, a country where 80 percent of citizens are experiencing economic challenges and only 40 percent of people in rural areas have access to the internet, struggled to adequately create a remote learning option for students (Lozano, 2019). In an attempt to remedy this situation, the Mexican government created a distance-learning program utilizing television and radio stations (Borgen Project, 2021). China also instituted a home-learning program using television and radio in the early stages of the pandemic. Its Home Study Initiative utilized high- and low-technology options, its national curriculum, and key technology partners to make lessons as accessible as possible (UNICEF, 2020). The Chinese initiative also included support for teachers as facilitators of distance learning, social-emotional learning, and psychosocial support for all age groups (UNICEF, 2020). Globally, many governments included extra funding for education in their COVID-19 stimulus packages, including Ethiopia, Tonga, Equatorial Guinea, Sweden, and Panama (International Monetary Fund, 2021; Al-Samarrai, Gangwar, & Gala, 2020).

Conclusion

As school communities continue their planning for the 2023 school year, K–12 stakeholders and research scholars are left to ponder how the pandemic has reshaped K–12 education systems globally. Already-exhausted teachers and administrators are readying themselves for a generation of students with greater disparities in academic readiness than expressed at the beginning of the previous year (Texas Education Agency, 2021), and students and parents await a return to normalcy in their schools amid early reports showing that children are at greater risk of infection from the variants of COVID-19 (Riley et al., 2021). The contemporaneous issues of fewer people entering preservice teacher programs nationally; fewer teachers entering or being retained in the field; and an increased number of teachers exiting the profession and leaving myriad vacancies across some school districts mean that the US educational system is far from seeing the light at the end of the tunnel. The ripple effect of COVID-19 on global educational systems will be felt for many years, potentially outlasting the current structures of COVID-19 relief support. National, state, and school policymakers must pay close attention to the physical and mental health, as well as the logistical and financial needs, of K–12 stakeholders during COVID-19 and in the post–COVID-19 school milieu recovery and be cognizant that student achievement is not the barometer for the health of the nation's schools, but rather a barometer for wider and more immediate needs. The pandemic has been catastrophically traumatic for US education and everyone who interacts with it. Recognizing that we have experienced trauma will provide the impetus for understanding, healing, and growth.

References

AACTE (American Association of Colleges for Teacher Education). (n.d.). *Teaching in the time of COVID-19: State recommendations for educator preparation programs and new teachers.* https://higherlogicdownload.s3-external-1.amazonaws.com/AACTE/3c00f6f6-80c9-4464-9acf-a10efffd93ae_file.pdf?AWSAccessKeyId=AKIAVRDO7IEREB57R7MT&Expires=1692297955&Signature=QXw2ZtD9X91kwBupkorzKq6JB4Q%3D

AACTE (American Association of Colleges for Teacher Education). (2020). *Educator preparation programs: In times of crisis recommendations.* https://f.hubspotusercontent40.net/hubfs/1818747/Education%20Preparation%20Program%20-%20In%20Times%20of%20Crisis.pdf

Achterberg, M., Dobbelaar, S., Boer, O. D., & Crone, E. A. (2021). Perceived stress as mediator for longitudinal effects of the COVID-19 lockdown on wellbeing of parents and children. *Scientific Reports, 11*(2971). https://doi.org/10.1038/s41598-021-81720-8

Al-Samarrai, S., Gangwar, M., & Gala, P. (2020). *The impact of the COVID-19 pandemic on education financing.* World Bank Group. https://thedocs.worldbank.org/en/doc/734541589314089887-0090022020/original/CovidandEdFinancefinal.pdf

American Academy of Pediatrics. (2022). *Children and COVID-19: State-level data report.* https://services.aap.org/en/pages/2019-novel-coronavirus-covid-19-infections/children-and-covid-19-state-level-data-report/

Associated Press. (2021, July16). COVID-19 spike not prompting mask mandate for Louisiana schools. https://apnews.com/article/health-religion-government-and-politics-louisiana-education-db618afcd25685120e00fc8d77feobda

Berger, M., Kuang, M., Jerry, L., & Freund, D. (2022). *Impact of the coronavirus (COVID-19) pandemic on public and private elementary and secondary education in the United States: Results from the 2020–21 national teacher and principal survey.* NCES 2022-019. National Center for Education Statistics, US Department of Education. https://nces.ed.gov/pubsearch/pubsinfo.asp?pubid=2022019

Berger, R., Abu-Raiya, H., & Benatov, J. (2016). Reducing primary and secondary traumatic stress symptoms among educators by training them to deliver a resiliency program (ERASE-Stress) following the Christchurch earthquake in New Zealand. *American Journal of Orthopsychiatry, 86*(2), 236–51.

Borgen Project. (2021, April 13). E-learning in Mexico: A path for poverty reduction. https://borgenproject.org/e-learning-in-mexico/

Boscarino, J. A., Figley, C. R., & Adams, R. E. (2004). Compassion fatigue following the September 11 terrorist attacks: A study of secondary trauma among New York City social workers. *International Journal of Emergency Mental Health, 6*, 57–66.

Bourne, K. (2021, May 28). Alberta announces $45M in funding to help young students struggling with reading, math. *Global News.* https://globalnews.ca/

Bowers, M. E., & Yehuda, R. (2016). Intergenerational transmission of stress in humans. *Neuropsychopharmacology, 41*(1), 232–44. https://doi.org/10.1038/npp.2015.247

Breslin, M. (2022, January 4). 1,000 Boston teachers, school staff out due to COVID-19, other reasons. *The Hill.* https://thehill.com/homenews/state-watch/588155 –1000-boston-teachers-school-staff-out-due-to-covid-19-other-reasons/

Busby, J., Tanberk, J., & Cooper, T. (2021, May 27). BroadbandNow estimates availability for all 50 states; confirms that more than 42 million Americans do not have access to broadband. BroadbandNow. https://broadbandnow.com/ research/fcc-broadband-overreporting-by-state

Calear, A. L., McCallum, S., Morse, A. R., Banfield, M., Gulliver, A., Cherbuin, N., Farrer, L. M., Murray, K., Rodney Harris, R. M., & Batterham, P. J. (2022). Psychosocial impacts of home-schooling on parents and caregivers during the COVID-19 pandemic. *BMC Public Health, 22*(119). https://doi.org/10.1186/ s12889-022-12532-2

Casselman, B. (2021, May 17). Rural areas are looking for workers. They need broadband to get them. *New York Times.* https://www.nytimes.com

CDC (Centers for Disease Control and Prevention). (2017, August 2). About rural health. https://www.cdc.gov/ruralhealth/about.html

CDC (Centers for Disease Control and Prevention). (2021a). COVID-19 in children and teens. https://www.cdc.gov/coronavirus/2019-ncov/daily-life-coping/ children/symptoms.html

CDC (Centers for Disease Control and Prevention). (2021b). SARS-CoV-2 variant classifications and definitions. https://www.cdc.gov/coronavirus/2019-ncov/ variants/variant-info.html

CDC (Centers for Disease Control and Prevention). (2021c, October 7). The hidden U.S. COVID-19 pandemic: Orphaned children. https://www.cdc.gov/media/ releases/2021/p1007-covid-19-orphaned-children.html#:~:text=The%20 study%20authors%20estimate%20that,COVID-19-associated%20death

CDC (Centers for Disease Control and Prevention). (2022). Anxiety and depression: Household pulse survey. https://www.cdc.gov/nchs/covid19/pulse/mental -health.htm

Charles Butt Foundation. (2021). *2021: How Texas teachers experience pandemic challenges; The 2021 poll on Texans' attitudes toward public education.* https:// charlesbuttfdn.org/wp-content/uploads/2022/01/2021_How-Texas-Teachers -Experience-Pandemic-Challenges.pdf

Cohen, M., Gagin, R., & Peled-Avram, M. (2006). Multiple terrorist attacks: Compassion fatigue in Israeli social workers. *Traumatology, 12*(4), 293–301.

Dooley, K. (2020, August 18). Educator certification flexibility in response to COVID-19. Human Resource Exchange. https://www.tasb.org/services/hr -services/hrx/hr-laws/educator-certification-flexibility-in-response-to -covid-19.aspx

Dorn, E., Hancock, B., Sarakatsannis, J., & Viruleg, E. (2021). COVID-19 and education: The lingering effects of unfinished learning. McKinsey & Company. https://www.mckinsey.com/industries/education/our-insights/ covid-19-and-education-the-lingering-effects-of-unfinished-learning

Economist Intelligence Unit. (2021, January 27). More than 85 poor countries will not have widespread access to coronavirus vaccines before 2023. https:// www.eiu.com/

Erikson, E. (1959). *Identity and the life cycle*. Psychological Issues Monograph. New York: International Universities Press.

Etchells, M. J., Brannen, L., Donop, J., Bielefeldt, J., Singer, E. A., Moorhead, E., & Walderon, T. (2021). Synchronous teaching and asynchronous trauma: Exploring teacher trauma in the wake of COVID-19. *Social Sciences & Humanities Open, 4*. https://doi.org/10.1016/j.ssaho.2021.100197

Fischer, C. B., Adrien, N., Silguero, J. J., Hopper, J. J., Chowdhury, A. I., & Werler, M. M. (2021). Mask adherence and rate of COVID-19 across the United States. *PLoS ONE, 16*(4), 1–10. https://doi.org/10.1371/journal.pone.0249891

Garcia, K. S. D., & Cowan, B. W. (2022). The impact of U.S. school closures on labor market outcomes during the COVID-19 pandemic. National Bureau of Economic Research Working Paper No. 29641. https://doi.org/10.3386/w29641

Gicheva, D. (2021). Teachers' working hours during the COVID-19 pandemic. *Educational Researcher, 51*(1), 85–87. https://doi.org/10.3102/0013189X211056897

Gopnik, A. (2016). *The gardener and the carpenter: What the new science of child development tells us about the relationship between parents and children*. Audible Studios on Brilliance Audio.

Green, E. L. (2022, February 20). New twist in pandemic's impact on schools: Substitutes in camouflage. *New York Times*. https://www.nytimes.com/2022/02/20/us/politics/substitute-teachers-national-guard-new-mexico.html

Gunn, M. (2022, February 9). Missouri school districts switching to four-day weeks to recruit and retain more teachers. KTVO. https://ktvo.com/news/local/missouri-school-districts-switching-to-four-day-weeks-to-recruit-and-retain-more-teachers?fbclid=IwAR0ULvgyEh_7fAX4Oj2jTs2NZAW-26091gE3NJIfz-fYWMycEf7hByGzaRI

Heim, J. (2021, April 22). As the school year ends, many districts expand summer school options. *Washington Post*. https://www.washingtonpost.com

Henderson, M. B., Houston, D., Peterson, P. E., & West, M. R. (2020, July 8). What American families experienced when Covid-19 closed their schools. Education Next, https://www.educationnext.org/what-american-families-experienced-when-covid-19-closed-their-schools/

Hillis, S., N'konzi, J. P. N., & Msemburi, W. (2022). Orphanhood and caregiver loss among children based on new global excess COVID-19 death estimates. *JAMA Pediatrics, 176*(11), 1145–48.

International Monetary Fund. (2021). Policy responses to COVID-19. https://www.imf.org/en/Topics/imf-and-covid19/Policy-Responses-to-COVID-19

Johnston, D. H., Foy, K., Mulligan, A., & Shanks, R. (2021). Teaching in a third space during national COVID-19 lockdowns: In loco magister? *Irish Educational Studies, 40*(2), 359–66.

Jotkoff, E. (2022, Februry 1). NEA survey: Massive staff shortages in schools leading to educator burnout; alarming number of educators indicating they plan to leave profession. National Education Association. https://www.nea.org/about-nea/media-center/press-releases/nea-survey-massive-staff-shortages-schools-leading-educator-burnout-alarming-number-educators

Kamenetz, A. (2021, February 23). States must test student learning this year, Biden administration says. National Public Radio. https://www.npr.org/sections/coronavirus-live-updates/2021/02/23/970520559/states-must-test-student-learning-this-spring-biden-administration-says

Kaur, H. (2021, February 3). Teachers have lost colleagues to COVID-19 and worry about being next. But, they say, no one's listening. CNN. https://www.cnn.com

KHOU-11. (2022, April 12). New teachers can qualify for $10,000 stipend from HISD: Qualified teachers will receive up to $10,000 as part of the RISE program. https://www.khou.com/

Kurtz, H. (2020, April 10). National survey tracks impact of coronavirus on schools: 10 key findings. *Education Weekly*. https://www.edweek.org/

Lambert, D. (2020, September 25). Waiting lists for home-school programs as parents grow weary of distance learning. EdSource. https://edsource.org/

Lambert, D. (2021, July 1). Pandemic drives sharp rise in California families opening their own home schools. EdSource. https://edsource.org/

Lozano, L. F. (2019, December 27). Mucho combate a la pobreza, pero en México 4 de cada 5 la padecen. *Forbes México*. https://www.forbes.com.mx

Maxouris, C., & Zdanowicz, C. (2022, February 5). Teachers are leaving and few people want to join the field. Experts are sounding the alarm. CNN. https://edition.cnn.com/2022/02/05/us/teacher-prep-student-shortages-covid-crisis/index.html?fbclid=IwAR0ULvgyEh_7fAX4Oj2jTs2NZAW-26091gE3NJIfz-fYWMycEf7hByGzaRI#Echobox=1644101774

McCann, I. L., & Pearlman, L. A. (1990). Vicarious traumatization: A framework for understanding the psychological effects of working with victims. *Journal of Traumatic Stress, 3*, 131–49.

McKegney, C. C. (2021). Understanding child development in the assessment of stress in children amidst the COVID-19 pandemic. *Pediatric Nursing, 47*(1), 48–54.

McMurdock M. (2022, February 20). School leader crisis: Overwhelmed by mounting mental health issues and public distrust, a "mass exodus" of principals could be coming. The 74. https://www.the74million.org/article/school-leaders-crisis-overwhelmed-by-mounting-mental-health-issues-public-distrust-mass-exodus-of-principals-could-be-coming/

Meyers, L. (2021). Feeling the strain: The effects of COVID-19 on children and adolescents. *Counseling Today, 63*(11), 22–27.

Morrison, N. (2021, April 2). These 17 countries have prioritized teachers for vaccinations. *Forbes*. https://www.forbes.com

Nietzel, M. T. (2021). New from U.S. Census Bureau: Number of Americans with a bachelor's degree continues to grow. *Forbes*. https://www.forbes.com/

Nissen, J. B., Højgaard, D. R. M. A., & Thomsen, P. H. (2020). The immediate effect of COVID-19 pandemic on children and adolescents with obsessive compulsive disorder. *BMC Psychiatry, 20*(511), 1–10.

Office of Elementary and Secondary Education, US Department of Education. (2021, May). Elementary and Secondary School Emergency Relief Fund. https://oese.ed.gov/offices/education-stabilization-fund/elementary-secondary-school-emergency-relief-fund/

Office of Postsecondary Education, US Department of Education. (2020, April 21). Higher Education Emergency Relief Fund. https://www2.ed.gov/about/offices/list/ope/caresact.html

Olson, L. (2020). A shifting landscape for state testing. *State Education Standard, 20*(3), 7–11.

Ontario Newsroom. (2021, April 14). Canada and Ontario invest in school infrastructure to respond to the impacts of COVID-19. https://news.ontario.ca/

Penuliar, M., Clark, C., Phillips, S., Curti, D., Hudson, C., & Philips, B. (2020). Simple COVID-19 susceptible-infected-recovered model with social distancing levels across time: A West Texas example. *Original Public Health Research, 74*(2), 15–20.

Reimers, F., & Scheicher, A. (2020). *A framework to guide an education response to the COVID-19 pandemic of 2020.* Organization for Economic Co-operation and Development (OECD). https://oecd.dam-broadcast.com/pm_7379_126_126988-t63lxosohs.pdf

Richards, E. (2021, April 5). Day camps, paying teens to study: Summer school looks different. Will it help kids catch up? *USA Today.* https://www.usatoday.com/story/news/education/2021/04/02/summer-school-changes-covid-federal-money-learning-loss/4808079001

Riley, S., Wang, H., Eales, O., Haw, D., Walters, C., Ainslie, K., . . . Elliott, P. (2021). *REACT-1 round 12 report: Resurgence of SARS-CoV-2 infections in England associated with increased frequency of the Delta variant.* Imperial College London.

Rosenblum, I. (2021, February 22). Letter to chief state school officer (letter). https://oese.ed.gov/files/2021/02/DCL-on-assessments-and-acct-final.pdf

Rundle, A. G., Park, Y., Herbstman, J. B., Kinsey, E. W., & Wang, Y. C. (2020). COVID-19-related school closings and risk of weight gain among children. *Obesity, 28*(6), 1008–9.

Saakvitne, K. W. (2002). Shared trauma: The therapist's increased vulnerability. *Psychoanalytic Dialogues, 12*(3), 443–49.

Saenz-Armstrong, P. (2020, April 16). Student teaching and initial licensure in the times of coronavirus. National Council on Teacher Quality (NCTQ). https://www.nctq.org/blog/Student-teaching-and-initial-licensure-in-the-times-of-coronavirus

Saenz-Armstrong, P. (2021, December 9). COVID-related incentives for teachers during the 2021–22 school year. National Council on Teacher Quality (NCTQ). https://www.nctq.org/blog/COVID--related-incentives-for-teachers-during-the-2021--22-school-year

Schwartz, S. (2021). Pay raises and pandemic bonuses: Can they keep teachers in classrooms? *Education Week.* https://www.edweek.org

Senate Bill No. 226. (2021). Relating to instruction in educator training programs regarding digital learning, virtual learning, and virtual instruction. S.B. No. 226, 87th Legislature. https://capitol.texas.gov/tlodocs/87R/billtext/pdf/SB00226I.pdf#navpanes=0

Siegler, K. (2020a, April 24). Even in crisis times, there is a push to wire rural America. National Public Radio. https://www.npr.org

Siegler, K. (2020b, September 28). In internet dead zones, rural schools struggle with distanced learning. National Public Radio. https://www.npr.org

Slay, L. E., Riley, J., & Miller, K. (2020). Facilitating a path to new teacher certification amid the COVID-19 pandemic: Unpacking states' "Unchanged-New Flex" guidelines. *Frontiers in Education, 5*(583896). https://doi.org/10.3389/feduc.2020.583896

Sparks, S. D. (2021, July 6). How does the Delta variant figure into schools' opening plans? *Education Week.* https://www.edweek.org

Swedo, E., Idaikkadar, N., Leemis, R., Dias, T., Radhakrishnan, L., Stein, Z., Chen, M., Agathis, N., & Holland, K. (2020). Trends in U.S. emergency department visits related to suspected or confirmed child abuse and neglect among children and adolescents aged <18 years before and during COVID-19 pandemic—United States, January 2019–September 2020. *Morbidity and Mortality Weekly Report, 69*(49), 1841–47.

Tal, C., Tish, S., & Tal, P. (2022). Parental perceptions of their preschool and elementary school children with respect to teacher-family relations and teaching methods during the first COVID-19 lockdown. *Pedagogical Research, 7*(1). https://doi.org/10.29333/pr/11518

Terlizzi, E. P, & Schiller, J. S. (2021, March). Estimates of mental health symptomatology, by month of interview: United States, 2019. National Center for Health Statistics, National Health Interview Survey. https://www.cdc.gov/nchs/data/nhis/mental-health-monthly-508.pdf

Texas Department of State Health Services, Center for Health Statistics. (2022, March 11). Texas public schools COVID-19 data. https://dshs.texas.gov/coronavirus/schools/texas-education-agency/

Texas Education Agency. (2021, June 28). TEA releases spring 2021 STAAR grades 3–8 and end-of-course assessment results; outcomes for in-person learners appreciably higher than for those who were remote. https://tea.texas.gov/about-tea/news-and-multimedia/news-releases/news-2021/tea-releases-spring-2021-staar-grades-3-8-and-end-of-course-assessment-results-outcomes-for-in-person-learners-appreciably-higher-than-for-those-who-were-remote

Thompson, C. (2021, June 7). Another COVID side effect: Many kids head to summer school. AP News. https://apnews.com

Tomlinson, M., Richter, L., & Slemming, W. (2021). What the science of child and adolescent development contributes to understanding the impacts of COVID-19. *Scientific Correspondence, 117*(1/2), 6–7.

Ujifusa, A. (2021, February 2). States still must give standardized tests this year, Biden administration announces. *Education Week.* https://www.edweek.org/

UNESCO (United Nations Educational, Scientific, and Cultural Organization). (2021a, February 2). COVID-19: Two-thirds of poorer countries are cutting their education budgets at a time when they can least afford to. https://www.unesco.org/en/articles/covid-19-two-thirds-poorer-countries-are-cutting-their-education-budgets-time-when-they-can-least

UNESCO (United Nations Educational, Scientific, and Cultural Organization). (2021b, May 31). UNESCO urges all countries to prioritize teachers in national COVID-19 vaccine rollout plans to ensure education can continue safely and

schools remain open. https://en.unesco.org/covid19/educationresponse/
teacher-vaccination

UNESCO (United Nations Educational, Scientific, and Cultural Organization).
(2021c, June). Education: From disruption to recovery. https://en.unesco.org/
covid19/educationresponse#schoolclosures

UNICEF (United Nations Children's Emergency Fund). (2020, May 17). UNICEF
education COVID-19 case study China—Distance learning and school
reopening. https://aa9276f9-f487-45a2-a3e7-8f4a61a0745d.usrfiles.com/ugd/
aa9276_0ec4d8cbe2ca4b24914b43bf1c7d6731.pdf

UNICEF (United Nations Children's Emergency Fund). (2021, March 2). COVID-19:
Schools for more than 168 million children globally have been completely closed
for almost a full year, says UNICEF. https://www.unicef.org/press-releases/
schools-more-168-million-children-globally-have-been-completely-closed

US Department of Education. (2021a, May 31). Education Stabilization Fund. https://
covid-relief-data.ed.gov/

US Department of Education. (2021b, May 31). *Frequently asked questions: Elementary
and secondary school emergency relief programs, governor's emergency education
relief programs.* https://oese.ed.gov/files/2021/05/ESSER.GEER_.FAQs_5.26.21_
745AM_FINALbocd6833f6f46e03ba2d97d30aff953260028045f9ef3b18ea602db4
b32b1d99.pdf

US Department of Education. (2021c, June 9). *Education in a pandemic: The disparate
impacts of COVID-19 on America's students.* https://www2.ed.gov/about/offices/
list/ocr/docs/20210608-impacts-of-covid19.pdf

Vargas-Tamez, C., & Wallet, P. (2021, March 15). Vaccinating teachers is crucial for
returning to school. Global Partnership for Education. https://www.global
partnership.org/blog/vaccinating-teachers-crucial-returning-school

WCVB. (2022, January 5). Boston public schools superintendent Brenda Cassellius
teaching 4th grade class as staff shortages rise. https://www.wcvb.com/article/
schools-struggling-to-stay-open-as-staff-absences-due-to-covid-19-climbs/
38672563

White House. (2021). The American Rescue Plan. https://www.whitehouse.gov/
wp-content/uploads/2021/03/American-Rescue-Plan-Fact-Sheet.pdf

Will, M. (2020, June 3). Teachers say they're more likely to leave the classroom
because of coronavirus. *Education Week.* https://www.edweek.org/teaching
-learning/teachers-say-theyre-more-likely-to-leave-the-classroom-because
-of-coronavirus/2020/06

Yard, E., Radhakrishnan, L., Ballesteros, M. F., Sheppard, M., Gates, A., Stein, Z.,
. . . Stone, D. M. (2021). Emergency department visits for suspected suicide
attempts among persons aged 12–25 years before and during the COVID-19
pandemic—United States, January 2019–May 2021. *Morbidity and Mortality
Weekly Report, 70*(24), 888–94. http://dx.doi.org/10.15585/mmwr.mm7024e1

Yarmuth, J. A. (2021, March 11). H.R.1319—American Rescue Plan Act of 2021,
117th Congress (2021–2022). Congress.gov. https://www.congress.gov/bill/
117th-congress/house-bill/1319

Yle News. (2021, April 17). Finland earmarks €68m for educational inequality
exposed during pandemic. https://yle.fi/a/3-11889547

PART FIVE

FUTURE PANDEMIC PREPAREDNESS

CHAPTER 12

A Pandemic Early Warning and Response System

ANDREW S. NATSIOS

AS THE SHOCK WAVES FROM COVID-19 AND ITS VARIANTS CONTINUE to cascade across the world, policymakers have begun asking what future arrangements can be made to avoid a repetition of this public health, social, and economic catastrophe. The focus on the early stages of the virus outbreak in China has inadvertently drawn attention to the timing problem during pandemics. Timing is one of the central challenges of disaster management: the natural order does not schedule its catastrophes for the convenience of human response institutions. Viruses have their own dynamics, which disaster managers must understand or risk failure. Emergency management professionals distinguish between fast-onset versus slow-onset disasters, the first category being more difficult to prevent than the latter. Pandemics are not fast-onset disasters; they begin as outbreaks, morph into epidemics, and then mutate into worldwide pandemics not over hours or even days, but over weeks and months. Sufficient early warning and proper preparedness may be able to stop the progression before the pandemic stage explodes.

Note: A condensed version of this chapter appeared in the online *Foreign Affairs* journal on July 14, 2020.

Political systems matter a great deal during disasters, particularly in disasters that threaten the survival of the incumbent governments. Fully functioning democracies, by their very nature, thrive on open-source information: it is very difficult to suppress stories of disease outbreaks even if leaders do not act in a timely fashion. This is particularly true in an age of instant electronic communication. Early warning is problematic in autocracies, which resist information on disease outbreaks that might be regime threatening. China has had an epidemic early warning system since the SARS outbreak in 2003, which is managed by able and dedicated scientists. These scientists, however, were ignored, muzzled, or arrested by government officials afraid of their warnings during the onset of the COVID-19 pandemic. All bureaucracies, but particularly those in autocratic systems, have incentives to avoid reporting bad news to superiors, which is why accountability systems in democracies are vastly superior at informing their chains of command of bad news, and when they fail, legislative branches, opposition parties, civil society, and the media quickly correct that failure.

The Success of the Famine Early Warning System

Suppression of information is not unique to any particular type of disaster. The same suppression of information occurs during famines as occurs during disease outbreaks. Nobel Prize–winning famine scholar Amartya Sen has famously argued that no famine has ever taken place in a democracy. Many of the worst famines in the twentieth century—the Ukrainian Holodomor under Stalin, Mao's Great Leap famine, the Cambodian Killing Fields, Mengistu's Ethiopian famine, Bashir's South Sudanese famines, and the North Korean famine—were well underway or over by the time the outside world knew what had happened. The development of the Famine Early Warning System (later called the Famine Early Warning System Network, or FEWS NET) by USAID in the late 1980s, however, changed autocracies' ability to hide famines. With the exception of the North Korean famine (which was not covered by the system), FEWS NET has accurately reported virtually all food crises before they have descended into famines. The system has been extremely valuable, saved untold lives, and can provide a blueprint for other types of early warning systems. But how does FEWS

NET overcome the inherent suppression of information on severe food distress under dictatorships or during civil wars?

To minimize uncertainty, FEWS NET uses a methodology known as scenario development to forecast food insecurity. This involves collaborating closely with partners around the world who participate in the network to gather the best available data on factors specific to food security in areas of concern. Partnering with the US Geological Survey, National Oceanic and Atmospheric Administration (NOAA), and others, FEWS NET uses remote sensing imagery and historical and current climate outlooks, alongside available nutrition surveys and regional market and trade data on staple foods and livestock. This tracking of high-risk areas, coupled with information from local field offices working with local governments—if they are cooperative—provides more nuanced information on what is happening in the country and helps verify areas of emerging concern.

USAID has contractual partnerships with commercial satellites to compare the color—green or brown—of the ground cover in agricultural areas from year to year during the same weeks and months. They produce Green Maps, which locate potential areas of severe nutritional distress. If the ground cover is brown when it should be green, crops have likely failed because of drought. Additionally, severe food insecurity, famine, and poverty are intimately connected to each other, so FEWS NET compares rates of poverty with agricultural distress and conflict to determine famine risk. Satellite analysis must be accompanied by ground-truthing teams of analysts, preferably people who live in the regions at risk. These teams gather market data inside the country and determine whether food prices are going up rapidly, particularly in relation to the price of animals and of people's labor. From these data it is possible to produce widely distributed and open-source analysis and maps of food-insecure areas of the world, which can show the onset of a food crisis. Thousands of development and humanitarian relief professionals around the world receive these open-source reports regularly, and this analysis plays a central role in famine mitigation efforts.

In his powerful 2018 book, *Mass Starvation: The History and Future of Famine*, Alex de Waal, a well-known scholar of famines, tracks famine deaths for the past 150 years and shows that mortality rates have noticeably declined since the mid-1980s. He attributes this to fewer totalitarian regimes, globalization (which has reduced poverty), and the evolution of the humanitarian response system, of which FEWS NET is an important part.

Creating a Pandemic Early Warning System

FEWS NET has been extremely successful in identifying oncoming famines, but can the FEWS NET model be adapted to pandemics to give policymakers advance warning before a disease outbreak mutates into a pandemic? Given that evidence of pandemics, like that of famines, threatens the stability of autocratic regimes, how can analysts gather information for advance warning of impending outbreaks? The answer to the first question is yes, and there are three important types of information that can provide input for a pandemic early warning system.

First, satellite photography can track the digging of mass graves. Mass graves do not necessarily mean that people have died from disease; they could also be the result of a famine or mass atrocities, particularly in a war zone, but they could serve as a preliminary indicator of severe stress. During the Bosnian civil war, US spy satellites were crucial in discovering the location of mass graves after the massacre in Srebrenica because the decomposing bodies created photographic heat signatures. Satellites can also track the existence and size of crowds outside health clinics in a defined geographic region from week to week and day to day. They do not prove an epidemic is occurring, but once again, this is a sign of severe health distress requiring further ground investigation. Satellite photography can capture information on the operation of crematoria (in urban areas in particular) from week to week. If they are functioning overtime, that implies excess mortality, which may be caused by disease.

Second, a number of electronic monitoring systems have been developed that track information on the internet from social media platforms such as Twitter and Facebook about reports of new illnesses. These data can be aggregated by geographic region in real time. Google Search can track the frequency of people's searches for certain disease symptoms, which is often a warning sign of an outbreak. It should be noted, however, that Google's flu tracker was discontinued because of its lack of accuracy. Thus, internet searches and social media information are just one data point to be used in conjunction with other inputs such as satellite photography. Cell phone communications can also be a source of information, which can be monitored remotely using newly developed innovative applications.

According to a study by scientists at Harvard University, satellites detected a marked increase in hospital traffic in Wuhan beginning in August 2019 at the same time that search engines using aggregated social media data recorded an uptick in searches in the Wuhan area for terms related to the specific and unique symptoms of COVID-19 (Nsoesie et al., 2020). Taken together, the study's authors argue, these two trends suggest that the coronavirus outbreak may have begun much earlier than previously thought.

Third, the Centers for Disease Control and Prevention (CDC) employs domestic outbreak monitoring systems to track annual influenza (flu) outbreaks by observing daily sales of pharmaceuticals used to treat high fevers, muscle pain, and other flu symptoms. During the George W. Bush administration, the US Department of the Interior monitored wild bird deaths in Alaska as billions of these birds migrated seasonally from Siberia to Latin America and back. The bodies were examined to determine whether they had died of one of the flu viruses.

All three of these approaches should be used to construct a pandemic early warning system (PEWS), given that a single dataset would likely prove inadequate. Using all these data inputs would reduce the likelihood that a serious new outbreak would slip by undetected until it was too late to control it. In countries that refuse to allow scientific research teams to ground-truth disease outbreak reports from this PEWS system, reporting from neighboring countries could be used to assess how severe and widespread the disease is. A properly constructed multitiered approach through PEWS would produce information for operators and policymakers in real time.

Most important, PEWS reports—like those of FEWS NET—must be available outside the US government, to civil society organizations around the world, research centers and think tanks, the news media, Congress and parliaments, and international organizations.

Response Logistics under a Pandemic Early Warning System

Information from PEWS will be of limited use without an early and rapid response system to take action on the data. Response teams should have seven critical characteristics:

- Be capable of mobilizing within a few days of an outbreak (and thus not require interagency coordination, which invariably slows down responses).
- Allow decentralized decision-making at the field level.
- Be exempt for purposes of grant making and equipment purchasing from oppressive federal contracting regulations, bureaucratic paperwork, and notifications, which bog down the response to any rapidly unfolding crisis.
- Be equipped with the proper protective gear to prevent the infection of aid workers.
- Have flexible, unearmarked funding readily available without supplemental appropriation, which can slow responses down.
- Have a rapidly expandable workforce of trained staff to be deployed overnight.
- Be expeditionary, which means that field staff are self-contained and can feed, house, transport, and care for themselves and communicate with each other and headquarters.

Such a system would require strategically located warehouses of vehicles (including armored vehicles to protect aid workers in war zones), means of water purification (for waterborne illnesses), equipment for large population clusters, shelter material for displaced camps (people will escape disease outbreaks by mass population movements), food rations, personal protective equipment (PPE) to protect health workers from disease, and medical supplies, including vaccines and syringes.

The next important question to address when building this system is, what would this emergency response system actually do operationally? It would conduct rapid assessments and evaluations; implement mass immunization campaigns of the most at-risk populations (if a vaccine exists); conduct mass distribution of pharmaceuticals to local health clinics to treat the disease (if effective treatments exist); work with community and religious leaders to inform the public about how the disease spreads and how transmission can be slowed or stopped by changes in behavior; build sentinel surveillance systems to monitor the incidence of disease and deaths to determine whether program interventions are working; and coordinate and immediately fund partner organizations such as the United Nations' World Food Programme (WFP), United Nations Children's Fund (UNICEF), United Nations High Commissioner for Refugees (UNHCR), and international nongovernmental organizations (NGOs), as well as groups such as the Red Cross.

Importantly, we do not need to create a system from scratch because a similar one already exists. The most powerful element of the international humanitarian response system has existed for decades within USAID, in what is now called the Bureau for Humanitarian Assistance (formerly the Office of US Foreign Disaster Assistance [OFDA] and Food for Peace, which were merged and streamlined by USAID administrator Mark Green). FEWS NET is managed by this bureau, which can deploy USAID's Disaster Assistance Response Teams (DARTs) around the world at a moment's notice. From the time the first DARTs were deployed in the summer of 1989, they have always included refugee program officers from the State Department, as well as CDC scientists. Thus, the teams are multidepartmental, but the funding, operational control, organizational structure, and reporting lines are centrally housed within USAID.

The Bureau for Humanitarian Assistance has a large discretionary budget ($5.7 billion, including food aid accounts) and a sizable crisis management staff of more than 450 funded, certified disaster operations officers who can be deployed in 72 hours. Historically, these programs have remarkable legal authorities that allow them to spend money quickly, which virtually no other federal program has. The USAID Disaster Assistance Program has had broad political support from both parties in the US Congress and the White House for 50 years (though the Office of Management and Budget unsuccessfully attempted cuts in 2017, which were restored by Congress), meaning that the program has enjoyed steadily increasing funding and staff every year. The Bureau for Humanitarian Assistance also has a large reserve surge force of trained disaster managers who can be quickly mobilized if needed. USAID has historically served as the federal coordinator for all international disaster responses under the Foreign Assistance Act, but it does not have a *specific* legal mandate to be responsible for pandemic detection and response—though the offices have served very effectively in this role for several decades in smaller-scale health emergencies.

Many proposals have recently been made for pandemic early warning systems, some international, some bilateral. Internationalists argue that a single centralized system in an international institution should be created to avoid redundancy and political interference from national governments in pandemic monitoring. What should be clear by now is that international organizations are no more able to withstand political pressure than national government institutions. The best way to reduce the risk of pandemic early warning system failure is to have multiple systems—some bilateral and some multilateral—instead of relying on a single system. All human-conceived and human-operated institutions are by nature flawed and cannot be trusted to function properly all the time and under all circumstances. Redundancy in the case of pandemic early warning is a good and desirable characteristic, not a weakness.

Conclusion

Gathering all these data under one roof would enable the United States to create a PEWS to function alongside the already successful FEWS NET. Such a system could furnish public health officials and policymakers with information in real time. It could also enable US administrators to distribute a PEWS report—like its FEWS NET counterpart—which could move the world to action. The possibilities of such a system bring up an important counterfactual question: If this system had already been in place, could it have prevented the COVID-19 pandemic? This PEWS system would have been an essential data stream to policymakers and operators had it been in place to warn of the impending crisis before it reached catastrophic levels. Importantly, collaboration on global health security kept some limited channels of communication open between scientists in China and the United States, even during the early days of the outbreak. However, it is still not known exactly when and where SARS-CoV-2 emerged other than the initial reporting in December 2019 of an unusual pneumonia cluster in Wuhan. It was incumbent on Chinese government officials to report in a timely way as much as they knew about this unusual outbreak that had significant global implications under international health regulations. Although China did report to the World Health Organization on December 31, 2019, it is now known that Beijing withheld essential information that delayed international preparedness and response efforts and led to the worldwide crisis. It is possible that a PEWS system could have provided enough information to convey the gravity of the situation to the world, reducing the reliance on accurate reporting from China.

COVID-19 is not a 100-year event. Emerging infectious diseases with pandemic potential are a new normal, requiring renewed emphasis on preparedness. More often than not, the next disease outbreak with pandemic potential will emerge in countries that lack public health infrastructure and effective disease surveillance systems, and that have authoritarian governments that may similarly withhold effective early reporting. The PEWS system, along with sustained international development support, will be an essential element of our international pandemic early warning and response system. This will require political will to make and sustain the needed investments to protect civilization from a potentially much more catastrophic pandemic.

References

Nsoesie, E. O., Rader, B., Barnoon, Y. L., Goodwin, L., & Brownstein, J. S. (2020). Analysis of hospital traffic and search engine data in Wuhan China indicates early disease activity in the fall of 2019. Digital Access to Scholarship at Harvard (DASH). http://nrs.harvard.edu/urn-3:HUL.InstRepos:42669767

Conclusion

CHRISTINE CRUDO BLACKBURN

History compels us not to look away lest we fail to learn the lessons paid for by our parents and our grandparents.

—BRUCE E. FLEURY

DISEASE, WHETHER COMMUNICABLE OR NONCOMMUNICABLE, IS consistently one of the greatest challenges faced by humanity. Each decade brings both new and old pathogens that must be confronted and contained. The 1918 influenza pandemic was the worst disease crisis in modern history, but equal or superior threats faced our ancestors. From cholera pandemics to the plague to smallpox, the fight against disease has been ongoing for centuries. With that in mind, every epidemic and pandemic of the twentieth and twenty-first centuries has offered societies opportunities to learn from both the successes and failures of their response. The influenza pandemics of 1957 and 1968, the HIV/AIDS pandemic of the 1980s and 1990s, and SARS and MERS in the early 2000s have each highlighted various aspects of the disease containment, economic, and social implications of response. The COVID-19 pandemic, however, is unique in modern history in both its scale and its length. Not since the 1918 flu has a pandemic caused significant disruptions and deaths throughout the entire world simultaneously. Additionally, not since the 1918 pandemic have those disruptions persisted for multiple years.

The unique nature of the COVID-19 pandemic and the unprecedented challenges it posed to an interconnected global population and policymakers offer a tremendous opportunity to study the impacts and lessons learned. This book brought together experts from academia, government, and the private sector to explore some of the pandemic challenges, impacts, and response successes to date.

This book has taken a broad look at all parts of society that the pandemic impacted. It examined the threat posed by the growing wildlife trade and human encroachment into wild spaces. It discussed the major scientific and policy achievement of Operation Warp Speed in developing and disseminating a vaccine for COVID-19 in less than 12 months. It investigated the economic and social impacts of the pandemic, touching on issues such as unemployment, supply chains, migration, and K–12 education. It analyzed the problem with media narratives and disinformation online. Finally, this book discussed the necessity of developing a pandemic early warning system to mitigate the impact of future outbreaks.

Examining and understanding the impacts of the COVID-19 pandemic in all these various realms is vital to understanding where the American and global response succeeded and where it failed. It is vital to creating better pandemic preparedness policy moving forward and directing support to needed scientific research. And most importantly, documenting these impacts is vital to preserving this knowledge for future generations. This will not be the last pandemic. It may not even be the last pandemic in our lifetime. Therefore, this book should be only the beginning of the analysis, both in the United States and globally, that will enable us to be better prepared for the next pandemic.

Contributors

DAMOLA ADESAKIN is a seasoned environmental, health, and safety (EHS) professional, boasting significant management expertise across both governmental and private sectors. She presently occupies the role of a regional workplace health and safety manager at Amazon, where she has been working diligently for nearly two years. Before joining Amazon, she made significant contributions to ExxonMobil as a public health advisor contractor, where she was pivotal in designing initiatives promoting wholesome lifestyles, disease prevention, and public health protection. Adesakin earned her MPH with an emphasis on environmental health from the University of Illinois.

SARA ALI is a recent graduate of Texas A&M University with a BS in public health. She is passionate about health access and equity across communities and has a keen interest in medicine. During her time at Texas A&M, Sara was involved in several research projects that focused on health disparities and access to care, particularly during the COVID-19 pandemic. She hopes to further her passion for health equity and access while pursuing a career in medicine.

NATALIE D. BAKER is an associate professor of strategy for the National War College at National Defense University. Baker is an interpretivist, qualitative researcher and expert in ethnography/co/autoethnography, and her primary research focuses on the importance of social order and the reestablishment of a sense of normalcy within instances of disruption, such as large-scale crises like disasters and war. Specific crises studied have included Hurricanes Katrina and Harvey, the 2014 Ebola situation in the US, the COVID-19 pandemic, and climate change.

Her research dispels social chaos mythologies in the context of large-scale crises and the role of mediated popular culture in perpetuating misconceptions of human behavior. Another way she studies the reestablishment of order is through alternative forms of governance, such as what can be thought of as "criminal insurgencies." Her most recent focus has been journalist safety issues and the murder of reporters in Mexico, and she has written on criminal factions in Brazil for *Small Wars Journal-El Centro*. She received her PhD from the University of California at Irvine in planning, policy, and design in addition to master's degrees in both international development and tropical medicine from Tulane University. Her bachelor's was from the University of Central Florida in psychology.

MIKE CRANFIELD was a renowned conservationist, veterinarian, and author of over 192 scientific publications. He passed away from Powassan virus and West Nile virus in August 2023 and leaves behind a legacy of contributions to global wildlife conservation, veterinary medicine, and the thousands of people and animals he touched through his work. Dr. Cranfield first came to the Maryland Zoo in 1982 as chief veterinarian and subsequently became the director of animal health, research, and conservation, responsible for the health and care of the zoo's more than 1,500 animals. In 1998, he became executive director of the world-renowned nonprofit Mountain Gorilla Veterinary Project (MGVP), which is dedicated to saving the lives of critically endangered mountain gorillas living in Rwanda, Uganda, and the Democratic Republic of Congo (DRC) as well as endangered eastern lowland gorillas in the DRC. Under Cranfield, MGVP expanded to include One Health programs for the mountain and Grauer's gorillas living in Uganda and the DRC, orphaned gorillas, and for the people and animals working in and living near gorilla habitat. MGVP was based at the Maryland Zoo until 2009, at which point MGVP partnered with the Wildlife Health Center at the University of California Davis School of Veterinary Medicine and became Gorilla Doctors. Under Cranfield's direction, Gorilla Doctors grew from a single American veterinarian to an organization with over 80 percent of its staff from African partner nations, including 13 veterinarians.

CHRISTINE CRUDO BLACKBURN is assistant professor in the Department of Health Policy and Management at Texas A&M University. She is also a faculty affiliate at the USA Center for Rural Public Health Preparedness in the School of Public Health at Texas A&M University. Her research examines how policies and social environments influence the health-seeking behavior of vulnerable populations and how health access barriers impact pandemic preparedness and response. She received an interdisciplinary PhD in the fields of political science, communication, and veterinary clinical sciences from Washington State University.

MALICK DIARA joined ExxonMobil in 2009 with more than 20 years of experience in international health and development. In 2010, he became the corporate public health manager of medicine and occupational health, focusing on infectious disease prevention and control in company workplaces. He has been instrumental in company preparedness and response for COVID-19, as well as for MERS, Coronavirus, Ebola, Zika, and outbreaks due to other infectious diseases. In 2023, Diara transitioned to the occupational health manager position leading related services for company operations in Mozambique. Prior to working for ExxonMobil, Malick worked with private nonprofit organizations in Washington, DC, for nine years and in West Africa for 12 years. With funding from USAID, the French Cooperation, or the European Union, and in partnership with local authorities and organizations such as UNICEF and WHO, Diara supported the design, implementation, and evaluation of global, national, and local public health programs. He is a former member of the Global Health Board of the National Academy of Medicine and present member of the American Society of Tropical Medicine and Hygiene. He holds an MD from Senegal School of Medicine, Dakar; an MBA from the Institut Superieur de Gestion, Paris; and an MPH from Tulane University, New Orleans.

JORDAN DONOP is an EC-6th certified educator, a Transformational Learning Fellow, and has an MEd in curriculum and instruction from Texas A&M University. Jordan engages in research with her colleagues from Texas A&M, and her first open access publication was on the impact of COVID-19 on teacher mental health, followed by a book chapter on the effects of COVID-19 on K–12 education. Her passion for research and lifelong learning led her to pursue a doctoral degree in educational psychology focusing on developmental sciences, and she is currently in her second year in the program.

MATTHEW J. ETCHELLS is the director of Education Outreach and International Partnerships for the Education Leadership Research Center & Center for Research and Development in Dual Language and Literacy Acquisition. He holds a PhD in curriculum and instruction from Texas A&M University. His research agenda includes teacher identity, shadow education, comparative education, and teacher education. Matthew has published over thirty articles and book chapters and is a coauthor and coeditor of three books: *A Companion to Interdisciplinary STEM Project-Based Learning: For Educators by Educators* (2nd edition), *Cultural Impact on Conflict Management in Higher Education*, and *Drawn to the Flame: Teachers' Stories of Burnout*.

MUHAMMAD (MOE) FAZAIL is an accomplished registered nurse with over six years of experience, specializing in trauma, critical care, and occupational health. Currently serving as the occupational health nurse manager for a renowned Fortune 500 company, he is responsible for integrating and implementing corporate occupational health service programs aimed at enhancing employee health, wellness, and safety. His areas of expertise include public health, case management, occupational medicine, emergency care, and primary care. Fazail has conducted thorough data analysis, developed comprehensive health reports, and provided valuable expertise in travel health. He also has made significant contributions to the development of educational materials and e-learning modules for employee training on global public health practices. Fazail obtained his BS in nursing from Lamar University and achieved induction into the prestigious Sigma Theta Tau honor society of nursing. He is certified by the National Institute for Occupational Safety and Health, the Council for Accreditation in Occupational Hearing Conservation, and holds Drug and Alcohol DOT certification.

RICHARD H. GELATT is currently the global program manager for medicine and occupational health in ExxonMobil responsible for the centers of excellence for infectious disease, clinical processes, alcohol and drug administration, culture of health, and occupational health information systems. His experience spans 32 years and covers a broad base of industrial hygiene as well as environmental and operations assignments supporting ExxonMobil Downstream, Chemical, Fuels, and Oil and Gas operations. His previous positions include global industrial hygiene manager and other roles in ExxonMobil Biomedical Sciences as exposure science section head and as research director for occupational health managing research programs for exposure science, epidemiology, and data quality. Richard has an MPH from Tulane University and a bachelor's degree from Louisiana State University and is a certified industrial hygienist.

ERICA MOORHEAD HENSCHEL is a middle school English teacher specializing in English language arts. She holds a master's in curriculum and instruction from Texas A&M University. She is actively involved in curriculum design and development within her district and has an interest in how schools work to retain high-quality teachers after the COVID-19 pandemic shifted the educational field. Her research has led her to become a campus leader and continue to advocate for teachers.

PETER HOTEZ is a professor of pediatrics and molecular virology and microbiology at Baylor College of Medicine where he is also dean of the National School of Tropical Medicine and codirector of the Texas Children's Hospital Center for Vaccine Development. His major interest is in the development of vaccines for neglected diseases of poverty, in addition to coronavirus vaccines. Together with his science copartner, Dr. Maria Elena Bottazzi, they led the development of a low-cost patent-free COVID-19 vaccine technology that led to the production and distribution of CORBEVAX (India) and INDOVAC (Indonesia) vaccines administered to almost 100 million people to date. For this work they were nominated for the 2022 Nobel Peace Prize. In addition to his vaccine development efforts, Hotez has led national and global efforts to combat antivaccine activism. This began when he wrote about his daughter with autism and intellectual disabilities in his book with Johns Hopkins University Press, *Vaccines Did Not Cause Rachel's Autism*. Hotez is the author of more than 650 scientific papers and five single-author books. He is an elected member of the National Academy of Medicine and American Academy of Arts and Sciences, and he has been honored by the AMA and AAMC, among other organizations. He previously served as US Science Envoy in the Obama Administration. During the pandemic he appeared regularly on cable news and radio outlets and podcasts to educate the public about COVID-19 and vaccinations. Hotez is a Fellow of the American Society of Tropical Medicine & Hygiene and Fellow of the American Academy of Pediatrics. He holds an MD from Weill Cornell Medical College, a PhD in biochemical parasitology from Rockefeller University, a bachelor's in molecular biophysics from Yale University, and honorary doctorates from City University of New York and Roanoke College.

LILLIAN BRANNEN JUREK is a middle school English teacher and campus leader who specializes in gifted education. She has a master's degree in curriculum and instruction from Texas A&M University. Her research interests include curriculum design—particularly incorporating technology—and the impact of COVID-19 on educators, students, and the global field of education, as can be seen in her first publication on teachers' traumatic experiences in the initial onset of COVID-19.

TODD JEFFERY LEFKO is president of the United Filtration Company, an import-export firm dealing with water purification equipment, art, linen, kilns, and new technologies. He has worked in Russia for 35 years and has homes in both Moscow and Minnesota. He was the weekly columnist for *Rossiske Vesti*, the political newspaper of the Russian Presidential Administration for eighteen years, and has written 700 articles in *Rossiske Vesti* and other newspapers and magazines. Lefko is on the editorial board for the *Russian Historical Reporter* and has been the English editor for four Russian books. He is Chairperson of East-West Connections, an international nonprofit, focused on citizen diplomacy. He has taught at the University of Minnesota and other Minnesota colleges and lectured at universities in Russia, Germany, China, Belarus, Kazakhstan, and Turkmenistan. He is a Fellow for the

Caux International Roundtable and serves on the Technical Advisory Committee for the Innovation Center at the Almaty Management University in Kazakhstan. He holds a BA in history, an MA in public administration, and a PhD in urban history from the University of Minnesota. He has also studied public policy as a Bush Fellow at Harvard University and urban planning at the University of Manchester, England.

CANDACE MCALESTER is currently the infectious disease control program officer for medicine and occupational health (MOH) in ExxonMobil, a global support role in which she applies evidence-based public health knowledge, techniques, and skills to mitigate infectious disease and environmental health threats in ExxonMobil locations. She also serves as cochair for the global travel team for MOH's clinical center of excellence, in which she develops travel health processes and infectious disease mitigation measures for occupational travelers. She has been in healthcare for over 30 years in a variety of positions, is an advanced practice registered nurse and board-certified family nurse practitioner. Candace obtained a BS in nursing from Prairie View A&M University and earned an MS with specialty as family nurse practitioner, a post-master certificate in nursing education, and DNP from Texas Women's University.

ANDREW S. NATSIOS is an executive professor of international affairs and director of the Scowcroft Institute of International Affairs at the George H. W. Bush School of Government at Texas A&M University. He was Distinguished Professor in the Practice of Diplomacy at the Walsh School of Foreign Service at Georgetown University from 2006–2012 and former administrator of the US Agency for International Development from 2001–2006. He serves as cochairman emeritus of the Committee on Human Rights in North Korea, a research center in Washington, DC. He also served as US Special Envoy to Sudan in 2006–2007 to deal with the Darfur crisis and the implementation of the South Sudan peace agreement. Retired from the US Army Reserves as a lieutenant colonel after 23 years, Natsios is a veteran of the Gulf War. From 1993 to 1998, he was vice president of World Vision US, the international nongovernmental organization. Natsios is the author of three books: *U. S. Foreign Policy and the Four Horsemen of the Apocalypse, The Great North Korean Famine,* and *Sudan, South Sudan, and Darfur: What Everyone Needs to Know.* He has also contributed to 13 other books, including two on North Korea. His areas of research are in food security, famines, and humanitarian assistance during conflict, human rights, and foreign aid.

ERIN NGUYEN is an ecologist and educator interested in the nexus between science and policy. She received her PhD in ecology and evolutionary biology from Texas A&M University in 2022 and her BS in biological studies from the University of Notre Dame in 2018. Her work focuses on questions of freshwater resource management and conservation.

SUSAN NGUNJIRI is the global public health manager for ExxonMobil Corporation. Ngunjiri's expertise and focus on global health spans from infectious disease control, travel health, and corporate wellness. A medical doctor and public health professional by training, Ngunjiri has an extensive background in global health, workplace health and safety, and project health management (primarily focusing on projects' remote settings). She has more than 18 years of experience in infectious diseases management and control, community-based healthcare systems research, and clinical trials, and she is a published author of several research papers in various peer-reviewed publications. A member of the American Public Health Association and National Academies of Sciences, Engineering, and Medicine, Ngunjiri received her MD from Moi University's College of Health Sciences in Kenya and her master's in global health sciences from the University of Oxford, UK.

GERALD W. PARKER JR. is the associate dean for Global One Health in the Texas A&M University School of Veterinary Medicine and Biomedical Sciences and director of the Pandemic Preparedness and Biosecurity Policy Program at the Scowcroft Institute of International Affairs within the Bush School of Government and Public Service at Texas A&M University. He is a member of several advisory boards, including the Texas Task Force on Infectious Disease Preparedness and Response, Texas Experts COVID Vaccine Advisory Panel, ex officio member for the Bipartisan Commission for Biodefense, and chairperson for the National Science Advisory Board for Biosecurity at the National Institutes of Health. He also served as a senior advisor to the assistant secretary for preparedness and response at the Department of Health and Human Services (HHS) from August 2020 to February 2021 during the COVID-19 response. Prior to his arrival at Texas A&M University, Parker held technical to executive leadership positions throughout 36 years of public service at the federal level as a recognized defense and civilian interagency leader in biodefense, high consequence emerging infectious diseases, global health security, and all-hazards public health/medical preparedness and response. This included coordinating the federal public health and medical responses to Hurricanes Katrina through Alex, to the 2009 H1N1 Pandemic and Haiti Earthquake. His service includes more than 26 years on active duty leading military medical research and development programs and organizations. He is a former commander and deputy commander with the United States Army Medical Research Institute of Infectious Diseases. After his military career, Parker held senior executive level positions at the Department of Homeland Security, HHS, and the Department of Defense (DOD). This includes serving as the principal deputy assistant secretary for preparedness and response at HHS and deputy assistant secretary of defense for chemical and biological defense at DOD. He holds a DVM and BS in veterinary medicine from Texas A&M University's College of Veterinary Medicine, a PhD in molecular physiology from Baylor College of Medicine Graduate School of Biomedical Sciences, and an MS in resourcing the national strategy from the Industrial College of the Armed Forces.

RAYMOND ROBERTSON is a professor and holder of the Helen and Roy Ryu Chair in Economics and Government in the Department of International Affairs at the Bush School of Government and Public Service at Texas A&M University and director of the Mosbacher Institute for Trade, Economics, and Public Policy. He is a research fellow at the Institute for the Study of Labor in Bonn, Germany, and a senior research fellow at the Mission Foods Texas-Mexico Center. He was named a 2018 Presidential Impact Fellow by Texas A&M University. Robertson earned a BA in political science and economics from Trinity

University in San Antonio, Texas, and an MS and PhD in economics from the University of Texas at Austin. He has taught at the Maxwell School of Citizenship and Public Affairs at Syracuse University and was a visiting professor in the department of economics at the Graduate School of Administration, Monterrey Institute of Technology's Mexico City campus. Widely published in the field of labor economics and international economics, Robertson previously chaired the US Department of Labor's National Advisory Committee for Labor Provisions of the US Free Trade Agreements and served on both the State Department's Advisory Committee on International Economic Policy and the Center for Global Development's advisory board.

LESLIE E. RUYLE is a conservation ecologist, innovative educator, and creative team builder for interdisciplinary problem solving. She holds a PhD in ecology from the School of Ecology at the University of Georgia, served as a Peace Corps Volunteer in Ghana, West Africa, and has managed university-based initiatives for the National Science Foundation and the United States Agency for International Development. Her research program focuses on the intersection of conservation, natural resources, gender, and development, particularly focusing on conflict regions. Living in four countries and having traveled to over eighty in her career, she has been a key leader or participant in multiple development, biodiversity research, and education initiatives around the world.

LIDIA AZURDIA SIERRA is a dedicated public health professional with a passion for improving health outcomes and promoting health equity in underserved communities. Sierra has garnered extensive research experience across a range of public health domains, affiliating herself with esteemed institutions and research centers. She earned her MPH from Texas A&M University School of Public Health and is pursuing a PhD at the University of Arizona's College of Public Health. Her research focuses on understanding the health impacts of neglected infectious diseases on migrant populations. Her work revolves around understanding these complex health issues, aiming to develop evidence-based interventions and sustainable programs. Sierra embraces a holistic One Health approach, recognizing the interconnectedness of human, animal, and environmental health, to effectively address the challenges faced by marginalized communities.

ERIN A. SINGER has been in education for over 25 years and received her PhD in curriculum and instruction from Texas A&M University. As the lead coordinator for Project Massive Open Online Professional Individualized Learning at the Education Leadership Research Center (ELRC) at Texas A&M University, Singer creates and distributes online professional development for teachers, administrators, and parents of English language learners. She currently serves as the coordinator of online professional development for two other grants in the ELRC. Her research interests include mentoring and coaching of teachers and administrators, online professional development, and teacher stress and burnout.

TAMRA WALDERON works in the Center for Research & Development in Dual Language & Literacy Acquisition as the Curriculum Development Coordinator where she helped develop two research-based dual language curriculums for English Learners as well as a graduate assistant researcher for Project RAISE in the Educational Leadership Research Center. She holds associate's and bachelor's degrees in elementary education, a master's degree in curriculum and instruction, and is currently pursuing a doctoral degree in bilingual/ESL education at Texas A&M University. Her research interests include teacher and school leader education and professional development, burnout in education, the impact of COVID-19 on K–12 education, critical consciousness in education, and culturally sustaining pedagogy.

VICTORIA (VICKI) M. WELDON is the global medical director for medicine and occupational health for ExxonMobil, where she has held a wide range of positions during her 30 years of service. During COVID-19 pandemic, she was a key member of the corporate preparedness and response mechanism while coordinating the medical department support provided to all sites and affiliates across the globe. She has a strong interest in preventive medicine/public health and its application in the workplace. In partnership with human resources design, safety, and the business sectors, she has developed and implemented ExxonMobil's wellbeing program, culture of health, enterprise wide. Additional areas of focus have been emergency response, fitness for duty, development of business service models for occupational health, global implementation of IT platform for occupational health services and managing effective interfaces for health and safety in a matrixed corporate environment. She earned her medical degree through the University of Missouri–Kansas City School of Medicine combined BA/MD program. She is board certified in internal medicine, achieved an MPH with emphasis in occupational medicine, and is a Fellow of the American College of Occupational and Environmental Medicine. She is a member of the IOGP/IPIECA Health Working Group and a past board member of National Business Group for Health subcommittee on health and human capital.

LILIANNA WOLF is a biologist whose earlier work explored disease dynamics of bat populations, but her time is now devoted to countering natural resource and wildlife trafficking. Her writing focuses on ecological conservation, policy, zoonotic disease, and the illicit wildlife trade. Originally from Houston, Texas, she now lives in Washington, DC.

Index

origin of, 18–23, 73; preventing the next pandemic, 31–45; Prisoner's Dilemma and, 73–75; private and public costs of, 155; risk factors for, 8; in US media, 266–68

COVID-19 response: about, 69; in Brazil, 84–85; in China, 86–87; in Germany, 81–82; in Italy, 83–84; in New Zealand, 80–81; shortcomings of the, 5–6; in Taiwan, 82–83; in United States, 85–86

Cowan, B., 144

cowboy culture, 147

Cox's Bazar refugee camp, 223

crises: civic perspectives on major, 265; Hobbes on, 268–70

Crisis and Emergency Risk Communication (CERC), 258

critical care capacity, communication and, *189*

Critical Operations phase, for ExxonMobil during pandemic, *175*

Cronin, C., 149

crop damage, 40

CRRSA (Coronavirus Response and Relief Supplemental Appropriations Act), 293

CSR (corporate social responsibility), 154–55

Cuba, pandemic management in, 14

culling wildlife, 39–41

cultural occurrences, human activities and, 56–57

cyclones, 75–76

Cyprus, pandemic management in, 14

DARPA (Defense Advanced Research Projects Agency), 19–20, 23, 106

DART (Disaster Assistance Response Teams), 313

Daszak, Peter, 20

data privacy, communication and, *185*

Davis, S., 142, 143

deaths, during pandemic, 6, 267–68

Debord, Guy, 268

debt trap, 206

deepfakes, 243

de-escalation, during pandemic, 173, 176

Defense Advanced Research Projects Agency (DARPA), 19–20, 23, 106

Defense Production Act (DPA), 102, 110

deglobalization, 198

Delaware, plastic bag use in, 86

Del Boca, D., 143

Delta variant, 118, 119, 120, 128, 225, 282, 289

demand expansion, dangers of, 35

demand planning processes, supply chain resilience and, 200

Democratic Republic of Congo (DRC), Ebola virus in, 104

demographic groups: effect of pandemic on, 18; unemployment across, 141–45

De Niro, Robert, 16

Denmark, mink farms in, 40–41

Department of Agriculture (USDA), 100, 255

Department of Defense (DoD), 100, 107, 108, 111, 124, 127

Department of Energy, 127–28

Department of Homeland Security (DHS), 100

deplatforming, 257

depressive disorder, *289*

Detroit (Michigan), as a vaccine hesitancy epicenter, 16

DeVos, Betsy, 294

de Waal, Alex, 309–10

Dewan, S., 210–11

DHS (Department of Homeland Security), 100

Ding, W., 154

Dingel, J., 145

direct cash assistance program, 232

Disaster Assistance Response Teams (DART), 313

disease: detection and prevention of, 61–62; surveillance of, as a prevention safeguard, 177–78

Disease emergence and spillover. *See* spillover

disinformation: about, 242–43; detection of, 257; vulnerability to, 245–46

Disinformation Dozen, as a source of spuriousness, 245
distribution ecosystems, 129
distribution planning, 101
diversified portfolios, as a success factor for OWS, 125
DMF (electromagnetic frequency) spectrum, 248
DNA viruses, 60
DoD (Department of Defense), 100, 107, 108, 111, 124, 127
Dominican Republic, 209–10
Dorius, S.F., 255
Dorn, E., 288
DPA (Defense Production Act), 102, 110
DRC (Democratic Republic of Congo), Ebola virus in, 104
drills, conducting, 192
drug trafficking, research into, 43–44
due diligence regulatory approach, 202
DuoProSS Meditech Corp., *117*
"Duty of Vigilance Law," 203–4

E2E (end-to-end) supply chain integration, supply chain resilience and, 200
early diagnosis/treatment, as a prevention safeguard, 181
early warnings, centralized systems for, 190
early warning system: creating for pandemics, 310–11; famine, 308–10; response logistics under, 312–14
East Asia: economic development in, 207; vaccine priority for teachers in, 296
Ebola virus, 33, 51–52, 56, 98, 103–6, 165, 171, 271
EcoHealth Alliance, 19–20, 21
"ecologically clean" alternative, 255
economic impacts: about, 137–39; of COVID-19 pandemic, 10–13; nontypical nature of COVID-19 crisis, 139–48; policy and, 148–55; what does work?, 155–56
ecosystem, 55, 58
edge habitat, 59

education: about, 278–79; global impact of COVID-19, 295–97; impact on, 18, 279–80; impact on child development, 285–86; impact on educators, 280–83, 288–90; impact on K-12 school funding and policy, 292–94; impact on parents, 286–90; impact on schooling, 290–92; impact on students, 283–86; as a prevention safeguard, 178
Education Stabilization Fund, 293–94
educators: deaths among, 282; impact of COVID-19 on, 280–83, 288–90
effectiveness, of vaccines, 115, 117–21
efficacy, of vaccines, 115, 117–21
efficiency, of supply chains, 205–6
Egypt, spread of COVID-19 in, 73
Eichenbaum, M., 155
EIDs (emerging infectious diseases): about, 52; human-wildlife interface and, 54; reservoir for, 58–59
Ekberg, M., 269
electromagnetic frequency (EMF) spectrum, 248
electronic monitoring systems, using in early warning systems, 310–11
electronics, disruption of global supply chains in, 11
El Salvador, 209–10
emergency support groups (ESGs): about, 165, 171–72; implemented by ExxonMobil, 167, *168*; objectives of, 172
emergency use authorization (EUA), 95–96, 109, 110, 117, 121, 122
Emergent BioSolutions, *116*
emerging diseases, infectious diseases compared with, 52
emerging infectious diseases (EIDs): about, 52; human-wildlife interface and, 54; reservoir for, 58–59
Emerging Pandemic Threats (EPT) program, 61, 63
emissions, reducing, 77
emotional factors, disinformation and, 245–46

end-to-end (E2E) supply chain integration, supply chain resilience and, 200

engagement, at all corporation levels, 190

environmental conservation: as a prevention safeguard, 181–82; TCM and, 36; wildlife health and, 53–54

Environmental Protection Agency (EPA), 85–86

environmental survival times, of spillover pathogens, 60

Epoch Times, 19

EPT (Emerging Pandemic Threats) program, 61, 63

Equatorial Guinea, stimulus packages in, 297

ESGs (emergency support groups): about, 165, 171–72; implemented by ExxonMobil, 167, *168*; objectives of, 172

Eslava, M., 150

Etchells, M. J., 279–80

Ethiopia, stimulus packages in, 297

EU (European Union), demand for wildlife trade in, 56–57

EUA (emergency use authorization), 95–96, 109, 110, 117, 121, 122

Europe: COVID-19 peak in, 167; ExxonMobil ESGs in, 167, 172; vaccine priority for teachers in, 296; Volkswagen in, 207

European Centre for Disease Prevention and Control, 169

European Union (EU), demand for wildlife trade in, 56–57

Evans, W., 149

evolutionary jump. *See* wildlife infectious disease spillover

Executive Council, 10

external experts, using for workplace disease prevention and control, 191–92

external systems, for site preparedness and response, 191

ExxonMobil case study: about, 12, 164–66; challenges *vs.* implementation approach, 182–83; communication, 184; early response by, 166–69;

global health perspectives, 169–71, *170*; leadership, 183, *184*; local site prevention and mitigation, 171–72; looking forward, 193; medical-clinical capacity, 186, *186–89*; pandemic phases and triggers, 173–82, *174–75*; take-home message, 190–92

Eysenbach, Gunther, 256

Facebook, 243, 245, 310

face masks, 246–47

facility management, communication and, *191*

Fairlie, R. W., 139, 142, 143

fake news, 243, 257

Families First Coronavirus Response Act, 151

Famine Early Warning System (FEWS NET), 308–10, 313

Fan, Y., 150, 156

Fauci, Anthony, 23

FDA (Food and Drug Administration), 9, 12, 95, 98–99, 100, 101, 108, 109, 111, 113, 121, 124, 247

federally funded R&D center (FFRDC) network, 127–28

FEWS NET (Famine Early Warning System), 308–10, 313

Finland, financial and government aid for education in, 296

5G network, 247–48

fixed effects specification, 211–12

Florida: climate adaptation structures in, 86; education funding in, 294

flying foxes, 40

flying geese model, of economic development, 207, 209–10, 211, 212

Food and Drug Administration (FDA), 9, 12, 95, 98–99, 100, 101, 108, 109, 111, 113, 121, 124, 247

Food for Peace, 313

food system, disruption of global supply chains in, 11

Foreign Affairs, 20

forest clearing, climate change and, 76

Forsythe, E., 142

fossil fuels, increased use of, 58

France: consequences of social stigmatization in, 221; Constitutional Council, 204; "Duty of Vigilance Law," 203–4; health care for migrants in, 221; pandemic management in, 13; regulatory push in, 203–4; spread of COVID-19 in, 73

French National Assembly, 203–4

Frith, J., 248

furin cleavage site, 23

G7 Build Back Better World (B3W) global initiative, 206

GAD (general anxiety disorder), 289

Gadot, Gal, 266–67, 271–72

gain-of-function research, 19

Gates, Bill, 248

GAVI, 123

Gaza Strip, 224–25

GDP (gross domestic product), contraction of, 138

general anxiety disorder (GAD), 289

genetically modified organisms (GMOs), 243, 255

geographic location, as a characteristic of reservoir hosts, 58

George Washington, 16

Georgia, standardized tests in, 288

Germany: carbon emission reductions in, 78; COVID-19 response in, 79, 81–82; "Lieferkettengesetz," 204; pandemic management in, 14; regulatory push in, 204; spread of COVID-19 in, 73, 137, 138

Ghebreyesus, Tedros Adhanom, 9–10

GHSA (Global Health Security Agenda), 165, 169, 171

gill nets, 35–36

GlaxoSmithKline, 111

global approach, 192

Global Health Security Agenda (GHSA), 165, 169, 171

global impact: of COVID-19 on education, 295–97; of COVID-19 on migrant communities, 222–27

globalization, containment and, 61

global migration, 217–20

Global Polio Eradication Initiative, 253

global resource mapping, 64

global supply chains, 11, 138, 139, 155, 197–99

global value chains, 153, 154–55

Global Virome Project, 63

GMOs (genetically modified organisms), 243, 255

Goldbelt Security, LLC, 116

Goldberg, Suzanne B., 280

Gold Coast Medical Supply, L.P., 117

Golding, William, 265

Google Meet, 290

Goolsbee, A., 149

Gorodnichenko, Y., 144, 152

governance, as a success factor for OWS, 124–25

government, public-private partnership between industry and, 15–17

Graeber, David, 272

Granja, J., 151

Great Influenza pandemic, 4–5, 11

The Great Influenza (Barry), 11

Green, Mark, 313

Greene, Doyle, 266

greenhouse gases, 75, 78

Green Maps, 309

Grisham, Michelle Lujan, 282

gross domestic product (GDP), contraction of, 138

Guatemala, 209–10

Guerrieri, V., 151

Guinea, Ebola virus in, 103

Gulf of California, 35–36

Gupta, S., 149–50

H1N1 flu, 82, 98, 126

H5N1 Pandemic Influenza National Strategy and Implementation Plan, 100–101

habitat fragmentation, 54

Hala Al Shwa Primary Healthcare Center, 224

Hamas, 224

Hansen, Lene, 269

hashtag hijacking, 244

Hassan, T., 152, 153

Japan: spread of COVID-19 in, 73; technology evolution in, 207; vaccine priority for teachers in, 296

Marburg virus, as an example of zoonotic spillover, 33
masks, 246–47
Massachusetts, National Guard as classroom support in, 282–83
mass graves, 310
Mass Starvation: The History and Future of Famine (de Waal), 309–10
Mauritius, culling in, 40
Mauritius Food and Agricultural Research and Extension Institute, 40
Mayo Clinic, 120
Mbembe, Achilles, *Necropolitics*, 269
MCMs (medical countermeasures), 99, 100, 106, 107–8, 109, 111
MCM task force, 107–8, 109
measles, 252–53
measles, mumps, and rubella (MMR) vaccine, 254
media crises: COVID-19 in US media, 266–68; COVID-19 zombie apocalypse, 270–72; Hobbes, Thomas, 264–66, 268–70; lessons learned, 272–74; Rousseau, Jean-Jacques, 264–66
Medicaid, 228–29
medical-clinical capacity, 166, 186
medical countermeasures (MCMs), 99, 100, 106, 107–8, 109, 111
medical countermeasures preparedness, risks and challenges for, 125–29
Medicine and Occupational Health (MOH) group, 167–69
Medline Industries, *117*
Meese, J., 248
Meissner, C., 149, 150
men, US monthly unemployment for, 141, 143, 144
mental health: impact of COVID-19 on educator and parent, 288–90; in students, 283–84
mercantilist policies, 209
Merck, 104, 105
Merkel, Angela, 81–82
MERS (Middle East respiratory syndrome), 98, 165, 171, 316

Mexico: air transportation system and, 14–15; barriers to efficiency-enhancing integration with Central America and, 210; evolution of, 208; financial and government aid for education in, 296; maquiladora program, 208, 209; pandemic management in, 14; production-sharing investments in, 208; supply chain performance and, 210; wages in, 210
Microsoft Teams, 12
Middle East, ExxonMobil ESGs in, 167, 172
Middle East respiratory syndrome (MERS), 98, 165, 171, 316
migrant communities: COVID-19 and, 217–34; obstacles and limitations to health care access among, 221–22
migration routes, climate change and, 76
mink farms, 40–41
Minnesota, 120
misinformation, 242–43
Missouri, educators in, 282
mitigation: climate change, 78–87; safeguards, 181
MMR (measles, mumps, and rubella) vaccine, 254
MNCs (multinational corporations), 197–98, 200, 202, 204–7
mobile populations, health care needs of, 63–64
mobility, policies to reduce, 149
Moderna, 107
Moderna vaccine, 95, 98, 113–14, *115*, 115, 120, 121, 123
Modern Slavery Act, 204
MOH (Medicine and Occupational Health) group, 167–69
Mongey, S., 145, 156
Mongolia, national school closure in, 278
Monitoring phase, for ExxonMobil during pandemic, *174*
Monmouth University, 248
monocultures, 58

morbidity: elevated, for other diseases, 251–53; elevated, from pandemic agent, 249–50

mortality: from COVID-19 pandemic, 4–5; elevated, for other diseases, 251 53; elevated, from pandemic agent, 249–50; from Great Influenza, 4–5

mRNA vaccine platform, 106, 112, 113–14

multinational corporations (MNCs), 197–98, 200, 202, 204–7

multisystem inflammatory syndrome, 8

Murthy, B. P., 258

mutation, emergence of, 5–6

Muthukrishnan, P., 142–43, 155

Myanmar, 223

NAFTA (North American Free Trade Agreement), 208, 209–10

NASEM (Committee on Safeguarding the Bioeconomy at the National Academies of Sciences, Engineering, and Medicine), 253

National Academy of Medicine, 259

National Council on Teacher Quality, 281–82

national governance, Prisoner's Dilemma and, 77–78

National Health Coordination Centre (NHCC), 80

National Institutes of Health (NIH), 9, 19, 22, 23, 97, 100, 105, 107, 108, 111

National Laboratory Network, 127–28

National Oceanic and Atmospheric Administration (NOAA), 309

national security, infodemic and, 256

National Strategy for Pandemic Influenza Implementation plan, 102

natives, safety-net programs and, 146

natural resource extraction, disruption of global supply chains in, 11

Nature, 21

ND-GAIN (Notre Dame Global Adaptation Initiative), 79–80, 80, 82–86

Necropolitics (Mbembe), 269

negative labor supply shock, 146

Neilson, C., 151

Neiman, B., 145

Netherlands: health care for migrants in, 221; mink farms, 40–41

New Mexico: carbon emissions in, 86; National Guard as classroom support in, 282

"new normal," 272

Newsweek, 22–23

New York: education funding in, 294; plastic bag use in, 86

New York Magazine, 21–22

New York Times, 7, 22, 36

New Zealand: COVID-19 response in, 79, 80–81; pandemic management in, 14

Ng, S., 140

NGOs (international nongovernmental organizations), 313

NHCC (National Health Coordination Centre), 80

Nicaragua, 209–10

Nietzel, M. T., 287

Nigeria: pandemic management in, 14; Russian vaccine sales in, 13

NIH (National Institutes of Health), 9, 19, 22, 23, 97, 100, 105, 107, 108, 111

Nipah virus: as an example of zoonotic spillover, 32, 33; in Malaysia, 54

NOAA (National Oceanic and Atmospheric Administration), 309

nonstate actors, as a source of spuriousness, 244

North America: ExxonMobil ESGs in, 172; vision for integrated Central and, 206–12

North American Free Trade Agreement (NAFTA), 208, 209–10

North Carolina, educator bonuses in, 281

North Korea: famine in, 308; as a state actor, 244

Notre Dame Global Adaptation Initiative (ND-GAIN), 79–80, 82–86

Novavax vaccine, 103, 115, *115*

novel viruses, human exposure to, 52

Obama, Barack, 19

obesity, in United States, 15

pandemic depression, 139
pandemic early warning system
  (PEWS), 310–11
Pandemic Influenza Risk Management
  document (WHO), 173
pandemic preparedness: about, 307–8;
  creating an early warning system, 310–11; Famine Early Warning
  System, 308–10; response logistics
  under early warning system, 312–14
Pandemic Prevention Platform, 106
pandemics: management ranking by
  country, 13–14; preparing for the last,
  126–27; timeline for, 1–4
panic prescribing, 250–53
Papanikolaou, D., 145
parents, impact of COVID-19 on, 286–90
Parker, Gerry, 24
parrot smugglers, 44
pathogen diversity, as a characteristic of
  reservoir hosts, 58
pathogen transmission, mechanisms
  of, 55
Paycheck Protection Program (PPP)
  and Health Care Enhancement Act,
  151, 156
pedagogists, impact of COVID-19 on
  parents as, 286–88
people; environment; assets; and reputation (PEAR), 172
permeability, survival of pathogens and,
  54–55
permitting, for wildlife transport, 64
Perna, Gustave, 111
personal preventive measures, 178–79
personal protective equipment (PPE),
  246–47
Peru, refugees in, 219
PEWS (pandemic early warning system), 310–11
Pfizer-BioNTech vaccine, 95, 98, 113–14,
  115, 115, 118, 120, 121, 123
pharmaceuticals: disruption of global
  supply chains in, 11; as a national
  security issue, 12
Phase 1, of vaccine development, 108
Phase 2, of vaccine development, 108

Phase 3, of vaccine development, 108
phases, of pandemic for ExxonMobil,
  173–82, *174–75*
PHEIC (public health emergency of
  international concern), 164
PHEMCA (Public Health Emergency
  Medical Countermeasures Enterprise), 100
PHEMCE model, 108
phenotypes, continuous monitoring of,
  62–63
Philippines, technology evolution in,
  207
Picciotti, E., 144
Pilossoph, L., 145
Polaris, 210
polemics, Ebola virus and, 271
policy: economic impact and, 148–55; of
  ESGs, 172; role of, 148–50; stimulus,
  151–52
poliovirus, 253
political systems: impact of on pandemic response, 13–15; wildlife culls
  and, 40
politicization, of pandemic, 85
portfolio effect, 57
post-traumatic stress disorder (PTSD),
  288
PPE (personal protective equipment),
  246–47
PPP (Paycheck Protection Program)
  and Health Care Enhancement Act,
  151, 156
PREP (Public Readiness and Emergency
  Preparedness) Act (2005), 99, 110
Preparation phase, for ExxonMobil
  during pandemic, *174*
preparedness. *See* pandemic
  preparedness
*Preparing for Pandemics in the Modern
  World* (Scowcroft Institute of
  International Affairs), 5
preventive measures: considered for
  de-escalation, 176; infodemic and,
  246–47; promoting use of, 190–91;
  in schools, 295
primates, 55

stay-in-place orders: COVID-19 case reduction due to, 150–51; unemployment and, 149–50

stimulus policies/packages, 151–52, 293, 297

stock market, 138, 139

stockpiling, 101

Stop TB Partnership, 252

Strategic National Stockpile (SNS), 100

strip mining, climate change and, 76

STS (secondary traumatic stress), 288

students, impact of COVID-19 on, 283–86

Subramanian, S., 154

suicide, among students, 283

Supplemental Nutrition Assistance Program (SNAP), 229

supply chains: disruptions of, 125, 153, 154–55; efficiency of, 205–6; growth in, 153; resilience of, 199–202; sustainability of, 202–5

surge manufacturing, 101

surveillance, priority of for RNA viruses, 62–63

Susceptible-Exposed-Infectious-Recovered (SEIR) model, 156

"Suspension of Adverse Immigration Actions That Deter Immigrant Communities from Seeking Health Services in a Public Health Emergency" section, of proposed bill, 232–33

sustainability, of supply chains, 202–5

Sweden: carbon emission reductions in, 78; spread of COVID-19 in, 137, *138*; stimulus packages in, 297; vaccine priority for teachers in, 296

Swedish solution, 156

Switzerland, pandemic management in, 14

Syria: forcibly displaced persons from, 218; refugees in, 219

Syverson, C., 149

tai chi, 34

Taiwan: COVID-19 response in, 79, 82–83; pandemic management in, 14; technology evolution in, 207

TAMUS (Texas A&M University System) and Emergent BioSolutions, 103

TB (tuberculosis), 252

TCM (traditional Chinese medicine), 34–36

TEA (Texas Education Agency), 281, 288

teacher certifications, 293

teacher training, 293

technological development, priority of for RNA viruses, 62–63

telehealth, communication and, *189*

testing gaps, communication and, *188*

Texas: education funding in, 294; educator bonuses in, 281; restaurants in, 147; school closures in, 279; Senate Bill No. 226, 293; vaccinations in, 122; virus spread in, 290

Texas A&M University System (TAMUS) and Emergent BioSolutions, 103

Texas A&M University with Fujifilm Diosynth Biotechnologies, *116*

Texas Education Agency (TEA), 281, 288

Thailand: health care in, 233; pandemic management in, 13; spread of COVID-19 in, 73

3 Rs (Review, Recognize, and Respond) framework, 258

TikTok, 243

timeline, for pandemic, 1–4

toilet paper shortage, 199

Tonga, stimulus packages in, 297

totoaba, 35–36

TPP (Trans-Pacific Partnership), withdrawal of US from, 209

Trabandt, M., 155

traditional Chinese medicine (TCM), 34–36

trained workforce, as a challenge for OWS, 125

transmission, infodemic and, 247–48

regulatory push in, 204; reshoring policies, 155, 205–6; restaurants in, 145–48; school closures in Texas, 279; Seattle COVID-19 Disaster Relief Fund for Immigrants, 232; spread of COVID-19 in, 73, 137, *138*; standardized tests in, 288; stay-in-place orders in, 151; stimulus policies, 151–52; supply chain disruptions, 154–55; Texas, 122; Transparency in Supply Chains Act (2010), 204; US Customs and Border Protection (CBP), 204–5; vaccination statistics, 119, *120*; vaccine distribution and administration in, 121–22; vaccine priority for teachers in, 295–96; vaccines, 95–130; Virginia Department of Health, 119–20; virus spread in Texas, 290; vision for integrated North and Central America, 206–12; withdrawal from Trans-Pacific Partnership of, 209

United States-Mexico-Canada Agreement (USMCA), 209–10

US Agency for International Development (USAID), 61, 63, 123, 308, 309, 313, 314

US Army Materiel Command, 111

US Bureau of Labor Statistics, 139–40

US Customs and Border Protection (CBP), 204–5

US Department of Agriculture (USDA), 100, 255

US Department of Education. *See* education

US Department of the Interior, 311

US Fish and Wildlife Service (USFWS), 57

US Geological Survey, 309

US government offices, infighting amongst, 9

US labor markets, spread of COVID-19 and, 138

USMCA (United States-Mexico-Canada Agreement), 209–10

Utah, educator bonuses in, 281

VA (Veterans Administration), 100

vaccine development: in China, 12–13; global, 122–23; Operation Warp Speed (OWS), 7, 15, 113–21; timelines for, 108, *109*; urgency of, 126

vaccine hesitancy: about, 128, 250; spread of movement in, 17; US epicenters of, 16

vaccine messaging, 128

vaccines: about, 95–96; adapting to availability of, 192; availability and distribution of, 17; clinical trials during an outbreak response, 105–6; communication and, *187–88*; contract value of, *115–17*; Defense Advanced Research Projects Agency (DARPA) grand challenges, 106; Defense Production Act (DPA), 102; distribution and administration of in US, 117, 121–22; Ebola (2014-2016, and 2018), 103–5; global access to, 128–29; H5N1 Pandemic Influenza National Strategy and Implementation Plan, 100–101; infodemic and, 248; Joint Program Executive Office for Chemical Biological, Radiological, and Nuclear Defense (JPEO-CBRND), 100; lessons learned from Anthrax, 96–97; manufacturing and distribution ecosystems, 129; Operation Warp Speed (OWS), 107–29; Pandemic and All-Hazards Preparedness Act (PAHPA), 99; priority for teachers, 295; Project BioShield, 97–99; promoting use of, 190–91; Public Health Emergency Medical Countermeasures Enterprise (PHEMCE), 100; Public Readiness and Emergency Preparedness (PREP) Act, 99; severe acute respiratory syndrome (SARS), 97; summary of lessons learned, 106–7; 2009 H1N1 Influenza Pandemic, 102–3; urgency of research on, 126; in US, 119, *120*, 129–30; vaccine platform technology research, 105

variants, 118–20, 128, 225–26, 281, 282, 289
vector control, as an intervention strategy, 64
veneer theory, 265
Venezuela, refugees in, 219–20
Veterans Administration (VA), 100
Vietnam: pandemic management in, 13; spread of COVID-19 in, 73; technology evolution in, 207
viral genetics, continuous monitoring of, 62–63
viral load, as a characteristic of reservoir hosts, 58
Virginia Department of Health, 119–20
virtual online platforms, 290–91
virus spread, air transportation system and, 14–15
visibility, supply chain resilience and, 200
volatile, uncertain, complex, and ambiguous (VUCA) environment, 198
Volkswagen, 207
VUCA (volatile, uncertain, complex, and ambiguous) environment, 198

Wakefield, Andrew, 254
Wakefield, Stephen, 16
Wall Street Journal, 11, 22–23
Wani, Riyaz, 227
War Power Acts (1941 and 1942), 102
Washington Post, 16, 21, 22–23
water use, climate change and, 76
Weber, M., 144, 152
Weinberg, A., 145
Wengrow, David, 272
Wenliang Shi, 86
wet markets, 17–18, 21, 56
WFP (World Food Programme), 313
White House COVID-19 Task Force, 109, 111
white people, US monthly unemployment for, 141
WHO (World Health Organization), 9–10, 32, 42, 73, 95, 164, 169–71, 173, 182, 223–24, 233–34, 242, 253

wildfires, 75–76
wildlife bans, effect on conservation of, 44
wildlife health, environmental factors and, 53–54
wildlife infectious disease spillover: about, 51–53; biodiversity, 57–58; disease detection and prevention, 61–62; future of, 62–64; globalization and containment, 61; human activities and cultural occurrences, 56–57; human-wildlife interface, 54–55; recipient host characteristics, 59–60; reservoir host characteristics, 58–59; viral characteristics, 60; wildlife health and environmental factors, 53–54
wildlife markets, reasons for existence of, 34–36
wildlife reservoirs, 57
wildlife trade/trafficking: about, 36–39, 41–43; as a human activity affecting wildlife-human interactions, 56–57; research into, 44; as a risk for zoonotic spillover, 33–34
Wilken, R., 248
Wilson, Woodrow, 11
Withhold Release Orders, 204–5
women: economic impacts of COVID-19 on, 144–45; unemployment for, 141, 143, 154
woolly mammoths, 43
worksite plans, support for, 190
World Bank, 139
World Development Report, 153
World Food Programme (WFP), 313
World Health Organization (WHO), 9–10, 32, 42, 73, 95, 164, 169–71, 173, 182, 223–24, 233–34, 242, 253
World Trade Organization (WTO), 197–98, 208
Wuhan Institute of Virology, 19, 20

Xie, T., 156
Xi Jinping, 23
Xu, H., 139, 142

Yanzhong Huang, 20
Yao Ming, 38
Yeoh, Michelle, 38
Yeşim, A. Y., 150, 156
ye wei (wild taste), 35

zebras, 37
Zika virus, 84, 98
zombie mythologies, 270–72

Zoom, 12, 290
zoonoses, human contact with, 43
zoonotic emerging diseases, 17–18, 51, 52
zoonotic spillover: about, 31–32; drivers of, 32–33; future suggestions for mitigating, 41–43; prevalence of, 32–33; probability of, 52; subsistence markets for wildlife protein and, 39